W9-CXN-408

Overcoming Barriers to Eliminate Hepatitis C

Editors

CAMILLA S. GRAHAM
STACEY B. TROOSKIN

INFECTIOUS DISEASE CLINICS OF NORTH AMERICA

www.id.theclinics.com

Consulting Editor
HELEN W. BOUCHER

June 2018 • Volume 32 • Number 2

ELSEVIER

1600 John F. Kennedy Boulevard • Suite 1800 • Philadelphia, Pennsylvania, 19103-2899.
http://www.theclinics.com

INFECTIOUS DISEASE CLINICS OF NORTH AMERICA Volume 32, Number 2
June 2018 ISSN 0891-5520, ISBN-13: 978-0-323-58403-6

Editor: Kerry Holland
Developmental Editor: Donald Mumford

Infectious Disease Clinics of North America (ISSN 0891-5520) is published in March, June, September, and December by Elsevier Inc., 360 Park Avenue South, New York, NY 10010-1710. Periodicals postage paid at New York, NY and additional mailing offices. Subscription prices are $319.00 per year for US individuals, $629.00 per year for US institutions, $100.00 per year for US students, $379.00 per year for Canadian individuals, $785.00 per year for Canadian institutions, $428.00 per year for international individuals, $785.00 per year for international institutions, and $200.00 per year for Canadian and international students. To receive student rate, orders must be accompanied by name of affiliated institution, date of term, and the *signature* of program/residency coordinator on institution letterhead. Orders will be billed at individual rate until proof of status is received. Foreign air speed delivery is included in all *Clinics* subscription prices. All prices are subject to change without notice. **POSTMASTER**: Send address changes to *Infectious Disease Clinics of North America*, Elsevier Health Sciences Division, Subcription Customer Service, 3251 Riverport Lane, Maryland Heights, MO 63043. **Customer Service: 1-800-654-2452 (US). From outside of the US and Canada, call 1-314-447-8871. Fax: 1-314-447-8029. E-mail: JournalsCustomerService-usa@elsevier.com (print support) or JournalsOnlineSupport-usa@elsevier.com (online support).**

Infectious Disease Clinics of North America is also published in Spanish by Editorial Inter-Médica, Junin 917, 1er A 1113, Buenos Aires, Argentina.

Reprints. For copies of 100 or more, of articles in this publication, please contact the Commercial Reprints Department, Elsevier Inc., 360 Park Avenue South, New York, New York 10010-1710. Tel. 212-633-3874, Fax: 212-633-3820, E-mail: reprints@elsevier.com.

Infectious Disease Clinics of North America is covered in *MEDLINE/PubMed (Index Medicus), Current Contents/Clinical Medicine, Science Citation Alert, SCISEARCH,* and *Research Alert.*

Printed in the United States of America.

BRYN GAY
Treatment Action Group, New York, New York, USA

RACHEL I. GONZALEZ, MPH
Research Health Care Group, VA Long Beach Health Care System, Long Beach, California, USA

STUART C. GORDON, MD
Henry Ford Health System, Detroit, Michigan, USA

CAMILLA S. GRAHAM, MD, MPH
Co-Director, Viral Hepatitis Center, Division of Infectious Disease, Beth Israel Deaconess Medical Center, Assistant Professor of Medicine, Harvard Medical School, Boston, Massachusetts, USA

JASON GREBELY, BSc, PhD
Associate Professor, Viral Hepatitis Clinical Research Program, The Kirby Institute, UNSW Sydney, Sydney, New South Wales, Australia

BEHZAD HAJARIZADEH, MD, MPH, PhD
Viral Hepatitis Clinical Research Program, The Kirby Institute, UNSW Sydney, New South Wales, Australia

SCOTT D. HOLMBERG, MD, MPH
Division of Viral Hepatitis, Centers for Disease Control and Prevention (CDC), Atlanta, Georgia, USA

MICHAEL A. HORBERG, MD, MAS, FACP, FIDSA
Mid-Atlantic Permanente Medical Group, PC, Mid-Atlantic Permanente Research Institute, Rockville, Maryland, USA

EMALIE HURIAUX, MPH
Project Inform, San Francisco, California, USA

M. CABELL JONAS, PhD
Mid-Atlantic Permanente Medical Group, PC, Rockville, Maryland, USA

ROBERT T. LAWRENCE, MD, MEd
Alaska Department of Corrections, Anchorage, Alaska, USA

BENJAMIN P. LINAS, MD, MPH
Associate Professor, Department of Medicine, Section of Infectious Diseases, Boston Medical Center, Boston University School of Medicine, Department of Epidemiology, Boston University School of Public Health, Boston, Massachusetts, USA

ALAIN H. LITWIN, MD, MS, MPH
Albert Einstein College of Medicine, Montefiore Medical Center, Bronx, New York, USA

BERNADETTE LOFTUS, MD
Mid-Atlantic Permanente Medical Group, PC, Rockville, Maryland, USA

MEI LU, PhD
Henry Ford Health System, Data Coordinating Center, Detroit, Michigan, USA

ANNIE LUETKEMEYER, MD
Division of HIV, Infectious Diseases and Global Medicine, Zuckerberg San Francisco General Hospital, University of California, San Francisco, San Francisco, California, USA

COLLEEN S. LYNCH, MD, MPH
Clinical Practice, Clinician, Southeast Health Center, Medical Director of Care
Coordination for Primary Care, San Francisco Health Network, San Francisco Department
of Public Health, Associate Physician Diplomate, University of California, San Francisco,
Zuckerberg San Francisco General Hospital, San Francisco, California, USA

ELISE S. MARA, MPH
Epidemiologist, ARCHES Branch, San Francisco Department of Public Health,
San Francisco, California, USA

NATASHA K. MARTIN, DPhil
Associate Professor, Division of Infectious Diseases and Global Public Health,
Department of Medicine, University of California, San Diego, San Diego, California, USA;
School of Social and Community Medicine, University of Bristol, Bristol, England

THOMAS C.S. MARTIN, MD
Infectious Disease Fellow, Division of Infectious Diseases and Global Public Health,
Department of Medicine, University of California, San Diego, San Diego, California, USA

MARIANNE MARTINELLO, MBBS, FRACP, PhD
Viral Hepatitis Clinical Research Program, The Kirby Institute, UNSW Sydney, Sydney,
New South Wales, Australia

GAIL V. MATTHEWS, MBChB, MRCP (UK), FRACP, PhD
Associate Professor, Viral Hepatitis Clinical Research Program, The Kirby Institute,
UNSW Sydney, Sydney, New South Wales, Australia

ANNE C. MOORMAN, BSN, MPH
Division of Viral Hepatitis, Centers for Disease Control and Prevention (CDC), Atlanta,
Georgia, USA

TIM R. MORGAN, MD
Division of Gastroenterology, VA Long Beach Health Care System, Long Beach,
California, USA

MICHAEL MUGAVERO, MD, MHS
Professor of Medicine, Division of Infectious Diseases, The University of Alabama at
Birmingham, Birmingham, Alabama, USA

SUSANNA NAGGIE, MD, MHS
Associate Professor of Medicine, Division of Infectious Diseases, Duke University Medical
Center, Duke Clinical Research Institute, Durham, North Carolina, USA

SHAYLA NOLEN, MPH
Research Associate, Section of Infectious Diseases, Boston Medical Center, Boston,
Massachusetts, USA

BRIANNA L. NORTON, DO, MPH
Assistant Professor of Medicine and Infectious Diseases, Albert Einstein College of
Medicine, Montefiore Medical Center, Bronx, New York, USA

ANGELA M. PARK, PharmD
New England Veterans Engineering Resource Center, Department of Veterans Affairs,
Boston, Massachusetts, USA

ANDRI RAUCH, MD
Professor, Institute for Infectious Diseases, University of Bern, Bern, Switzerland

DAVID B. ROSS, MD, PhD, MBI
HIV, Hepatitis and Related Conditions, Office of Specialty Care Services, Department of Veterans Affairs, Washington, DC, USA

LORALEE B. RUPP, MSE
Henry Ford Health System, Detroit, Michigan, USA

JILIAN A. SACKS, PhD
HIV/HCV Scientist, Clinton Health Access Initiative, Boston, Massachusetts, USA

LUISA SALAZAR-VIZCAYA, PhD
Postdoctoral Researcher, Institute for Infectious Diseases, University of Bern, Bern, Switzerland

MARK A. SCHMIDT, PhD
Center for Health Research Northwest, Kaiser Permanente Northwest, Portland, Oregon, USA

MIKE SELICK, MSW
Harm Reduction Coalition, New York, New York, USA

AARON A. SMITH, BS
HCV Project Coordinator, Community Health Equity and Promotion Branch, San Francisco Department of Public Health, San Francisco, California, USA

ANNE C. SPAULDING, MD, MPH
Department of Epidemiology, Rollins School of Public Health, Emory University, Morehouse School of Medicine, Atlanta, Georgia, USA

PHILIP R. SPRADLING, MD
Division of Viral Hepatitis, Centers for Disease Control and Prevention (CDC), Atlanta, Georgia, USA

EYASU H. TESHALE, MD
Division of Viral Hepatitis, Centers for Disease Control and Prevention (CDC), Atlanta, Georgia, USA

WILLIAM VON OEHSEN, JD
Powers Pyles Sutter & Verville PC, Washington, DC, USA

REED VREELAND
Housing Works, Brooklyn, New York, USA

PHIL WATERS, JD
Center for Health Law and Policy Innovation of Harvard Law School, Boston, Massachusetts, USA

JULIUS M. WILDER, MD, PhD
Associate Professor, Department of Medicine, Duke Division of Gastroenterology, Duke Clinical Research Institute, Durham, North Carolina, USA

JIAN XING, PhD
Division of Viral Hepatitis, Centers for Disease Control and Prevention (CDC), Atlanta, Georgia, USA

PHILIPPE J. ZAMOR, MD
Carolinas Healthcare System, Charlotte, North Carolina, USA

YUNA ZHONG, MSPH
Division of Viral Hepatitis, Centers for Disease Control and Prevention (CDC), Atlanta, Georgia, USA

Contents

Chronic Hepatitis Cohort Study (CHeCS) publications using data from "real-world" patients with hepatitis C virus (HCV) have described demographic disparities in access to care; rates of advanced liver disease, morbidity, and mortality (2.5%–3.5% per year during 2006–10, although only 19% of all CHeCS decedents, and just 30% of those with deaths attributed to liver disease, had HCV listed on death certificate); substantial comorbidities, such as diabetes, advanced liver fibrosis (29% prevalence), renal disease, and depression, and partial reversal of all these with successful antiviral therapy; patient risk behaviors; and use of noninvasive markers to assess liver disease.

Australia is on track to achieve World Health Organization hepatitis C virus (HCV) elimination targets. An active HCV screening program led to 82% of HCV-infected population being diagnosed. An unrestricted direct-acting antiviral (DAA) program, launched in March 2016, resulted in an estimated 58,500 individuals (26% of total HCV-infected population, including 70% of those with cirrhosis) initiating treatment through 2017. Treatment uptake was high among subpopulations at greater HCV transmission risk, with 22% of people injecting drugs and >60% of those with HIV/HCV coinfection initiating DAA treatment in 2016. A monitoring and evaluation program will inform strategies required to achieve HCV elimination targets.

The Department of Veterans Affairs (VA) has made significant progress in treating hepatitis C virus, experiencing more than a 75% reduction in veterans remaining to be treated since the availability of oral direct-acting antivirals. Hepatitis C Innovation Teams use lean process improvement and system redesign, resulting in practice models that address gaps in care. The key to success is creative improvements in veteran access to providers, including expanded use of nonphysician providers, video telehealth, and electronic technologies. Population health management tools monitor and identify trends in care, helping the VA tailor care and address barriers.

therapy. Although people who inject drugs carry the highest burden, few have initiated treatment. The authors present a comprehensive review of the evidence on the efficacy of HCV medications, drug–drug interactions, and barriers to and models of care. Studies have demonstrated comparable efficacy for individuals who are on opioid agonist therapy compared with those who are not. We propose that a strategy of treatment and cure-as-prevention is imperative in this population to curb the hepatitis C epidemic.

Reinfection after direct-acting antiviral therapy may pose a challenge to hepatitis C virus elimination efforts. Reinfection risk is cited as a reason for not offering treatment to people who inject drugs. As treatment scale-up expands among populations with risks for reacquisition, acknowledgment that reinfection can and will occur is essential. Efforts to prevent and manage reinfection should be incorporated into individual- and population-level strategies. The risk of reinfection after successful treatment emphasizes the need for education, harm reduction, and post-treatment surveillance. Reinfection must not be considered an impediment to treatment, if hepatitis C virus elimination is to be achieved.

Hepatitis C virus reinfection rates among men who have sex with men are high. Factors associated with infection point to varied sexual and drug-related risks that could be targeted for interventions to prevent infection/reinfection. Modeling indicates that tackling increasing incidence and high reinfection rates requires high levels of hepatitis C virus treatment combined with behavioral interventions. Enhanced testing strategies and prompt retreating of reinfection may be required to promptly diagnose re-infections. Behavioral interventions studies addressing reinfection are required. Other interventions include traditional harm reduction interventions, adapted behavioral interventions, and interventions to prevent harms related to ChemSex and other risk factors.

This article considers how existing human immunodeficiency virus (HIV) infrastructure may be leveraged to inform and improve hepatitis C virus (HCV) treatment efforts in the HIV-HCV coinfected population. Current gaps in HCV care relevant to the care continuum are reviewed. Successes in HIV treatment are then applied to the HCV treatment model for coinfected patients. Finally, the authors give examples of HCV treatment strategies for coinfected patients in both domestic and international settings.

INFECTIOUS DISEASE CLINICS OF NORTH AMERICA

ISSUE OF RELATED INTEREST

Clinics in Liver Disease, August 2017 (Vol. 21, Issue 3)
Hepatitis C Infection as a Systemic Disease: Extra-Hepatic Manifestation of Hepatitis C
Zobair M. Younossi, *Editor*

THE CLINICS ARE AVAILABLE ONLINE!
Access your subscription at:
www.theclinics.com

INFECTIOUS DISEASE CLINICS
OF NORTH AMERICA

FORTHCOMING ISSUES

September 2018
Management of Infections in Solid Organ
Transplant Recipients
Sherif Beniameen Mossad, Editor

December 2018
Device-Associated Infections
Vivian H. Chu, Editor

March 2019
Updates in Tropical Medicine
Michael Libman and Cédric Yansouni,
Editors

RECENT ISSUES

March 2018
Infections in Children
Jennifer E. Schuster and
Jason G. Newland, Editors

December 2017
Infections in Older Adults
Robin L.P. Jump and David H. Canaday,
Editors

September 2017
Complex Infectious Disease Issues in the
Intensive Care Unit
Naomi P. O'Grady and Sameer S. Kadri,
Editors

ISSUE OF RELATED INTEREST

Clinics in Liver Disease, August 2017 (Vol. 21, Issue 3)
Hepatitis C Infection as a Systemic Disease: Extra-Hepatic Manifestation of Hepatitis C
Zobair M. Younossi, Editor

Preface

Removing the Barriers from the Path to Eliminate Hepatitis C

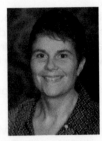 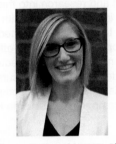

Camilla S. Graham, MD, MPH   Stacey B. Trooskin MD, PhD
Editors

Major organizations, including the World Health Organization and the United States National Academy of Medicine, Science, and Engineering, and many other individual countries have created plans to eliminate hepatitis C virus (HCV) infection as a public health threat by 2030. This will require expanding screening, diagnosis, linkage to care, and antiviral treatment, as well as liver cancer screening and monitoring persons for reinfection. It is easy to list all the challenges that will make this goal difficult to achieve. This group of authors was asked to focus on how to actually achieve HCV elimination.

The Centers for Disease Control and Prevention has been at the forefront of defining the seriousness of hepatitis C in the United States and starts this issue with a summary of a remarkable collection of studies derived from following a cohort of persons living with HCV for over a decade. This is followed by a series of examples of implementation programs to eliminate HCV in a country (Australia), in a major health care system (US Veterans Administration), by local/state US advocacy coalitions, and by a program to expand HCV care capacity in primary care. Common themes include strong clinical guidelines, comprehensive policies, and advocacy for adequate funding to pay for antiviral treatment.

Elimination of hepatitis C will not succeed if the needs of vulnerable populations are not addressed. The next section starts with an analysis of the US justice system. If federal and state prisons and state and city jails do not address HCV, this infection will never be eliminated in the United States because up to a third of persons living with HCV pass through the justice system every year. These authors offer a unique analysis of how this financially constrained system might be able to afford antiviral treatment. Subsequent articles address challenges in treating people who inject drugs and reducing the risk of reinfection in people who inject drugs and men who have sex with other men.

Infect Dis Clin N Am 32 (2018) xv–xvi
https://doi.org/10.1016/j.idc.2018.03.001
0891-5520/18/© 2018 Published by Elsevier Inc.

id.theclinics.com

The HCV elimination movement can learn valuable lessons from global strategies to address other diseases of public health significance. Models of care for HIV could be expanded to address HCV, and in extension, could leverage a robust care system for HIV to improve HCV care and treatment. The major challenge facing most countries is a low rate of HCV diagnosis. There are global efforts to implement high-quality and affordable diagnostics with a focus on the "holy grail" point-of-care diagnostic that will detect the presence of HCV infection. Global advocacy will be required to encourage ongoing investment and research into this initiative.

Most programs will have to implement plans with very limited resources. Models can help determine how best to direct these limited resources and guide the data that must be generated to support the advocacy efforts. Finally, in many countries, reimbursement by payers determines who gets treated and with what drugs, so it is important to understand how decision making occurs.

We are delighted to share this outstanding collection of articles and hope it inspires all of you to join in the global campaign to eliminate HCV.

Camilla S. Graham, MD, MPH
Viral Hepatitis Center
Division of Infectious Disease
Beth Israel Deaconess Medical Center
Harvard Medical School
110 Francis Street, LMOB Suite GB
Boston, MA 02215, USA

Stacey B. Trooskin, MD, PhD
Philadelphia FIGHT Community Health Centers
Viral Hepatitis Program
1233 Locust Street, 5th floor
Philadelphia, PA 19107, USA

E-mail addresses:
cgraham@bidmc.harvard.edu (C.S. Graham)
Strooskin@fight.org (S.B. Trooskin)

Long-Term Liver Disease, Treatment, and Mortality Outcomes Among 17,000 Persons Diagnosed with Chronic Hepatitis C Virus Infection

Current Chronic Hepatitis Cohort Study Status and Review of Findings

Anne C. Moorman, BSN, MPH[a],*, Loralee B. Rupp, MSE[b],
Stuart C. Gordon, MD[b], Yuna Zhong, MSPH[a], Jian Xing, PhD[a],
Mei Lu, PhD[c], Joseph A. Boscarino, PhD, MPH[d],
Mark A. Schmidt, PhD[e], Yihe G. Daida, PhD[f],
Eyasu H. Teshale, MD[a], Philip R. Spradling, MD[a],
Scott D. Holmberg, MD, MPH[a], for the CHeCS Investigators

KEYWORDS

- Hepatitis C • Comorbidities • Cirrhosis • Sustained viral response
- Direct-acting antiviral • Mortality • Real-world cohort

Conflict of Interest: The authors have made the following disclosures: S.C. Gordon receives grant/research support from AbbVie Pharmaceuticals (M15-410, M13-576, M15-942, M14-222, M13-590, M14-227, M14-868), Conatus (IDN-6556-14, IDN-6556-120), CymaBay (CB8025-21629, CB8025-31731), Gilead Pharmaceuticals (GS-US-330-1508, GS-US-320-4018, GS-US-367-1170, GS-US-367-1171, GS-US-367-1172, GS-US-367-1173, GS-US-334-0154, GS-US-337-4063, IN-US-337-3957), Intercept Pharmaceuticals (747-303, 747-301, 747-302, 747-207, [Master agreement dated Nov 9, 2015, with Statements of Work 1–3 for Fibrotic Liver Diseases (FOLD) study]), and Merck (MK5172-017, MK5172-062, MK3682-035, MK3682-041, MK3682-012, MK3682-021). He is also a consultant/advisor for Abbvie, Gilead, Intercept, and Merck. L.B. Rupp, M. Lu, J.A. Boscarino, M.A. Schmidt, and Y.G. Daida receive research grant support from Gilead Pharmaceuticals (IN-US-337-3957) and Intercept (Master agreement dated Nov 9, 2015, with Statements of Work 1–3 for Fibrotic Liver Diseases (FOLD) study).

Financial Support: Henry Ford Health System receives funding for CHeCS from the Centers for Disease Control and Prevention (1U18PS005154) and from Gilead Sciences. CHeCS was previously funded through May 2016 by the CDC Foundation (MOA-481-09 and MOA-481-15), which received grants from AbbVie; Genentech, A Member of the Roche Group; Gilead Sciences; Janssen Pharmaceuticals, Inc; and Vertex Pharmaceuticals. Past partial funders include Bristol-Myers Squibb. Granting corporations do not have access to CHeCS data and do not contribute to data analysis or writing of articles.

Disclaimer: The findings and conclusions in this report are those of the authors and do not necessarily represent the official position of the Centers for Disease Control and Prevention.

Infect Dis Clin N Am 32 (2018) 253–268
https://doi.org/10.1016/j.idc.2018.02.002
0891-5520/18/Published by Elsevier Inc.

id.theclinics.com

KEY POINTS

- The Chronic Hepatitis Cohort Study (CHeCS) was established to improve the understanding of chronic viral hepatitis in "real-world" US patients and the impact of their screening, care, and treatment.
- This report summarizes CHeCS results to date and updates the clinical experience among more than 17,000 current HCV cohort patients.
- The more than 40 CHeCS publications have described access to care, status of hepatic disease, and comorbidities in this population. Current activities center on comorbidities, impact, and access to new therapies.

INTRODUCTION

Accurately delineating the progression and rates of liver disease and death in patients with chronic viral hepatitis infection requires following many affected patients for a long period. The Chronic Hepatitis Cohort Study (CHeCS), an ongoing dynamic, retro-spective/prospective observational cohort study, was launched in 2008 to study the natural history of chronic viral hepatitis with and without antiviral treatment in the United States.[1] It is one of the largest cohorts of "real world" chronic hepatitis patients in the world. CHeCS currently includes a geographically and demographically diverse population of more than 4300 persons with chronic hepatitis B virus (HBV) infection and more than 17,000 persons with chronic hepatitis C virus (HCV) infection. Major objectives of the study are to determine the health burden and mortality associated with chronic viral hepatitis, monitor the implementation and effectiveness of recommended screening and care practices, understand the costs and potential savings of appropriate care and treatment, monitor access to care and treatment, and better understand the epidemiology of currently infected persons. This report summarizes CHeCS HCV cohort study findings to date and updates the clinical experience among current cohort patients.

METHODS

Criteria for inclusion and composition of the CHeCS cohort as well as details of the database created have been summarized in previous reports.[1-4] Briefly, the cohort was based on analysis of electronic health records (EHR) and administrative data of about 2.7 million patients aged $\geq$18 years who had a clinical service (ie, outpatient or inpatient, emergency department, or laboratory) visit provided on or after January 1, 2006 at 1 of 4 integrated health care systems: Geisinger Health System in Danville,

[a] Division of Viral Hepatitis, Centers for Disease Control and Prevention (CDC), Mailstop G-37, Atlanta, GA 30329, USA; [b] Division of Gastroenterology and Hepatology, Henry Ford Health System, 2799 West Grand Boulevard, Detroit, MI 48202, USA; [c] Public Health Sciences, Henry Ford Health System, 1 Ford Place -3A, Detroit, MI 48202, USA; [d] Department of Epidemiology and Health Services Research, Geisinger Clinic, 100 North Academy Avenue, Danville, PA 17822, USA; [e] Kaiser Permanente-Center for Health Research, Northwest, Kaiser Permanente Northwest, 3800 North Interstate Avenue, Portland, OR 97227-1098, USA; [f] Kaiser Permanente–Center for Health Research, Hawaii, Kaiser Permanente Hawaii, 501 Alakawa Street, Suite 201, Honolulu, HI 9681, USA
* Corresponding author. Division of Viral Hepatitis, Centers for Disease Control and Prevention (CDC), 1600 Clifton Road, Mailstop G-37, Atlanta, GA 30329.
E-mail addresses: Amoorman@cdc.gov

Pennsylvania that serves approximately 2.6 million Pennsylvania residents in 44 counties; Henry Ford Health System in Detroit that serves more than one million southeastern Michigan residents; Kaiser Permanente-Northwest in Portland, Oregon that serves approximately 500,000 members; and Kaiser Permanente of Honolulu, Hawaii that serves about 220,000 persons or approximately one-sixth of Hawaii residents. The study protocol was approved by an Institutional Review Board registered with the Department of Health and Human Services Office for Human Research Protections at each participating site.

Extensive review, by algorithm, was undertaken to specify and characterize chronic patients with HBV and HCV. Patients were identified principally by laboratory results and secondarily by International Classification of Diseases, Ninth Revision, Clinical Modification (ICD-9-CM) criteria.[1–4] Health system patients seen since 2006 who have met cohort eligibility criteria have been enrolled in the cohort; during 2014 to 2016, only newly eligible patients with HCV prescribed direct-acting antiviral (DAAs) were enrolled as a subset of the cohort, with data collection on the remainder of 2014 to 2016 eligible (untreated) patients planned for 2018. For all enrolled patients, once chronic viral hepatitis infection is confirmed by data abstractors[1,4] or an electronically available test that detects hepatitis C nucleic acid, all electronically available retrospective EHR and administrative data on medical encounters, diagnoses, procedures, hepatitis treatment, and laboratory tests back to the first health system visit are collected. Collection of prospective longitudinal follow-up data continues for all HCV cohort patients.

Electronically available data were supplemented with individual EHR chart review of text fields by trained data abstractors. Data on hepatitis treatment, external laboratory tests, and biopsy results were abstracted following a standard procedure and manual.[1,4] Abstractors reviewed all charts for patients enrolled based on 2006 to 2008 data collection. Because of capacity and funding constraints, patients newly identified as meeting HCV cohort criteria after these dates were selected by simple random sampling (enhanced by cohort-based adaptive criteria for the year 2012)[2] for chart abstraction as funding allowed.[3] In 2014, retrospective and prospective records for all patients prescribed HCV therapy and those coinfected with HBV were abstracted as well to enhance ascertainment of treatment data. Of all 17,893 enrolled in the CHeCS at the 4 health systems, 11,858 (66%) have had extensive chart abstraction. Behavioral data were collected from a one-time cross-sectional survey in 2011 to 2012.[5] To enhance ascertainment of deaths among cohort patients and obtain causes of death from death certificate data, each health system performs a yearly comparison of the records of patients with no health system contact in the previous 2 years, or with a known date of death, with the most recent National Death Index, Social Security Death Index, or electronic state death registries.[1,6] An algorithm to detect decompensated cirrhosis through ICD-9 codes was developed and validated with chart review by gastroenterology fellows using standard diagnosis guidelines provided by a senior hepatologist.[7]

Current patient demographic and clinical status as of January 1, 2016 among 2006 to 2013 HCV cohort-eligible patients are presented as well as a review of CHeCS publications to date.

RESULTS
Study Source Population

Among the 1.6 million adults in the 4 health systems as of the end of 2009 from which the initial CHeCS cohort was drawn, only 57% of predicted patients with

HCV had been identified from testing and less than half of those with 2 or more abnormal alanine aminotransferase (ALT) levels had received HCV testing.[8] In this initial study source population, only 61% of persons with a positive HCV antibody test had documentation of a follow-up RNA test indicative of clinical follow-up by the end of 2011.[9] The current cohort is sourced from more than 2.8 million patients aged ≥18 years with health care utilization during 2006 to 2013 at the 4 participating health systems.

Mortality Data

CHeCS analyses revealed high rates of morbidity and mortality in the era before the availability of DAA therapy. Analyses of mortality 2006 to 2010 found very high death rates, about 2.5% to 3.5% per year.[1] Mean age of death was 59 years, 15 years younger than in age-adjusted nationally representative data, with an age-adjusted mortality for liver disease 12 times higher than the national average.[6] This study also found that only 19% of all CHeCS decedents, and just 30% of those with deaths attributed to liver disease, had HCV listed on their death certificates, even though most had biopsy, biomarker, or other evidence of advanced liver disease. Applying this to the 20,000 death certificates a year listing HCV indicates that more than 100,000 patients with HCV a year are dying of or with HCV: this is an estimate projected only from those who have been diagnosed. In current data, achievement of sustained viral response to therapy (SVR) was associated with a reduction in all-cause mortality and risk of death, but continued mortality risk was associated with severe fibrosis and cirrhosis, and older age.[10] Further analyses showed that although prevalence of cirrhosis has increased over the past decade, particularly among non–white patients, overall mortality may be decreasing.[11]

Hospitalization Data

Compared with other patients in the health systems from which the cohort was drawn in the pre-DAA era, patients with HCV overall not only were more likely to be hospitalized from liver-related conditions but also had an approximately 3.7-fold higher likelihood of all-cause hospitalization, with 27.4 hospitalizations per 100 person-years versus 7.4 per 100 person-years for other health system patients.[12] However, the relatively small number of patients with HCV who achieved SVR following treatment in the pre-DAA era experienced a posttreatment reduction in all-cause hospitalization of about 25%.[13] These findings highlight the incremental costs and health care burden of patients with chronic HCV infection.

Advanced Liver Fibrosis and Hepatocellular Carcinoma

CHeCS analyses showed that serum/blood assays (eg, ALT, aspartate aminotransferase [AST], and platelet count) and patient age can be calculated in an index (FIB-4 or aspartate aminotransferase platelet ratio index [APRI] score) that accurately distinguishes advanced fibrosis and cirrhosis from no to moderate levels of hepatic fibrosis as measured by liver biopsy, to reduce the need for doing biopsy.[14,15]

As of 2012, almost one-fifth of CHeCS patients had been diagnosed "late," that is, with advanced liver disease concurrent with their initial HCV diagnosis, despite many years of prior engagement with the health care system; these patients had high rates of hospitalization (59%) and mortality (33%), highlighting the severe consequences of missed opportunities for earlier diagnosis.[16] In this analysis, advanced liver disease was defined as having one or more of the following: a biopsy indicating cirrhosis; FIB-4 score >5.88 predictive of biopsy stage F4[15]; or an

ICD-9 or procedure code indicating liver transplant, hepatocellular carcinoma (HCC), liver failure, hepatic encephalopathy, portal hypertension, esophageal varices, other gastroesophageal hemorrhage, ascites, or other sequelae of chronic liver disease. Among data from biopsied CHeCS patients before 2013, analyses showed that about two-thirds of currently active patients would meet criteria for urgent HCV treatment based on American Association for the Study of Liver Diseases/Infectious Diseases Society of America/International Antiviral Society-USA guidelines,[17] and among these patients, there were substantial rates of disease progression to hepatic decompensation, HCC, liver transplant, and death.[18] Patients and their providers may not be aware of advanced liver fibrosis despite the substantial (29%) prevalence as measured by biopsy, noninvasive markers, and/or diagnoses consistent with cirrhosis or hepatic decompensation.[19] Of note, in this study only 46% of even those patients with biopsy-confirmed cirrhosis were not assigned *ICD-9* codes for cirrhosis, suggesting that cirrhosis may be underdocumented and underdiagnosed.

Given the inherent challenge in identifying when patients with longstanding HCV infection become cirrhotic and at risk for HCC, CHeCS investigators devised a simple clinical scoring system to estimate the 1-, 3-, and 5-year probabilities of developing HCC before and after SVR, based on APRI score, age, sex, alcohol abuse history, and prior (interferon-based) treatment history (Xing and colleagues 2017).[20] Patients who were male, were older (ie, aged >50 years), had higher APRI scores (including post-SVR values), had a history of alcohol abuse, and had a history of interferon treatment failure had the highest probability of HCC.[20] In an earlier CHeCS study, failure of interferon-based therapy was associated with increased rates of HCC.[21] The same study found that those with genotype 3 did have a greater risk of HCC than those with genotype 1. SVR appeared to induce long-term regression of hepatic fibrosis based on FIB-4 scores collected over 10 years; patients receiving no treatment or with treatment failure had progressive increases in FIB-4 scores.[22] In this study, men and patients with HCV genotype 3 infections had higher FIB-4 scores than women or patients with HCV genotype 2 infections. Additional studies found that highly elevated ALT (>2 times the upper limit of normal) was significantly more common in patients with genotype 3 and that FIB-4 scores indicative of cirrhosis were most common in the patients with genotypes 4 and 6, with overall cohort distribution of genotypes and subtypes more variable than suggested by previous national-level estimates and single-center studies.[23]

Nonhepatic Comorbidities

Substantial comorbidities, such as kidney disease,[24] diabetes, and coronary artery disease,[25,26] are likely to affect clinical course and may complicate HCV care management. Although the prevalence of severe renal impairment and diagnosed extrahepatic manifestations was low (about 2%), mild to moderate renal impairment was common (about 33%) in patients with HCV, across all levels of hepatic fibrosis.[24] In addition to the expected excess of liver cancers that was 48.6 times higher than the national average, investigators found significantly elevated age-adjusted incidence of pancreatic, kidney, non-Hodgkin lymphoma, and lung cancers in the CHeCS cohort over a comparable nationally representative comparison group.[27]

Contributions to National Disease Estimates

Significant national disease estimates incorporated data from CHeCS and other sources. Based on information from CHeCS and the National Health and Nutrition Examination Study as well as other sources, investigators were able to estimate the rate at which US residents were tested for HCV, referred for specialist care, treated and achieved SVR before the availability of DAAs.[28] Only about half of the chronic cases had been identified, and of these, only 5% to 6% were successfully treated. CHeCS data were also used to estimate the number of people infected with HCV in 2014 in the United States who would qualify for immediate treatment according to 2014 treatment guidance, finding that as many as 813,000 persons nationwide were in need of urgent treatment.[29] Similar analyses determined that immediate treatment of HCV-infected patients with moderate and advanced fibrosis appears to be cost-effective, and immediate treatment of even patients with minimal or no fibrosis can be cost-effective.[30]

Access to Care

Analyses of access to care from the pre-DAA era showed that only 57% had ever received liver specialist care with high variation in rates by health system[31] and that many patients lacked recommended protection against other forms of viral hepatitis: 35% had been neither tested nor vaccinated for hepatitis A and 32% neither tested nor vaccinated for hepatitis B.[32] Recently updated data as of 2016 showed that a little over one-half the cohort appeared susceptible to either infection.[33]

Patient Survey

The extensive cross-sectional survey of almost 5000 HCV-infected CHeCS patients during 2010 to 2011 provided a novel source of data on risk behaviors, physical and psychosocial functioning, demographics, and clinical history. About half of surveyed patients reported past injection drug use, 34% were current smokers, 18% had abused alcohol in the previous year, 30% met criteria for current depression, and one-quarter were in poor physical health.[5] Achieving a 12-week SVR was found to be protective for depression. A substantial proportion reported having been tested for HCV only after clinical indications that their infection had progressed and became symptomatic.[34]

Current Analyses

Current analyses focus on the impact of and access to new therapies and comorbidities, including their reversal with current effective therapies. For instance, to test the hypothesis that antiviral treatment may have an impact on long-term extrahepatic outcomes, investigators examined incidence of type 2 diabetes and found that SVR significantly reduces this incidence in analyses controlling for demographic and clinical factors, including race and body mass index.[25] In addition, among patients under treatment for type 2 diabetes, the achievement of SVR led to reduced rates of end-stage renal disease and acute coronary syndrome, and to temporary reductions in hemoglobin A1c levels.[26] Additional studies are examining health outcomes by survey self-reported behavioral risks and measures of physical and psychosocial functioning[35] as well as describing substantial rates of depression and alcohol misuse whether measured by ICD-9 code or survey.[36] In 2016, the prevalence of HBV current coinfection (1.1%) and past resolved infection (40% of tested, 15% of entire cohort as more than half were untested) was similar to other US studies, with no hepatitis B reactivation identified in almost 700 (31%) of CHeCS patients with a history of (mostly resolved) hepatitis B infection who were treated with DAAs.[37] Despite improvements in care, barriers remain: black race, Medicaid coverage, and care at one of the sites were associated with noninitiation of DAA therapy during 2014 to 2015.[38] In addition, the prevalence of consistent surveillance for HCC (screening at least every 6 months) in cirrhotic patients with chronic HCV infection remains low (11.8%) (Abara WE, Spradling P, Zhong Y, et al. Surveillance for hepatocellular carcinoma in a cohort of

Table 1
Chronic Hepatitis Cohort Study hepatitis C virus cohort patient status on January 1, 2016

Variables	Overall N (Column%)	Died (All Cause) n (row%)	Liver Transplant[a] n (row%)	Achieved SVR[b] n (row%)	Still HCV Infected n (row%)	HCV Status Cannot Be Determined n (row%)
	17,893	3871 (21.6%)	555 (3.1%)	3378 (18.9%)	8906 (49.8%)	1183 (6.6%)
Birth year						
1965 through 1984	5985 (33.4)	1054 (17.6)	190 (3.2)	1231 (20.6)	3129 (52.3)	381 (6.4)
1945 through 1964	6682 (37.3)	1882 (28.2)	292 (4.4)	1305 (19.5)	2933 (43.9)	270 (4.0)
Birth year ≤1944	1467 (8.2)	657 (44.8)	46 (3.1)	180 (12.3)	550 (37.5)	34 (2.3)
Gender						
Male	10,862 (60.7)	2684 (24.7)	420 (3.9)	1941 (17.9)	5108 (47.0)	709 (6.5)
Female	7031 (39.3)	1187 (16.9)	135 (1.9)	1437 (20.4)	3798 (54.0)	474 (6.7)
Race						
Non-Hispanic white	11,308 (63.2)	2109 (18.7)	357 (3.2)	2403 (21.3)	5518 (48.8)	921 (8.1)
Non-Hispanic black	4022 (22.5)	1247 (31.0)	115 (2.9)	544 (13.5)	1982 (49.3)	134 (3.3)
Other	2563 (14.3)	515 (20.1)	83 (3.2)	431 (16.8)	1406 (54.9)	128 (5.0)
Insurance status						
Private	8824 (49.3)	1362 (15.4)	179 (2.0)	1959 (22.2)	4641 (52.6)	683 (7.7)
Medicaid	2054 (11.5)	499 (24.3)	38 (1.9)	208 (10.1)	1165 (56.7)	144 (7.0)
Medicare	5538 (31.0)	1612 (29.1)	326 (5.9)	1054 (19.0)	2365 (42.7)	181 (3.3)
Other/unknown	1477 (8.3)	398 (26.9)	12 (0.8)	157 (10.6)	735 (49.8)	175 (11.8)

(continued on next page)

Table 1
(continued)

Variables	Overall N (Column%)	Died (All Cause) n (row%)	Liver Transplant[a] n (row%)	Achieved SVR[b] n (row%)	Still HCV Infected n (row%)	HCV Status Cannot Be Determined n (row%)
	17,893	3871 (21.6%)	555 (3.1%)	3378 (18.9%)	8906 (49.8%)	1183 (6.6%)
Income (estimated census tract geocode)						
<$30,000	4258 (23.8)	1172 (27.5)	80 (1.9)	578 (13.6)	2137 (50.2)	291 (6.8)
$30,000 to <50,000	8201 (45.8)	1700 (20.7)	237 (2.9)	1585 (19.3)	4110 (50.1)	569 (6.9)
≥$50,000	4850 (27.1)	872 (18.0)	212 (4.4)	1159 (23.9)	2345 (48.4)	262 (5.4)
Not available	584 (3.3)	127 (21.7)	26 (4.5)	56 (9.6)	314 (53.8)	61 (10.4)
Study site						
Portland, OR	4329 (24.2)	577 (13.3)	53 (1.2)	809 (18.7)	2633 (60.8)	257 (5.9)
Honolulu, HI	1564 (8.7)	222 (14.2)	25 (1.6)	292 (18.7)	969 (62.0)	56 (3.6)
Detroit, MI	7402 (41.4)	2288 (30.9)	423 (5.7)	1345 (18.2)	3158 (42.7)	188 (2.5)
Danville, PA	4598 (25.7)	784 (17.1)	54 (1.2)	932 (20.3)	2146 (46.7)	682 (14.8)
Observation time in years[c]						
Median	5.9	4.8	6.6	2.9	7.5	4.4
Range	0.0–25.4	0.0–20.5	0.0–20.5	0.0–25.4	0.0–23.0	0.0–22.8
Mean (SE)	6.8 (0.0)	5.8 (0.1)	7.6 (0.2)	4.6 (0.1)	8.2 (0.1)	5.5 (0.1)

[a] Liver transplant status identified by at least one of the following *ICD-9* diagnosis or procedure codes: 996.82, 50.5, 50.51, 50.59, 47135, or 47136.
[b] Defined as having more negative HCV RNA tests at least 12 wk after treatment as evidenced by available EHR laboratory data or provider documentation.
[c] Observation defined as time from the first diagnosis of hepatitis C within the health system to the date of the first endpoint (death, liver transplant, SVR) or last encounter in the health system.

Table 2
Demographic and clinical characteristics of patients still infected with hepatitis C virus in 2016,[a] by Chronic Hepatitis Cohort Study site

Variables	Overall N = 8906 (Column%)	Portland, OR n = 2633 (29.6%)	Honolulu, HI n = 969 (10.9%)	Detroit, MI n = 3158 (35.4%)	Danville, PA n = 2146 (24.1%)
				CHeCS Study Site	
Age (median on 1/1/16)	58.8	58.8	61.0	61.4	49.9
Birth year					
1965 through 1984	2294 (25.8)	573 (21.8)	114 (11.8)	475 (15.0)	1132 (52.7)
1945 through 1964	6062 (68.1)	1949 (74.0)	779 (80.4)	2365 (74.9)	969 (45.2)
Birth year ≤1944	550 (6.2)	111 (4.2)	76 (7.8)	318 (10.1)	45 (2.1)
Male	5108 (57.4)	1556 (59.1)	610 (63.0)	1867 (59.1)	1075 (50.1)
Previous treatment attempt[b]					
Yes	3963 (44.5)	945 (35.9)	466 (48.1)	1430 (45.3)	1122 (52.3)
No	4943 (55.5)	1688 (64.1)	503 (51.9)	1728 (54.7)	1024 (47.7)
Genotype distribution					
Genotype 1	4010 (77.2)	980 (69.7)	533 (74.5)	1735 (84.6)	762 (74.8)
Genotype 2	565 (10.9)	219 (15.6)	94 (13.1)	135 (6.6)	117 (11.5)
Genotype 3	498 (9.6)	176 (12.5)	79 (11.0)	146 (7.1)	97 (9.5)
Genotype 4, 5, or 6	97 (1.9)	30 (2.1)	8 (1.1)	33 (1.6)	26 (2.6)
Genotype mixed	22 (0.4)	2 (0.1)	1 (0.1)	2 (0.1)	17 (1.7)

(continued on next page)

Table 2
(continued)

Variables	Overall N = 8906 (Column%)	CHeCS Study Site			
		Portland, OR n = 2633 (29.6%)	Honolulu, HI n = 969 (10.9%)	Detroit, MI n = 3158 (35.4%)	Danville, PA n = 2146 (24.1%)
Had liver biopsy during 2004-15	1764 (19.8)	741 (28.1)	226 (23.3)	418 (13.2)	379 (17.7)
Latest biopsy stage distribution[c]					
Metavir F0/1	724 (45.5)	248 (34.8)	60 (28.3)	201 (57.8)	215 (67.4)
Metavir F2	518 (32.6)	332 (46.6)	68 (32.1)	85 (24.4)	33 (10.3)
Metavir F3	186 (11.7)	91 (12.8)	42 (19.8)	35 (10.1)	18 (5.6)
Metavir F4	163 (10.2)	41 (5.8)	42 (19.8)	27 (7.8)	53 (16.6)
Latest FIB-4, score category[11,12,d] during 2004-2015					
<1.6	4005 (49.2)	1088 (46.1)	359 (41.1)	1204 (42.4)	1354 (65.8)
1.6–2.5	1855 (22.8)	630 (26.7)	224 (25.6)	712 (25.1)	289 (14.0)
2.5 to <3.25	720 (8.9)	194 (8.2)	94 (10.8)	306 (10.8)	126 (6.1)
≥3.25	1554 (19.1)	450 (19.1)	197 (22.5)	618 (21.8)	289 (14.0)
Latest APRI score category[11,12,e] during 2004-2015					
<1.5	6852 (82.3)	1971 (82.2)	710 (80.2)	2362 (79.4)	1809 (87.3)
≥1.5	1476 (17.7)	426 (17.8)	175 (19.8)	611 (20.6)	264 (12.7)
Viral load from latest test[f]					
<1.5 million	2249 (54.0)	378 (39.6)	306 (61.3)	813 (52.9)	752 (63.9)
≥1.5 to <6 million	1192 (28.6)	312 (32.7)	132 (26.5)	453 (29.5)	295 (25.1)
≥6 million	726 (17.4)	265 (27.7)	61 (12.2)	271 (17.6)	129 (11.0)
Decompensated cirrhosis or portal hypertension[g]					
Yes	612 (6.9)	183 (7.0)	70 (7.2)	237 (7.5)	122 (5.7)
No	8294 (93.1)	2450 (93.0)	899 (92.8)	2921 (92.5)	2024 (94.3)

HCC[h]					
Yes	115 (1.3)	35 (1.3)	12 (1.2)	50 (1.6)	18 (0.8)
No	8791 (98.7)	2598 (98.7)	957 (98.8)	3108 (98.4)	2128 (99.2)
Platelet count below normal[i]					
Yes	1872 (21.6)	466 (18.3)	167 (17.8)	827 (27.0)	412 (19.5)
No	6790 (78.4)	2079 (81.7)	772 (82.2)	2240 (73.0)	1699 (80.5)
HIV coinfection	293 (3.3)	65 (2.5)	17 (1.8)	150 (4.7)	61 (2.8)
Ever had hepatitis B surface antigen or HBV DNA test	5847 (74.4)	1682 (72.8)	708 (85.9)	2007 (71.7)	1450 (75.1)
Among those tested, one or more tests positive	94 (1.3)	25 (1.5)	2 (0.2)	38 (1.9)	29 (2.0)
Charlson comorbidity score (excluding liver diseases)[j]					
0	5824 (65.4)	1710 (64.9)	652 (67.3)	1969 (62.3)	1493 (69.6)
1	1347 (15.1)	445 (16.9)	153 (15.8)	409 (13.0)	340 (15.8)
2 or more	1735 (19.5)	478 (18.2)	164 (16.9)	780 (24.7)	313 (14.6)

[a] Among patients alive but without documented liver transplant or SVR as of January 1, 2015.

[b] Treatment defined as having been prescribed at least 1 day of antiviral therapy.

[c] Biopsy reports from different scoring systems (International Association for the Study of the Liver, Batts-Ludwig, Metavir, Ishak, Knodell, Scheuer) were mapped to an F0–F4 equivalency scale and ranked as follows: F0, no fibrosis; F1, portal fibrosis without septa; F2, portal fibrosis with few septa; F3, numerous septa without cirrhosis; and F4, cirrhosis.[1]

[d] Among 8928 (93%) patients with available laboratory data for calculation of FIB-4, excluding laboratory results during hospitalization.

[e] AST/platelet ratio, calculated among 8829 (93%) patients with available same-day AST and platelet count data, excluding laboratory results during hospitalization.

[f] Among 6631 (70%) patients with available viral load data.

[g] The development of decompensated cirrhosis was ascertained based on the presence of an ICD-9 diagnosis or procedure codes in the following groups: hepatic encephalopathy (572.2), portal hypertension (572.3, 37140, 37160, 37180, 37181, 37182, 37183), esophageal varices with bleeding (456.0, 456.20, 42.91, 44.91, 96.06, 43204, 43205, 43244, 43400, 43401), ascites (789.5, 789.59, 54.91, 49080, 49081), liver failure with hepato-renal syndrome (572.4).

[h] Primary HCC as determined from validated tumor registry reports.[27]

[i] Among 9289 (97%) patients with available platelet count data.

[j] Calculated from standard diagnosis codes, while omitting liver diseases in inpatient, outpatient, and claims data[5] during the last 2 y of observation before January 1, 2015.

cirrhotic patients chronically infected with hepatitis C virus, 2006-2014. Submitted for publication, 2018).

Current Hepatitis C Virus Cohort Status

From more than 2.8 million adult patients seen during 2006 to 2013 at participating sites, 23,603 were identified that met criteria for potential inclusion before chart review. Patients whose chronic HCV status was ruled out or could not be confirmed were excluded.[1–3] Of 17,893 patients finally included in the cohort, comparing the 12465 (70%) sampled for chart review with the 5428 (30%) whose charts were not abstracted showed that differences were small and not statistically significant. Among those sampled for data abstraction, 61% were men, mean year of birth was 1961, and mean FIB-4 score was 3.3; among those not sampled and abstracted, 60% were men, mean year of birth was 1956, and mean FIB-4 score was 3.4.

As of the beginning of 2016, cohort patients had been observed for an average of 6 years and 22% (3871) had died, ranging from 13% to 31% by site; most deaths were among those born between 1945 and 1964 (**Table 1**). Three percent (555) had undergone liver transplant (ranging from 3% to 4% by site). Nineteen percent (3378) of the total cohort had achieved SVR after antiviral therapy. Achievement of SVR varied widely by demographic factors, with lowest rates among those with lowest census tract estimated income, nonprivate insurance, black race, and the oldest age group (born ≤1944). The 50% (8906) of cohort patients who remained infected because of either no treatment or treatment failure had a mean observation time of 7.5 years (see **Table 1**). In **Table 2**, the demographic and clinical characteristics of patients who were still infected by the beginning of 2016 are shown by study site. Mean age of these patients ranged from 50 to 61 years. Overall, 6.9% (612) patients had received a diagnosis of decompensated cirrhosis or portal hypertension, 1.3% (115) had received a diagnosis of HCC, and 44.5% (3963) had a prior unsuccessful treatment attempt. Of these persons still infected at last follow-up, 27.0% (2400) had no health system visits during 2014 to 2016 after the availability of DAA therapy, but did not appear in the death registries.

DISCUSSION

CHeCS has provided a wealth of highly impactful information about HCV epidemiology, outcomes such as long-term liver disease, comorbidities, and mortality, and access to and outcomes of treatment with a current cohort of almost 18,000 persons diagnosed with chronic HCV. As one measure of CHeCS's impact, per the Science Citation Index, CHeCS publications have been referenced more than 900 times by others. An early analysis of viral hepatitis testing in the health system populations from which CHeCS was drawn[8] was used as a basis for the Centers for Disease Control and Prevention (CDC) and U.S. Public Health Service *Recommendations for One-time Screening of Persons Born 1945 to 1965*, critical to the cost-effectiveness analyses that underlay and supported those recommendations. CHeCS contributions to national disease estimates include developing a national HCV care cascade to quantify the number of persons getting diagnosed and moving along the care continuum and the numerous benefits of treatment.[28] In addition, data from CHeCS were used to estimate the number of persons infected with HCV in the United States who would qualify for immediate treatment according to 2014 treatment guidance,[29] which were shared with the Center for Medicare and Medicaid Services that, in turn, advised and urged state partners to expand treatment. CHeCS studies were used for the National Academies of Sciences, Engineering, and Medicine report on the feasibility of eliminating HCV in the United States.[39] Cost-effectiveness analyses, including data from CHeCS, are increasingly cited in the argument to treat all hepatitis C patients, including those early in infection or with no or minimal liver disease.[30] CHeCS analyses indicating that more than 100,000 HCV-infected persons per year are dying, 75% with evidence of moderate or worse liver disease,[6] dramatically changed perceptions of HCV as a benign chronic condition and highlighted the urgent need for treatment.

The lack of attribution of HCV to liver-related deaths on death certificates is particularly striking in light of current findings that mortality attributed to chronic HCV infection on death certificates recently surpassed mortality attributable to 60 other nationally notifiable infectious conditions in the United States combined.[40] In current data as of January 1, 2016, among more than 17,000 HCV cohort patients observed for an average of 6 years, the authors found that 1 in 5 had died or had achieved treatment-induced SVR, which varied widely by demographic factors, and 1 of every 2 cohort patients remained infected (ranging by site from 43% to 62%).

Although CHeCS is among the largest long-term observational studies to date of persons with chronic viral hepatitis infection, this analysis has several unavoidable limitations. Some comorbid conditions that confer high priority for HCV treatment, such as debilitating fatigue, could not be included because of lack of reliable measures. Differential mortalities by site may be due to greater number of patients with end-stage liver disease in the 2 sites with transplant centers, in Detroit and Pennsylvania. Also, results from these large integrated health systems may not be generalizable to other populations. Demographic differences between abstracted and nonabstracted cohort patients were modest, so sampling of charts for full supplementary data abstraction due to budget constraints in later years was unlikely to have introduced bias. All electronically derived data (eg, mortality dates and causes, health system laboratory results, and hospitalizations) were available for both abstracted and nonabstracted patients.

Current cohort characteristics may be rapidly changing in the current era of highly effective therapy. More than one-quarter of patients who remained HCV infected at last health system visit had no further follow-up visits during 2014 to 2016 after the availability of DAA therapy, which may indicate loss to follow-up and missed opportunity for treatment, although in some cases could also indicate change to a new health provider. Efforts are underway within all 4 health systems to reengage patients who appear lost to follow-up.

Among current cohort patients, clinical management may be complicated for the 3% who had been transplanted, and the 7% of untreated, still-infected patients who had already progressed to hepatic decompensation. Among these patients alive and without previous SVR, almost one-half had experienced treatment failure, primarily with prior interferon-based therapy, which some data suggest may confer additional morbidity risk.[20] At least 30% of cohort patients are at a high priority for treatment as defined by laboratory-derived fibrosis score; of the small proportion (20%) who underwent liver biopsy, more than 50% were stage F2 or higher. Treatment will be essential for these remaining cohort patients to avoid the substantial morbidity and mortality demonstrated in this cohort in the era before the widespread availability of highly effective DAA therapy. More than one-half the cohort was without documented protection from hepatitis A or B infection, with potentially serious consequences in the event of exposure. CHeCS data are continuing to provide unique, population-based insights into the changing dynamics of hepatitis C in the United States.

ACKNOWLEDGMENTS

The CHeCS Investigators include the following investigators and sites: Scott D. Holmberg, Eyasu H. Teshale, Philip R. Spradling, Anne C. Moorman, Jim Xing, and

Yuna Zhong, Division of Viral Hepatitis, National Centers for HIV, Viral Hepatitis, STD, and TB Prevention (NCHHSTP), Centers for Disease Control and Prevention (CDC), Atlanta, Georgia; Stuart C. Gordon, David R. Nerenz, Mei Lu, Lois Lamerato, Jia Li, Loralee B. Rupp, Nonna Akkerman, Nancy Oja-Tebbe, Talan Zhang, Sheri Trudeau, and Yueren Zhou, Henry Ford Health System, Detroit, Michigan; Joseph A. Boscarino, Zahra S. Daar, and Robert E. Smith, Center for Health Research, Geisinger Health System, Danville, Pennsylvania; Yihe G. Daida, Connie Mah Trinacty, and Carmen P. Wong, The Center for Health Research, Kaiser Permanente-Hawaii, Honolulu, Hawaii; Mark A. Schmidt and Judy L. Donald, The Center for Health Research, Kaiser Permanente-Northwest, Portland, Oregon.

REFERENCES

1. Moorman AC, Gordon SC, Rupp LR, et al. Baseline characteristics and mortality among people in care for chronic viral hepatitis: the Chronic Hepatitis Cohort Study (CHeCS). Clin Infect Dis 2013;56:40–50.
2. Lu M, Rupp LB, Moorman AC, et al. Comparative effectiveness research of Chronic Hepatitis B and C Cohort Study (CHeCS): improving data collection and cohort identification. Dig Dis Sci 2014;59:3053–61.
3. Abara WE, Moorman AC, Zhou Y, et al. The predictive value of International Classification of Disease Codes for chronic hepatitis C virus infection surveillance: the utility and limitations of electronic health records. Popul Health Manag. [Epub ahead of print].
4. Mahajan R, Moorman A, Liu S, et al. Use of the International Classification of Diseases, 9th revision, coding in identifying chronic hepatitis B virus infection in health system data: implications for national surveillance. J Am Med Inform Assoc 2013;20:441–5.
5. Boscarino JA, Lu M, Moorman AC, et al. Predictors of poor mental and physical health status among patients with chronic hepatitis C infection: the Chronic Hepatitis Cohort Study (CHeCS). Hepatology 2015;61:802–11.
6. Mahajan R, Xing J, Liu SJ, et al. Mortality among persons in care with hepatitis C virus infection: the chronic hepatitis cohort study (CHeCS), 2006–2010. Clin Infect Dis 2014;58:1055–61.
7. Lu M, Chacra W, Rabin D, et al, for the Chronic Hepatitis Cohort Study (CHeCS) Investigators. Validity of an automated algorithm using diagnosis and procedure codes to identify decompensated cirrhosis using electronic health records. Clin Epidemiol 2017;9:369–76.
8. Spradling PR, Rupp L, Moorman A, et al. Hepatitis B and C virus infection among 1.2 million persons with access to care: factors associated with testing and infection prevalence. Clin Infect Dis 2012;55:1047–55.
9. Spradling PR, Tong X, Rupp L, et al. Trends in HCV RNA testing among HCV antibody positive persons in care, 2003-2010. Clin Infect Dis 2014;59:976–81.
10. Xu F, Xing J, Moorman A, et al. Cause of death in HCV patients who achieved sustained virologic response: chronic hepatitis cohort study (CHeCS), 2006-2012. Presented at the 66th Annual Meeting of the American Association for the Study of Liver Diseases (AASLD), San Francisco, November 13–17, 2015.
11. Lu M, Li J, Rupp L, et al. Changing trends in complications of chronic hepatitis C. Liver Int 2018;38(2):239–47.
12. Teshale E, Xing J, Moorman A, et al. Higher all-cause hospitalization among patients with chronic hepatitis C: the Chronic Hepatitis Cohort Study (CHeCS), 2006-2013. J Viral Hepat 2016;10:748–54.

13. Teshale E, Xing J, Moorman AC, et al. Effect of HCV treatment outcome on hospitalization rate: Chronic Hepatitis Cohort Study (CHeCS). Presented at the 66th Annual Meeting of the American Association for the Study of Liver Diseases (AASLD), San Francisco, November 13–17, 2015.
14. Holmberg S, Lu M, Rupp LB, et al. Use of non-invasive serum markers for staging hepatitis C virus (HCV) in the Chronic Hepatitis Cohort Study (CHeCS). Clin Infect Dis 2013;57:240–6.
15. Li J, Gordon SC, Rupp LB, et al. The validity of serum markers for fibrosis staging in chronic hepatitis B and C. J Viral Hepat 2014;21:930–7.
16. Moorman AC, Xing J, Ko S, et al. Late diagnosis of hepatitis C virus (HCV) infection among patients in the Chronic Hepatitis Cohort Study (CHeCS): missed opportunities for intervention. Hepatology 2015;61:1479–84.
17. American Association for the Study of Liver Disease (AASLD). Recommendations for testing, management, and treatment of persons with HCV. Available at: http://www.hcvguidelines.org/full-report-view. Accessed January 17, 2018.
18. Xu F, Moorman AC, Tong X, et al. All-cause mortality and progression risks to hepatic decompensation and hepatocellular carcinoma in patients infected with hepatitis C virus. Clin Infect Dis 2016;62:289–97.
19. Gordon SC, Lamerato LE, Rupp LB, et al. Prevalence of cirrhosis in hepatitis C patients in the Chronic Hepatitis Cohort Study (CHeCS): a retrospective and prospective observational study. Am J Gastroenterol 2015;110:1169–77.
20. Xing J, Spradling PS, Moorman A, et al. A point system to forecast hepatocellular carcinoma risk before and after treatment among persons with chronic hepatitis C. Dig Dis Sci 2017;62:3221–4.
21. Lu M, Li J, Rupp LB, et al. Hepatitis C treatment failure is associated with increased risk of hepatocellular cancer. J Viral Hepat 2016;23:718–29.
22. Lu M, Li J, Zhang T, et al. Serum biomarkers indicate long-term reduction in liver fibrosis in patients with sustained virological response to treatment for HCV infection. Clin Gastroenterol Hepatol 2016;14:1044–55.
23. Gordon S, Trudeau S, Li J, et al. Race, age, and geography impact hepatitis C genotype distribution in the United States. J Clin Gastroenterol 2017 [Epub ahead of print].
24. Moorman AC, Tong X, Spradling PR, et al. Prevalence of renal impairment and associated conditions among HCV-infected persons in the Chronic Hepatitis Cohort Study (CHeCS). Dig Dis Sci 2016;61:2087–93.
25. Li J, Zhang T, Gordon SC, et al. Impact of sustained virological response on incidence of type 2 diabetes in hepatitis C patients. J Viral Hepat 2018. [Epub ahead of print].
26. Li J, Gordon SC, Rupp LB, et al. Does hepatitis C eradication lead to improved glucose metabolism, renal and cardiovascular outcomes in diabetic patients? Presented at the 68th Annual Meeting of the American Association for the Study of Liver Diseases (AASLD), Washington, DC, October 20–24, 2017.
27. Allison RD, Tong X, Moorman AC, et al, for the Chronic Hepatitis Cohort Study (CHeCS). Increased incidence of cancer and cancer-related mortality among persons with chronic hepatitis C infection, 2006-2010. J Hepatol 2015;63:822–8.
28. Holmberg SD, Spradling PR, Moorman AC, et al. Hepatitis C in the United States. N Engl J Med 2013;368:1859–61.
29. Xu F, Leidner AJ, Tong X, et al. Estimating the number of patients infected with chronic HCV in the United States who meet highest or high-priority treatment criteria. Am J Public Health 2015;105:1285–9.

30. Leidner AJ, Chesson HW, Xu F, et al. Cost-effectiveness of hepatitis C treatment for patients in early stages of liver disease. Hepatology 2015;61:1860–9.

31. Foster MA, Xing J, Moorman AC, et al. Frequency of and factors associated with receipt of liver-related specialty care among patients with hepatitis C in the Chronic Hepatitis Cohort Study. Dig Dis Sci 2016;61:3469–77.

32. Henkle E, Lu M, Rupp LB, et al, for the CHeCS Investigators. Hepatitis A and B immunity and vaccination in chronic hepatitis B and C patients in a large United States cohort. Clin Infect Dis 2015;60:514–22.

33. Moorman AC, Xing J, Nelson N, for the CHeCS Investigators. Increasing HAV vaccination among patients infected with HBV and HCV. Gastroenterology, in press.

34. Centers for Disease Control and Prevention. Locations and reasons for initial testing for hepatitis C infection–Chronic Hepatitis Cohort Study, United States, 2006-2010. MMWR Morb Mortal Wkly Rep 2013;62:645–8. Reported by: Boscarino J, Gordon S, Rupp L, Schmidt M, Vijayadeva V, Moorman A, Xu F. Corresponding contributor: Ko S.

35. Hofmeister MG, Xing J, Moorman AC, et al. Health outcomes among patients infected with hepatitis C in the Chronic Hepatitis Cohort Study. Presented at the 68th Annual Meeting of the American Association for the Study of Liver Diseases (AASLD), Washington, DC, October 20–24, 2017.

36. Boscarino J, Moorman A, Rupp L, et al. Comparison of ICD-9 codes for depression and alcohol misuse to survey instruments suggests these codes should be used with caution. Dig Dis Sci 2017;62:2704–12.

37. Moorman A, Xing X, Rupp L, et al. Hepatitis B virus (HBV) infection and hepatitis C virus (HCV) treatment in a large cohort of HCV-infected patients in the United States. Gastroenterology 2018;154:754–8.

38. Spradling P, Xing J, Rupp L, et al. Uptake of and factors associated with direct-acting antiviral therapy among patients infected with hepatitis C virus in the Chronic Hepatitis Cohort Study, 2014-2015. J Clin Gastroenterol 2017. [Epub ahead of print].

39. National Academies of Sciences, Engineering, and Medicine. A national strategy for the elimination of hepatitis B and C: phase two report. Washington, DC: The National Academies Press; 2017.

40. Ly KN, Hughes EM, Jiles RB, et al. Rising mortality associated with hepatitis C virus in the United States, 2003-2013. Clin Infect Dis 2016;62:1287–8.

Elimination of Hepatitis C Virus in Australia

Laying the Foundation

Gregory J. Dore, BSc, MBBS, MPH, FRACP, PhD*,
Behzad Hajarizadeh, MD, MPH, PhD

KEYWORDS

- Hepatitis C, HCV • Elimination • People who inject drugs • Australia
- Direct acting antivirals, DAA, public health

KEY POINTS

- Australia has laid the foundation for hepatitis C virus elimination within the next decade.
- Key aspects of this foundation include high levels of screening and diagnosis, unrestricted access to direct-acting antiviral therapy, a diverse range of models of care, and high coverage of harm reduction strategies.
- Key features include government risk-sharing arrangement with the pharmaceutical companies, minimal out-of-pocket cost, no restrictions based on liver disease stage or drug/alcohol use, prescribing authorization for all registered medical practitioners; and retreatment is allowed.
- Although initial uptake of direct-acting antiviral therapy was high, more efforts are required to continue the momentum.
- An hepatitis C virus elimination monitoring and evaluation program is in progress to inform further strategies required to achieve hepatitis C virus elimination targets.

INTRODUCTION

The development of direct-acting antiviral (DAA) therapy for chronic hepatitis C virus (HCV) infection is one of the great advances in clinical medicine in recent decades. Involving simple (once daily oral dosing), tolerable, short duration (8–12 weeks), and highly efficacious (cure rates of >95%) regimens, DAA therapy has the potential to markedly increase HCV treatment uptake and turn around the escalating global disease burden associated with chronic HCV infection.[1] The transformative nature of DAA therapy underpinned the development of World Health Organization (WHO) goals to eliminate HCV as a public health threat, which include 80% of eligible patients treated, a 65% decrease in HCV-related mortality, and an 80% decrease in new HCV infections by 2030.[2]

Viral Hepatitis Clinical Research Program, Kirby Institute, Wallace Wurth Building, UNSW Sydney, NSW 2052, Australia
* Corresponding author.
E-mail address: gdore@kirby.unsw.edu.au

Infect Dis Clin N Am 32 (2018) 269–279
https://doi.org/10.1016/j.idc.2018.02.006
0891-5520/18/Crown Copyright © 2018 Published by Elsevier Inc. All rights reserved.

Major barriers to broadened DAA access have been low rates of HCV screening and diagnosis in most countries,[3] and restrictions driven largely by high drug pricing and related concerns of budget impact.[4,5] In contrast, Australia has had an active HCV screening program for more than 2 decades, with an estimated 81% of the HCV-infected population diagnosed,[6,7] and the development of an unrestricted DAA access program, launched in March 2016.[8] The development of the Australian Government-funded DAA access program is described, along with key features that strengthen the foundation for achieving the WHO HCV elimination targets.

KEY FEATURES OF RESPONSE TO HEPATITIS C VIRUS OVER THE LAST 2 DECADES

There are several key features that have driven the successful HCV response. Australia has a history of national HCV strategic development, with the First National Hepatitis C Strategy launched in 2000, is in a Fourth Strategy (2013–2017),[9] and is developing a Fifth Strategy. This strategic development has been underpinned by partnerships between government, clinical, academic, and civil society stakeholders. Government funding for national and state-based hepatitis and drug user community organizations has been pivotal to these partnerships, and has driven community-based education and advocacy. HCV education and training for primary care and addiction medicine physicians from the early 2000s has facilitated high levels of screening, and laid the foundation for the current major involvement of these groups in DAA prescribing.[8] The broad implementation of harm reduction strategies for people who inject drugs (PWID), from the early 1990s, maintained a low prevalence of human immunodeficiency virus (HIV) infection (around 1% among PWID),[10] prevented many HCV infections[11] (although the chronic HCV prevalence was 45% before the DAA scale-up),[12] and provided the public health interface to enable a highly marginalized population to have high levels of HCV screening (around 90%).[12,13] Finally, as with the HIV response in Australia, bipartisan support (from both major political parties) and political leadership have been crucial to the development of HCV public health strategies that are pragmatic, highly cost effective, and generally well-accepted by the broader community.

MAJOR MILESTONES IN THE DEVELOPMENT OF THE UNRESTRICTED DIRECT-ACTING ANTIVIRAL ACCESS PROGRAM

A pivotal meeting was convened in 2014 by Dr Sue Hill, Chair of the Pharmaceutical Benefits Advisory Committee (PBAC), an independent body that evaluates applications for government subsidization of therapeutic agents. Representatives from the government, clinical, academic, civil society groups, and the pharmaceutical industry were present. The hepatitis and drug user community-based organization representatives were particularly vocal in advocating "access to all," rather than a liver disease stage-restricted access strategy that most high-income countries were pursuing.

In July 2014, the PBAC rejected the initial application for subsidization of sofosbuvir plus ribavirin (for genotypes 2 and 3) by Gilead, on cost-effectiveness grounds. In March 2015, the PBAC reevaluated sofosbuvir plus ribavirin (for genotypes 2 and 3), and further DAA regimens, including sofosbuvir/ledipasvir (for genotype 1), and sofosbuvir plus daclatasvir (for genotypes 1 and 3). The committee recommended access for all patients with chronic HCV infection aged 18 years or older. Importantly, the public minutes of the PBAC meeting stated that the cost effectiveness of these therapies should be at the $AUD 15,000 ($US 12,000) per incremental cost-effectiveness ratio level, rather than the generally accepted benchmark for therapeutic interventions of $AUD 40,000 to 50,000 ($US 32,000–40,000) per incremental cost-effectiveness ratio level, thus sending a clear message to the pharmaceutical companies (Gilead, and Bristol-Myers Squibb) that lower prices would be required to enable an unrestricted DAA access program.

Several months of price negotiations between the Australian government and the pharmaceutical companies ensued (PBAC is not directly involved in these negotiations), with the announcement by the Australian Government Health Minister, Sussan Ley, in December 2015 of an investment of $AUD 1 billion ($US 800 million) over the 2016 to 2020 period for DAA treatment.

KEY FEATURES OF UNRESTRICTED DIRECT-ACTING ANTIVIRAL PROGRAM, LAUNCHED IN MARCH 2016

Some details of DAA drug pricing and the Australian Government risk-sharing arrangement with the pharmaceutical companies remain confidential. There are, however, several features that together make the program relatively unique and clearly highly cost effective. The initial DAA regimens were subsidized from March 2016, with additional regimens added in May 2016 (paritaprevir/ritonavir/ombitasvir plus dasabuvir with or without ribavirin), January 2017 (grazoprevir/elbasvir), and August 2017 (sofosbuvir/velpatasvir) (Table 1). The Australian recommendations for the management of hepatitis C infection: A consensus statement 2016 were developed by the key stakeholder groups in Australia, released for the DAA program launch in March 2016, and updated on January 2017 and August 2017.[14]

From the start of the DAA program, there were no restrictions based on liver disease stage or drug/alcohol use. There is no cap on the number of patients able to be treated per year, but the risk-sharing arrangement between the Australian government and the pharmaceutical companies capped the annual expenditure (probably $AUS 250–300 million). Thus, the greater the number of patients treated (assuming the cap is reached each year), the lower the overall price per patient course. There is minimal out-of-pocket cost for patients (copayment of $AUS 7–36 per month).

The Australian government made the crucial decision to allow prescribing by any registered medical practitioner. In the initial period (March to November 2016) a "consultation" between nonspecialists and a gastroenterology or infectious diseases

Table 1
Interferon-free direct-acting antiviral treatment regimens listed on PBS in Australia

Date of PBS Listing	Treatment Regimen	Eligible Hepatitis C Virus Genotypes	Eligible Durations (wk)
March 2016	Sofosbuvir/ledipasvir with or without ribavirin	1	8, 12, 24
	Sofosbuvir with daclatasvir with or without ribavirin	1, 3	12, 24
	Sofosbuvir with ribavirin	2, 3	12, 24
	Sofosbuvir with pegylated interferon with ribavirin	1, 3, 4–6	12
May 2016	Paritaprevir/ritonavir/ ombitasvir with dasabuvir with or without ribavirin	1	12, 24
January 2017	Elbasvir/grazoprevir	1, 4	12, 16
August 2017	Sofosbuvir/velpatasvir with or without ribavirin	1–6	12

Abbreviation: PBS, Pharmaceutical Benefits Scheme.

specialist was required. This generally involved completing a short pro-forma with demographic, HCV clinical, and planned regimen details, which was sent (usually via email) to a specialist. This consultation requirement was removed in November 2016 for nonspecialists who had gained experience in DAA-based treatment during the initial months of the program, but remains in place for less experienced prescribers. Successful primary care physician prescribing pilot programs had been undertaken in the interferon-based therapy era,[15] however, these programs involved a small number of clinicians. A DAA prescribing accreditation course was not required to be completed, but there has been considerable investment in education and training by the government and pharmaceutical companies over the last 2 years.

Unlike many settings, there is limited paperwork/administration required to gain patient authorization for DAA therapy, with only a short phone call (1–2 minutes) to an Australian government department (Pharmaceutical Benefits Scheme) to provide key information, including patient identifiers, HCV genotype, cirrhosis status, and planned regimen and duration. Importantly, DAA dispensing is allowed through both hospital-based and community (retail) pharmacies.

Specific provisions to ensure treatment for prisoners were included within the DAA program, with the Australian Government bearing the DAA therapeutic costs, despite this generally being a state government responsibility. The Australian Government Health Minister, Sussan Ley (member of the Liberal "Conservative" Party), made prison-based access a particular priority for the DAA program. Importantly, in the context of HCV elimination, retreatment of HCV reinfection is allowed in both community and prison settings.

DIRECT-ACTING ANTIVIRAL TREATMENT UPTAKE DURING 2016 AND 2017

A large number of patients (n = 43,360) have received DAA therapy through the Australian government-funded program from March 2016 to June 2017 (**Fig. 1**). An estimated 4,340 patients had received DAA therapy from late 2014 to February 2016, through pharmaceutical company compassionate access programs (estimated n = 1,930, the vast majority with cirrhosis), clinical trials (estimated n = 910), and generic importation (estimated n = 1,500).[8] With a preliminary estimate of 2017 DAA treatment of 21,560 patients (**Fig. 2**), this would bring a combined figure of 58,480 patients who have received DAA therapy, which is equivalent to 26% of the estimated chronic HCV population in 2015 (n = 227,000). The rapid DAA uptake in 2016 took Australia from a position behind most countries with major DAA programs, to a position at the international forefront in terms of the proportion of chronic HCV population treated (**Fig. 3**).

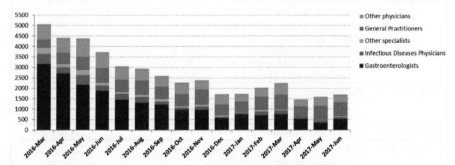

Fig. 1. Estimated monthly number of individuals initiating direct-acting antiviral treatment in Australia between March 2016 and June 2017, by prescriber type.

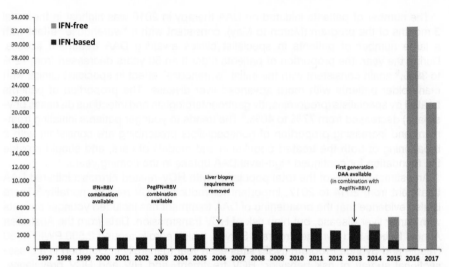

Fig. 2. Estimated annual number of individuals with chronic hepatitis C virus (HCV) infection initiating HCV treatment from 1997 to 2017 in Australia (2017 number is estimated based on the data of the first 6 months of 2017). IFN, interferon; PegIFN, pegylated interferon; RBV, ribavirin.

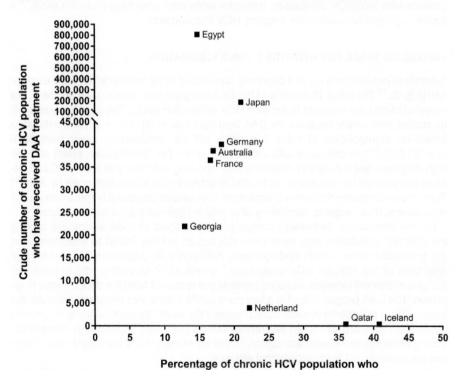

Fig. 3. The crude number and percentage of individuals with chronic hepatitis C virus (HCV), initiating direct-acting antiviral (DAA) therapy during 2015 to 2016 in 9 countries considered to be "on-track" for HCV elimination. (*Data from* Center for Disease Analysis. Polaris observatory. Available at: http://polarisobservatory.org/. Accessed December 18, 2017.)

The number of patients initiated on DAA therapy in 2016 was highest in the initial 3 months of the program (March to May), consistent with a "warehouse" effect with a large number of patients in specialist clinics awaiting DAA treatment access. During the year, the proportion of patients older than 50 years decreased from 72% to 39%,[8] again consistent with the initial "warehouse" effect in specialist clinics with many older patients with more advanced liver disease. The proportion of patients treated by specialists (predominantly gastroenterologists and infectious diseases physicians) decreased from 77% to 40%.[8] The trends to younger patients initiating treatment and increasing proportion of nonspecialists prescribing are consistent with a broadening of both the treated population and models of care, and should provide the foundation for continued high-level DAA uptake in the coming years.

An estimated 70% of the total population with HCV-related cirrhosis initiated DAA treatment from 2014 to 2017, important for reducing HCV-related mortality.[8] There is also evidence that the broadening of DAA treatment has included younger patients with earlier liver disease, but high risk of HCV transmission. Data from the Australian Annual Needle and Syringe Program Survey, which enrolls around 2,500 PWID at 50 Needle and Syringe Program (NSP) sites each year (generally in October) in a cross-sectional survey of risk behavior, HCV treatment, and HIV and HCV prevalence, showed that 22% of participants with HCV infection self-reported DAA initiation in 2016 (compared with 3% in 2015).[16,17]

Additional data indicate DAA treatment uptake in 2016 of greater than 60% among patients with HIV/HCV coinfection (predominantly men who have sex with men),[18] a further high-risk population for ongoing HCV transmission.

STAYING ON TRACK FOR HEPATITIS C VIRUS ELIMINATION

Australia is included in a list of 9 countries considered to be "on-track" for HCV elimination (**Fig. 3**).[19] The initial 16 months of the DAA program has been a great success, but renewed efforts are required to achieve HCV elimination goals. The next few years will be crucial, particularly because the DAA treatment rate in 2017 (n = 21,560, estimated based on extrapolation of initial 6 months) will be considerably lower than 2016 (n = 32,550).[8] This decrease was anticipated, given the "warehouse" effect and the high diagnosis rate in Australia. Mathematical modeling indicates that around 20,000 patients per year will be required to be treated to achieve HCV elimination goals by 2026.[20] These models assume that there is equivalent DAA uptake across HCV transmission risk populations; thus, ongoing monitoring of uptake in high-risk populations is crucial.

Further *community awareness campaigns* are needed to raise awareness among the affected population who have been diagnosed but not linked to treatment, and the population who remain undiagnosed. Although this proportion is estimated at only 19% of the chronic HCV population,[7] unless HCV screening efforts continue, this proportion will increase as cured patients are removed from the denominator population. The DAA program itself is a key community awareness program, because the large number of patients already cured "spread the word" through social and injecting networks. This word-of-mouth awareness raising has been important in counterbalancing the interferon-based era legitimate stories of major HCV treatment side effects and disappointment from suboptimal efficacy.

The continued *development of diverse models of care and broad prescriber involvement* is also required. The slowing in DAA treatment rates should provide the impetus to enhanced infrastructure for HCV assessment and delivery of therapy. Simplification of assessment and DAA treatment should also support continued uptake. A key example of this is within the Australian prison setting. An estimated 1,500 inmates were treated during the first year of DAA therapy (March 2016 to February 2017; personal communication with Professor Andrew Lloyd), but based on current trends, treatment uptake should rise significantly in 2017 and 2018. Part of the enhanced capacity in the prison setting is the move from predominantly directly observed therapy (daily dosing at prison clinic) to predominant monthly dispensing with inmates taking medications in their cells. The broad access to DAA therapy in the community and the lack of any mood-altering effects of DAA therapy seem to have negated potential issues of diversion in the prison setting.

Additional models of care are also required to reach more marginalized PWID, including those injecting stimulants (in Australia, predominantly methamphetamines). The NSP has provided a potential infrastructure for HCV assessment and delivery of therapy to PWID. The TEMPO study (TEst and treat hepatitis C aMong needle and syringe PrOgram clients) will soon evaluate DAA therapy delivery through NSP sites, with peer-based support.

Specific models of care will be required to provide equitable DAA access to Indigenous Australians. A recently funded NHMRC project called the SCALE-C (*Strategies for hepatitis C testing and treatment in Aboriginal communities that Lead to Elimination*) will evaluate a community-based model of care that includes point-of-care HCV testing and noninvasive liver disease assessment. The SCALE-C project incorporates evaluation of the community-level impact of rapid DAA scale-up on HCV viremic prevalence and HCV incidence.

An increasing number of nonspecialist prescribers are becoming involved in DAA treatment,[8] with an estimated 9,760 patients having been prescribed DAA by general practitioners by June 2017. This finding is extremely encouraging, but further efforts are required to encourage and train additional prescribers. The goal should be to have the large majority of primary care-based opioid substitution treatment prescribers involved in DAA prescribing, as well as many other practitioners with high caseloads of HCV patients.

Maintenance of a *harm reduction framework* is essential. High levels of DAA uptake could be undermined by a lack of HCV prevention services. Fortunately, Australia is one of the few countries that has both high NSP (400 needle-syringes distributed per PWID per year) and opioid substitution treatment (40 per 100 PWID) coverage.[21] The equivalent figures for the United States, which are around the global average for these measures, are 40 needle-syringes per PWID per year and 16 per 100 PWID on opioid substitution treatment.[21] Optimized harm reduction is crucial for 3 reasons. First, it reduces the risk of primary HCV infection among PWID.[22] Second, it should also reduce the risk of HCV reinfection among PWID cured through DAA therapy. Mathematical modeling clearly demonstrates how difficult (near impossible) it would be to achieve HCV elimination among PWID in a setting with poor harm reduction coverage and increasing HCV transmission,[23] a situation present in many areas of the United States.[23] Finally, a strong harm reduction framework is a vital engagement point for a highly marginalized population in terms of HCV screening, assessment, and potentially DAA therapy delivery.

KEY ELEMENTS OF MONITORING AND EVALUATION OF THE HEPATITIS C VIRUS ELIMINATION PROGRAM

To inform further strategies for HCV elimination in Australia, a program of monitoring and evaluation is essential (**Table 2**). The key elements should cover information on DAA uptake, treatment outcomes, and the population-level impact on HCV prevalence, incidence, and disease burden.

Table 2	
Key elements of monitoring and evaluation of HCV elimination program in Australia	
Area	Project (s)
DAA treatment uptake	Monitoring hepatitis C treatment uptake in Australia: Data on dispensed DAA prescriptions for a longitudinal cohort of individuals, representing a 10% random sample of the PBS database, are used to provide reports of DAA uptake numbers per month, and by jurisdiction, demographics, DAA regimen and duration, and prescriber type.[8] The reports are released as a regular newsletter series.[24]
DAA treatment outcome	Real world Efficacy of Antiviral therapy in Chronic Hepatitis C (REACH-C Study): A national observational cohort study of real-world DAA outcomes, with the data collected from tertiary, primary care, drug and alcohol, and prison-based clinics.[25]
Population-level impact of DAA treatment on HCV prevalence, incidence, and disease burden	• Australian Needle and Syringe Program Survey: An annual cross-sectional survey of ∼2,500 PWID, including HCV RNA testing to evaluate incidence and prevalence of HCV infection among PWID over time.[16] • National HCV surveillance: Monitoring of the rates of new HCV diagnosis among younger age groups (eg, 15–24 y) provides a surrogate measure of recent HCV transmission trend. • Data linkage studies: Notified HCV cases are linked with several administrative datasets (ie, Pharmaceutical Benefits Scheme, Admitted Patient Data Collection, Cancer Registry, and Registry of Births, Deaths, and Marriages), evaluating the population-level burden of HCV infection, including the rate of advanced liver disease and death over time.[30,32–35] • Mathematical modeling

Abbreviations: DAA, direct-acting antiviral; HCV, hepatitis C virus; PBS, Pharmaceutical Benefits Scheme; PWID, people who inject drugs.

From the start of the Australian Government-funded DAA program an evaluation of HCV treatment uptake has been undertaken, with regular *Monitoring hepatitis C treatment uptake in Australia* newsletters to inform stakeholders of progress.[8,24] These newsletters have covered DAA uptake numbers per month, demographic details (age and gender distribution), regimen types and durations, and prescriber pattern. The breakdown of HCV treatment rates (estimates of chronic HCV population treated) by jurisdictions (6 states and 2 territories) has provided an element of competitive spirit in the drive toward HCV elimination.

Australia has 2 *large-scale observational cohort studies* to evaluate real-world DAA outcomes: OPERA-C (Observational Prospective Epidemiological Registry in Australia of HCV) has largely recruited from tertiary care gastroenterology and liver clinics; and REACH-C (*Real world Efficacy of Antiviral therapy in Chronic Hepatitis C*), with data collected from tertiary care, primary care, drug and alcohol, and prison-based clinics. Initial DAA treatment outcomes among 1,618 patients from REACH-C have been reported,[25] with a per protocol sustained virologic response rate of 96.5%. Similar to many other real-world cohorts[26–29] there is a sizable rate of loss to follow-up between end of treatment and sustained virologic response at 12 weeks (19%), highlighting the need to optimize ongoing patient engagement. The REACH-C cohort will also evaluate rates and outcomes of HCV retreatment, both for virologic failure and reinfection.

A major component of disease burden monitoring will be through *data linkage studies*, linking notified HCV cases (mandatory in all Australian jurisdictions since the early 1990s) with several administrative datasets, including individual-level Pharmaceutical Benefits Scheme DAA treatment, hospitalization, cancer diagnoses, and death. These studies have characterized population-level burden of decompensated cirrhosis, HCC, and liver-related mortality,[30–35] and will continue to monitor this burden and the specific impact of DAA scale-up in Australia. These studies will inform progress in terms of the WHO HCV elimination target to reduce liver-related mortality by 65% by 2030. They will also provide essential information to validate and or adjust mathematical model-based estimates and projections of the impact of DAA therapy on advanced liver disease complications and mortality.

Ongoing surveillance through the *Australian Needle and Syringe Program Survey*, an annual cross-sectional survey of around 2,500 PWID incorporating risk behavior, self-reported HCV treatment uptake, and dried blood spot–based testing for HIV and HCV seroprevalence, will be a major component of HCV elimination monitoring. The inclusion from 2015 of HCV RNA testing on dried blood spot samples provides the ideal format for PWID-based HCV viremic estimates over time. A comparison of 2015 and 2016 samples demonstrated a reduction in HCV RNA prevalence from 45% to 33%,[17] strong evidence for a population-level impact of initial DAA uptake.

Further valuable information will come from *national HCV surveillance* data, particularly given that all new HCV diagnoses are reported to public health surveillance departments, with national collation from all Australian jurisdictions. Monitoring of rates of new HCV diagnosis among younger age groups (eg, 15–24 years), which have been stable over recent years, should provide a surrogate measure of recent HCV transmission trends. High rates of HCV screening among high-risk populations, particularly PWID, provide reassurance that this form of surveillance is valuable in terms of monitoring HCV transmission.

Ongoing *mathematical modeling* will also inform HCV elimination monitoring and evaluation, and associated strategic development. Preliminary modeling incorporating 2016 DAA treatment uptake (n = 32,550), has indicated that DAA treatment uptake of 27,770 in 2017, 23,143 in 2018, then 18,510 per year from 2019 would achieve WHO elimination targets in 2024 to 2026.[20]

SUMMARY

Australia has laid the foundation for HCV elimination within the next decade. Key aspects of this foundation include high levels of HCV screening and diagnosis, unrestricted access to DAA therapy, a diverse range of HCV models of care including broad prescriber involvement, and high coverage of harm reduction strategies for PWID. Despite this foundation, major initiatives are required to maintain the initial momentum, particularly to ensure DAA access in highly marginalized populations.

REFERENCES

1. Dore GJ, Feld JJ. Hepatitis C virus therapeutic development: in pursuit of perfectovir. Clin Infect Dis 2015;60(12):1829–36.
2. World Health Organization (WHO). Combating hepatitis B and C to reach elimination by 2030. Geneva (Switzerland): World Health Organization; 2016.
3. Dore GJ, Ward J, Thursz M. Hepatitis C disease burden and strategies to manage the burden. J Viral Hepat 2014;21(Suppl 1):1–4.
4. Barua S, Greenwald R, Grebely J, et al. Restrictions for Medicaid reimbursement of sofosbuvir for the treatment of Hepatitis C virus infection in the United States

Medicaid restrictions of sofosbuvir for hepatitis C. Ann Intern Med 2015;163(3): 215–23.

5. Marshall AD, Cunningham EB, Nielsen S, et al. Restrictions for reimbursement of interferon-free direct-acting antiviral drugs for HCV infection in Europe. Lancet Gastroenterol Hepatol 2018;3(2):125–33.

6. Hajarizadeh B, Grebely J, McManus H, et al. Chronic hepatitis C burden and care cascade in Australia in the era of interferon-based treatment. J Gastroenterol Hepatol 2017;32(1):229–36.

7. The Kirby Institute. HIV, viral hepatitis and sexually transmissible infections in Australia: annual surveillance report 2017. Sydney (Australia): The Kirby Institute, UNSW Sydney; 2017.

8. Hajarizadeh B, Grebely J, Matthews GV, et al. Uptake of direct acting antiviral treatment for chronic hepatitis C in Australia. J Viral Hepat 2018. [Epub ahead of print].

9. Australian Government Department of Health and Ageing. Fourth National Hepatitis C Strategy 2014–2017: Commonwealth of Australia; 2014. Available at: http://www.health.gov.au/internet/main/publishing.nsf/Content/ohp-bbvs-hepc.

10. Iversen J, Wand H, Topp L, et al. Extremely low and sustained HIV incidence among people who inject drugs in a setting of harm reduction. AIDS 2014; 28(2):275–8.

11. Kwon JA, Anderson J, Kerr CC, et al. Estimating the cost-effectiveness of needle-syringe programs in Australia. AIDS 2012;26(17):2201–10.

12. Iversen J, Grebely J, Catlett B, et al. Estimating the cascade of hepatitis C testing, care and treatment among people who inject drugs in Australia. Int J Drug Policy 2017;47:77–85.

13. Butler K, Day C, Sutherland R, et al. Hepatitis C testing in general practice settings: a cross-sectional study of people who inject drugs in Australia. Int J Drug Policy 2017;47(Supplement C):102–6.

14. Hepatitis C, Virus Infection Consensus Statement Working Group. Australian recommendations for the management of hepatitis C virus infection: a consensus statement (August 2017). Melbourne (Australia): Gastroenterological Society of Australia; 2017.

15. Baker D, Alavi M, Erratt A, et al. Delivery of treatment for hepatitis C virus infection in the primary care setting. Eur J Gastroenterol Hepatol 2014;26(9):1003–9.

16. Memedovic S, Iversen J, Geddes L, et al. Australian needle syringe program Survey National Data Report 2012-2016: prevalence of HIV, HCV and injecting and sexual behaviour among NSP attendees. Sydney (Australia): The Kirby Institute, UNSW Sydney; 2017.

17. Iversen J, Dore G, Catlett B, et al. Progress towards elimination: Rapid uptake of HCV treatment among people who inject drugs following broad access to DAA therapies. The 6th International Symposium on Hepatitis Care in Substance Users (INHSU); 6–8 September 2017; New York, USA.

18. Martinello M, Dore GJ, Bopage RI, et al. DAA treatment scale-up in HIV/HCV co-infection: characterising a population at risk for reinfection. J Hepatol 2017; 66(Supp 1):S495–6 [Abstract].

19. Center for Disease Analysis. Polaris observatory. Available at: http://polarisobservatory.org/. Accessed December 18, 2017.

20. Kwon A, Dore G, Grebely J, et al. Australia could meet the WHO HCV elimination targets if the current rollout of DAA treatment is continued. J Virus Eradication 2017; 3(Suppl 2):5 [Abstract]. Available at: http://viruseradication.com/supplement-

details/Abstracts_of_the_Australasian_Viral_Hepatitis_Elimination_Conference_
2017/.
21. Larney S, Peacock A, Leung J, et al. Global, regional, and country-level coverage
of interventions to prevent and manage HIV and hepatitis C among people who
inject drugs: a systematic review. Lancet Glob Health 2017;5(12):e1208–20.
22. Platt L, Minozzi S, Reed J, et al. Needle and syringe programmes and opioid substitution therapy for preventing HCV transmission among people who inject
drugs: findings from a Cochrane Review and meta-analysis. Addiction 2018;
113(3):545–63.
23. Fraser H, Zibbell J, Hoerger T, et al. Scaling-up HCV prevention and treatment
interventions in rural United States- model projections for tackling an increasing
epidemic. Addiction 2018;113(1):173–82.
24. The Kirby Institute. Monitoring hepatitis C treatment uptake in Australia (Issue 8).
Sydney (Australia): The Kirby Institute, UNSW Sydney; 2017. Available at: https://
kirby.unsw.edu.au/report/monitoring-hepatitis-c-treatment-uptake-australia-issue-
8-december-2017.
25. The Kirby Institute, UNSW Sydney. Real world efficacy of antiviral therapy in
chronic hepatitis C in Australia (Issue 1). Sydney (Australia): The Kirby Institute,
UNSW Sydney; 2017. Available at: https://kirby.unsw.edu.au/report/reach-c-
newsletter-issue-1-july-2017.
26. Backus LI, Belperio PS, Shahoumian TA, et al. Real world effectiveness of ledi-
pasvir/sofosbuvir in 4365 treatment-naïve genotype 1 hepatitis C infected patients. Hepatology 2016;64(2):405–14.
27. Calleja JL, Crespo J, Rincón D, et al. Effectiveness, safety and clinical outcomes
of direct-acting antiviral therapy in HCV genotype 1 infection: results from a Spanish real world cohort. J Hepatol 2017;66(6):1138–48.
28. Terrault NA, Zeuzem S, Di Bisceglie AM, et al. Effectiveness of ledipasvir-sofosbuvir
combination in patients with hepatitis C virus infection and factors associated of
sustained virologic response. Gastroenterology 2016;151(6):1131–40.e5.
29. Ioannou GN, Beste LA, Chang MF, et al. Effectiveness of sofosbuvir, ledipasvir/
sofosbuvir, or paritaprevir/ritonavir/ombitasvir and dasabuvir regimens for treatment of patients with Hepatitis C in the veterans affairs national health care system. Gastroenterology 2016;151(3):457–71.e5.
30. Waziry R, Grebely J, Amin J, et al. Trends in hepatocellular carcinoma among
people with HBV or HCV notification in Australia (2000–2014). J Hepatol 2016;
65(6):1086–93.
31. Alavi M, Janjua NZ, Chong M, et al. The contribution of alcohol-use disorder to
decompensated cirrhosis among people with hepatitis C: an international study.
J Hepatol 2018;68(3):393–401.
32. Aspinall EJ, Hutchinson SJ, Janjua NZ, et al. Trends in mortality after diagnosis of
hepatitis C virus infection: an international comparison and implications for monitoring the population impact of treatment. J Hepatol 2015;62(2):269–77.
33. Alavi M, Law MG, Grebely J, et al. Time to decompensated cirrhosis and hepatocellular carcinoma after an HBV or HCV notification: a population-based study.
J Hepatol 2016;65:879–87.
34. Waziry R, Grebely J, Amin J, et al. Survival following hospitalization with hepatocellular carcinoma among people notified with hepatitis B or C virus in Australia
(2000-2014). Hepatol Commun 2017;1(8):736–47.
35. Alavi M, Law MG, Grebely J, et al. Lower life expectancy among people with an HCV
notification: a population-based linkage study. J Viral Hepat 2014;21(6):e10–8.

Hepatitis C Care in the Department of Veterans Affairs: Building a Foundation for Success

Pamela S. Belperio, PharmD, BCPS[a], Maggie Chartier, PsyD, MPH[b],
Rachel I. Gonzalez, MPH[c], Angela M. Park, PharmD[d],
David B. Ross, MD, PhD, MBI[b], Tim R. Morgan, MD[e],
Lisa I. Backus, MD, PhD[a],*

KEYWORDS

- Veterans • Direct-acting antiviral • SVR • Hepatitis C • Population health
- Innovation • System redesign

KEY POINTS

- Since January 2014 the Department of Veterans Affairs (VA) has made significant progress in the treatment of veterans with hepatitis C virus (HCV) and, as of December 2017, more than 100,000 veterans have been treated.
- Special regional multidisciplinary Hepatitis C Innovation Teams were created that used lean process improvement and system redesign, resulting in innovative hepatitis C practice models that help to address gaps in care.
- The VA has expanded access and treatment capacity for HCV-infected veterans through the use of nonphysician providers (clinical pharmacists, nurse practitioners, and physician assistants), video telehealth, and electronic technologies.
- The VA continues to use population health management tools to effectively manage and track the treatment and care of veterans with HCV.

Disclosure Statement: P.S. Belperio, M. Chartier, R.I. Gonzalez, A.M. Park, D.B. Ross, and L.I. Backus have no personal or financial disclosures to report. Dr T.R. Morgan reports the following: clinical trial funding by AbbVie (NCT01089944, NCT02640482), GenFit (NCT02607735) and, Gilead (NCT02607800, NCT02639338, NCT02639247).
[a] Patient Care Services/Population Health, Department of Veterans Affairs, Palo Alto Health Care System, 3801 Miranda Avenue (132), Palo Alto, CA 94304, USA; [b] HIV, Hepatitis and Related Conditions, Office of Specialty Care Services (10P11I), Department of Veterans Affairs, 810 Vermont Avenue, Washington, DC 20420, USA; [c] Research Health Care Group, VA Long Beach Health Care System, 5901 East 7th Street, Long Beach, CA 90822, USA; [d] New England Veterans Engineering Resource Center, Department of Veterans Affairs, 150 South Huntingtin Avenue, Boston, MA 02130, USA; [e] Division of Gastroenterology, VA Long Beach Health Care System, 5901 East 7th Street, Long Beach, CA 90822, USA
* Corresponding author.
E-mail address: Lisa.Backus@va.gov

The introduction of direct-acting antivirals (DAAs) in 2014 led to transformational change in hepatitis C virus (HCV) care in the US Department of Veterans Affairs (VA). The substantial progress the VA has made in identifying and curing HCV infection has been multifactorial and spurred by several key aspects of the VA health care system.

The VA is the single largest HCV care provider in the United States and cares for a population with a high prevalence of HCV infection. Veterans are at a disproportionately high risk for HCV as evidenced by an estimated prevalence of 8.4%, a rate more than 3 times that of the general US population.[1–4] Veterans who served during the Vietnam War era, those with alcohol or substance use disorders, those with psychiatric conditions, and those who experience homelessness are particularly likely to be affected.[2,3,5] Although it is estimated that more than 90% of veterans in VA care with HCV infection have been diagnosed, it is projected that an additional 8,000 to 10,000 veterans in VA care remain to be diagnosed.

The VA operates the largest comprehensive health care system in the United States, with 170 medical centers, 950 community-based outpatient clinics, 135 living centers, 48 domiciliaries, and 300 readjustment counseling and outreach centers grouped into 18 Veterans Integrated Service Networks (VISNs) across the country, serving more than 9 million enrolled veterans.[6,7] The VA has a robust electronic medical record (EMR) used throughout the health care system.[8,9] Medical documentation and ordering have been fully computerized at all VA facilities for more than a decade.

The VA health care system includes comprehensive in-house pharmacy services. The VA has one national formulary and formulary decisions are evidence-based, not preference-based. This national formulary reduces geographic variability in utilization of pharmaceuticals across the VA system and promotes portability and uniformity. All HCV antivirals approved by the US Food and Drug Administration (FDA) are covered by VA pharmacy benefits and are available on the VA national formulary with no quantity limits. The VA does not require prior authorization approval of prescriptions; however, there are drug-specific Criteria for Use that generally follow FDA labeling. There are no retreatment restrictions, no restrictions based on liver disease stage, and no minimum length of abstinence from alcohol or substance use required before treatment. Copays are the same for all HCV medications and do not exceed $11 for a 1-month supply. Depending on a veteran's financial status and other eligibility criteria, this medication copay may be waived. Thus, veterans pay a maximum of $33 for a 12-week HCV treatment course. The low out-of-pocket cost contrasts with many private and Medicaid payers that use tiers or only cover certain medications, often with quantity limits, higher out-of-pocket costs, and restrictions based on patient or disease characteristics.

THE DEPARTMENT OF VETERANS AFFAIRS NATIONAL VIRAL HEPATITIS PROGRAM

The VA has had a National Viral Hepatitis Program since 2001 that has used a data-informed population health framework to coordinate and support HCV care across the health care system. Every veteran in VA care diagnosed with HCV is included in the VA's National Hepatitis C Clinical Case Registry, which uses data extracted from the EMR to identify and track veterans with HCV at the local and national level.[10] The National Viral Hepatitis Program has been responsible for developing tools, training, and resources for VA clinicians and patients; publishing standardized policies and guidelines for diagnosis, antiviral treatment, and management of advanced liver disease; adopting recommended birth cohort and high-risk testing policies; and promoting integrated care for HCV patients. Many of these resources are centrally available from the VA HCV Web site (available at: www.hepatitis.va.gov).[11]

In 2013 the National Viral Hepatitis Program established a working group of VA experts to develop VA recommendations for HCV treatment. These recommendations are consistently updated based on the most up-to-date evidence about HCV therapy and as new medications are approved by the FDA. The VA's Chronic Hepatitis C Treatment Considerations are nationally recognized as cutting-edge guidance on HCV treatment.[11]

In 2015, with the National Viral Hepatitis Program's establishment of Hepatitis C Innovation Teams (HITs), VISN-level system redesign was implemented to identify and rapidly address gaps in HCV testing, access, linkage to care, and treatment using lean processes improvement.[12,13] Increased drug funding, coupled with reduced drug prices, made treatment accessible, and efforts by VISN HITs provided the infrastructure to address treatment capacity and the impetus for many HCV clinical providers and staff to work on aggressive outreach.

IMPACT OF ALL-ORAL DIRECT-ACTING ANTIVIRAL TREATMENTS ON THE SPECTRUM OF CARE

Before January 2014, HCV treatment required weekly injections with pegylated interferon, had extended durations of therapy, and had significant physical and psychiatric side effects, which led to frequent early discontinuation and low cure rates (35%–55%) among veterans.[14] Veterans were generally referred from primary care to liver specialists for evaluation and treatment. All patients could be considered for treatment; however, contraindications were present in 30% to 50% of veterans evaluated. By December 2013, the VA had cumulatively treated approximately 39,000 veterans, or 24% of its HCV-infected population in care, of which only about 16,000 (10% of its HCV-infected population) achieved a cure.[15] Future treatment projections based on historical utilization from the triple-therapy, interferon-based era, with adjustments for anticipated increases, assumed an average of 200 starts per week and an annual treatment rate of approximately 16,000.

The availability of second-generation DAAs, sofosbuvir and simeprevir, in the VA in January 2014, and ledipasvir-sofosbuvir and ombitasvir-paritaprevir-ritonavir and dasabuvir in late 2014, led to dramatic changes in HCV antiviral uptake, given the shorter treatment durations, ease of administration, absence of psychiatric side effects, and high cure rates (**Fig. 1**). Interferon-free DAA regimens vastly increased the VA population willing and able to undergo antiviral treatment. Consequently, the VA experienced a surge in prescribing.[16] The number of veterans started on HCV antiviral treatment nationally increased from approximately 2800 per year in 2013, to 6500 in 2014, to 31,000 in 2015, and to 38,000 in 2016. In 2016, the VA averaged about 1000 treatment starts per week, representing a 40% increase over the average start rate in 2015, an 88% increase over 2014, and a 95% increase from 2013. Since the availability of second-generation DAAs in January 2014 through December 2017, the VA has treated more than 100,000 patients, more patients than any other health care system in the United States.[17]

Cure rates with all oral, second-generation DAAs in the veteran population are greater than 90%.[18,19] As a result, the VA has cured almost 60% of its total HCV population, compared with less than 15% for the United States as a whole.[20] As of December 2017, fewer than 42,000 veterans in VA care who were known to be HCV viremic were still awaiting treatment, compared with 168,000 3.5 years ago.[17]

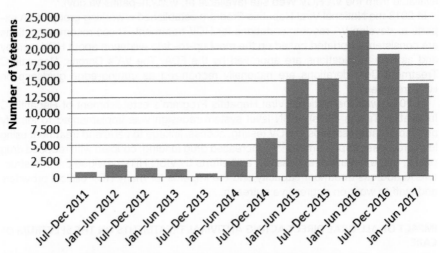

Fig. 1. Number of veterans starting a HCV DAA agent. Includes boceprevir, telaprevir, simeprevir, sofosbuvir, ledipasvir-sofosbuvir, ombitasvir-paritaprevir-ritonavir, dasabuvir, daclatasvir, elbasvir-grazoprevir, sofosbuvir-velpatasvir, sofosbuvir-velpatasvir-voxilaprevir, and glecaprevir-pibrentasvir.

Getting It Done

The largest barriers the VA encountered with the massive scale-up of treatment were provider capacity and patient access, aside from the high cost of HCV antivirals. To rapidly address both clinical capacity and access to HCV treatment providers, the VA intensified national, VISN, and facility-level efforts to expand staffing, infrastructure, administration support, and training, largely guided by VISN-level HITs.

Veterans Integrated Service Network Hepatitis C Innovation Teams

The development of the HIT infrastructure has leveraged and supported the implementation work of VA providers that has allowed the VA to respond to challenges in capacity, access, and outreach. Local operational barriers were most effectively addressed by HIT-initiated local systems redesign whereby creative solutions to address site-specific barriers were tested, implemented, and measured to assess improvement in care delivery. In this process, the HIT, consisting of facility and VISN multidisciplinary providers and managers, maps the current state process to target areas for improvement and identify strong practices. Team members subsequently map the ideal or future state to determine the path forward, developing programs and systems to remedy deficiencies and barriers, with a goal of creating a culture of continuous improvement. The HIT infrastructure has fostered rapid and widespread dissemination of these best practices across the VA system for local adaptation at other sites. HIT leadership encourages local facilities to set ambitious screening and treatment goals and to reassess how care is being delivered and where additional improvements could be made. National and facility-level data are paired and reported monthly to identify gaps in care and hold teams accountable to leading and lagging outcome measures for HCV care indices, including birth cohort screening, treatment initiation, sustained virologic response (SVR) or cure, and follow-up SVR testing. The use of existing electronic databases and the creation of real-time HCV population health management tools with drill-down and write-back capabilities allowed VA HCV staff to identify, track, and co-ordinate care for HCV-infected veterans.

Practice examples

Many successful models and activities have evolved in response to the HCV scale-up in the VA. Several examples are provided here.

Increased outreach Local programs raised awareness among providers and staff about the need for HCV testing and availability of treatment, and promoted direct outreach to at-risk veterans and the veteran community more broadly through national and local social media and advertising campaigns (available at: https://www.hepatitis.va.gov/campaign-test-treat-cure.asp; https://www.youtube.com/watch?v=sMXRbgIjB2I; https://www.youtube.com/watch?v=7UMez-o8flY; https://www.youtube.com/watch?v=4AJGRQPiK1g).

Increased access through increased clinic availability Some VA facilities have expanded clinic hours into evenings, added Saturday clinics, and brought on additional staff to share administrative duties and increase clinical care.

Group clinics or shared medical visits In the group clinic or shared medical visit model, clinical pharmacists or other advanced-practice providers organize visits for a group of 4 to 8 uncomplicated patients who will be starting the same treatment regimen. Information about the medication, administration, adherence, resources, and follow-up are provided in a group setting with facilitated discussion. Each patient is provided a card with their relevant personal clinical information and has the opportunity for individual consultation at the end of the group appointment. Patients are seen in the group setting monthly while on treatment, which provides the opportunity to share experiences with other veterans undergoing the same treatment.

Electronic consults The electronic consults (e-consult) model allows HCV clinicians to evaluate patients during off-clinic hours or from a remote location, such as another medical facility, using standardized electronic templates. HCV clinic staff use electronic databases to identify HCV-viremic patients. A clinician performs a chart review to determine treatment candidacy and provides recommendations for HCV therapy initiation via electronic notes directly to the providers. E-consults have helped the VA reach key populations of HCV-infected patients who lack convenient access to HCV specialists, simultaneously reducing time, distance, and transportation barriers by avoiding the need for additional appointments.

Virtual care technology Virtual care technology modalities include mobile phone applications, secure messaging, telemedicine, and clinical video telehealth or real-time video teleconferencing whereby HCV clinicians provide care to patients and/or consultation to other providers at another location. Such modalities provide access to HCV treatment expertise remotely, without subjecting patients to prolonged travel or separate appointments to see an HCV provider. As a modified version of the Extension for Community Healthcare Outcomes (ECHO) project, provider-to-provider teleconsultation has been expanded in the VA beyond primary care to also include homeless, mental health, and substance use clinic providers; urban settings; and a pharmacist-to-pharmacist consultation model.[21,22] The expanded HCV VA-ECHO program was associated with a 20% higher HCV treatment initiation rate and a 75% decrease in time to initiation of treatment compared with sites without this program.[22]

Clinical pharmacist management of hepatitis C virus treatment

Clinical pharmacist involvement with HCV care has been a key component in addressing critical gaps related to access and capacity. In the VA, clinical pharmacists maintain a scope of practice that authorizes them to act as advanced practice providers, autonomously or collaboratively, managing all aspects of a patient's disease, including prescribing medication.[23] The VA mobilized existing pharmacy infrastructure and developed a series of intensive HCV boot camps to train clinical pharmacists, and subsequently provided mentorship experiences with regional HCV clinical pharmacy experts. Since 2011, more than 700 pharmacists participated in the boot camps; as of 2017, 252 clinical pharmacists were managing HCV patients as part of their scope of practice. A spectrum of care is provided by clinical pharmacists, ranging from treatment of only those without cirrhosis to the treatment of all HCV patients regardless of the stage of liver disease. Some VA sites have developed decision-flow maps to triage patients directly to clinical pharmacists for treatment.

The impact of advanced practice providers, and clinical pharmacists in particular, on the VA's care capacity has been substantial. The percentage of veterans started on DAA regimens by clinical pharmacists in the VA has increased from 11.5% of treatment starts in 2014 to 25.4% of starts in 2017, accounting for a total of almost 18,000 veterans. Nurse practitioners and physician assistants accounted for 22.9% and 11.3% of new starts, respectively, in 2017; and, combined since 2014, have started more than 34,000 veterans on DAA regimens. These providers are recognized as delivering the same quality of care and providing more timely access to HCV treatment.[24,25]

Clinical pharmacists assuming greater responsibility for HCV treatment has resulted in greater access to liver specialists by offloading specialist time, thereby allowing them to focus on more complex cases. The expanded clinical pharmacist role has also increased awareness of HCV in primary care clinics, improved identification of patients who may be eligible for treatment, increased population health management activities, and allowed flexibility in patient scheduling. Additional cost-avoidance may be realized in salary offset because pharmacist's salaries are lower than physician specialists, reduced drug costs from optimization of regimens, reduced drug-drug interactions, the facilitation of timely medication refills, and closely monitored adherence. This has been a highly successful and effective practice. The VA experience suggests that expansion of the clinical pharmacist practice model in the community, through collaborative drug therapy management agreements, could greatly improve capacity in the community.[23,26]

Increased hepatitis C virus screening

The VA's commitment to HCV screening has been longstanding and has always included risk-based testing recommendations.[27–29] As part of the VA's risk-based testing, veterans who served during the Vietnam era (1964–1975), a group mostly born in the 1940s and 1950s, were considered at increased risk for HCV and were targeted for HCV screening.[2,26] Thus, the testing rate in the 1945 to 1965 birth cohort, even before the Centers for Disease Control and Prevention recommendation, was already 51%.[27]

Since 2009, the VA has had a policy mandating reflex confirmatory testing to ensure that all patients with positive serologic test results for HCV are automatically tested for the presence of chronic HCV infection with nucleic acid testing. The VA now performs confirmatory testing on more than 97% of individuals who have a positive HCV antibody test result.

The VA's ongoing efforts to increase 1945 to 1965 birth cohort testing have been substantial and highly effective. Since the adoption of 1945 to 1965 birth cohort testing, the VA has (1) disseminated a national HCV testing electronic clinical reminder, (2) charged regional HITs with a primary goal of increasing birth cohort testing, (3) made HCV testing a national and regional VA quality performance metric, and (4) provided quarterly reporting of HCV birth cohort testing rates. Two national point-of-care clinical reminders, *"HCV Risk Screening"* and *"Testing for HCV,"* were released in May 2015. Although not mandated, local facilities were encouraged to use these national reminders or to modify their local clinical reminders to align with the VA screening policy. Most recently, the VA removed the requirement for documentation of oral consent for HCV testing. As an innovative practice disseminated through the HITs, numerous VA facilities have automated outreach to untested veterans in the 1945 to 1965 birth cohort. This process leverages data available in the EMR to automate mailing of letters that recommend patients be tested for HCV and, after testing, generates a notification to the patient if the test is negative or a notification to their provider to contact the patient for treatment if the test is positive. At some facilities, the letter to the patient also dually serves as a laboratory order for HCV antibody and reflex testing when presented to a VA laboratory, thus increasing efficiency and eliminating office visits.

The combination of these efforts has resulted in 4% to 5% increases in testing rates per year. By December 2017, the VA had screened 81.4% of the 2.89 million veterans in the 1945 to 1965 birth cohort nationally in VA care; these testing rates are higher than that of any other US health care system.[30–32]

DIFFICULT TO ENGAGE POPULATIONS

Recently, the VA has entered a new era in HCV treatment with more focus on more difficult to engage populations. As a larger percentage of infected veterans are treated, initiation rates have begun to decline. This is due to an increasing proportion of untreated HCV-infected veterans who are more difficult to link to and retain in care and, therefore, are more difficult to start in treatment, as well as those who are currently uninterested in treatment. The VA estimates that as many as 30% of veterans remaining to be treated may be more difficult to engage. To adequately address these barriers, different resources may be required. Although some factors are not modifiable, many are potentially modifiable.

The VA is adapting to these challenges and addressing potentially modifiable barriers by (1) encouraging more difficult to reach veterans to enter into treatment using targeted media outreach via social media, advertising, external communications, and education; (2) increasing availability of appropriate staff to provide care for treatment-limiting comorbidities and issues of homelessness; (3) effectively assessing alcohol and substance use and matching a patient's use with the actual risk of nonadherence; (4) ensuring the necessary care coordination, case management, transportation, mental health services, and substance use services are in place to reach and continue to reassess Veterans' treatment candidacy; (5) direct outreach by HCV clinic staff to patients via personal calls or letters; (6) adding directly observed HCV treatment with opioid substitution therapy in buprenorphine or methadone clinics; and (7) collaborations with the Housing and Urban Development–VA Supportive Housing (HUD-VASH) programs to allow for closer contact and observed HCV treatment programs (**Table 1**).

Per VA policy, ongoing substance use involving alcohol, illicit drugs, and/or marijuana, or participation in an opioid replacement program, should not be an automatic exclusion criterion for HCV treatment. There are no published data supporting a minimum length of abstinence or showing that these patients are less likely to achieve SVR with HCV treatment if they remain adherent. VA studies have shown cure rates

Table 1
The Department of Veterans Affairs solutions addressing barriers to hepatitis C virus care and treatment

Clinical Need	Issues or Obstacles	Solutions
Identification of undiagnosed veterans	1. Nonstandardized approaches to risk assessment and test ordering 2. Variation in laboratory capacity, resources, and availability 3. Burdensome consent requirements 4. High-risk patient awareness	1. Implementation of birth cohort and risk factor clinical reminder, automated letter for testing and laboratory orders 2. Site or regional coordination, centralized reference laboratories for testing and confirmatory testing, reflex testing 3. Remove written consent requirement 4. Partner with Housing and Urban Development or homeless care providers, engagement of mental health or substance use disorder treaters
Linkage to care	1. Patient uninterested in treatment or loss of diagnosed patients to follow-up 2. Geographic and transportation barriers 3. Capacity issues (personnel and space) 4. Loss of high-risk patients (ie, substance use or alcohol use disorders) to follow-up	1. Proactive identification and outreach to HCV patients with dashboards and registries, educate patients about available treatment, social media and advertising campaigns, use of telehealth and ECHO models for meeting treatment needs and ease of access 2. Mapping of HCV patient locations and resources, expand VA-ECHO and telehealth modalities 3. Expand the scope of practice for advanced practice providers, hire new personnel, night or weekend clinics, telehealth, group appointments 4. Integrated care for mental health or substance use disorders, nurse navigators focusing on high-risk patients, peer support specialists
Evaluation and risk stratification	1. Missing processes or responsibility for evaluation, risk stratification, laboratory testing and referral 2. Gaps in provider knowledge on evaluation and risk stratification 3. Gaps in patient education 4. Psychosocial determinants such as homelessness, substance or alcohol abuse, or untreated mental health	1. Standardized procedures or algorithms for evaluation, risk stratification, and referral; consult templates with order sets 2. Clinical resources and education for providers 3. Use of and expansion of patient education materials, veteran peer educators, support groups, and marketing and media campaigns 4. Processes and resources for addressing mental health and substance use issues, rapid referral of patients to address co-morbidities, effectively assessing alcohol and substance use, matching a patient's use with the actual risk of nonadherence, eliminating non–evidence-based abstinence policies for HCV treatment, partnering with homeless programs and mental health and substance use clinics, treatment of psychiatric comorbidities

(continued on next page)

Table 1 *(continued)*		
Clinical Need	**Issues or Obstacles**	**Solutions**
Treatment of appropriate veterans	1. Shortage of trained providers 2. Inefficient delivery of care 3. Limitations in capacity and/or clinic space 4. Lack of access to rapid laboratory turnaround for deciding whether to continue treatment 5. Treatment of rural or highly rural veterans 6. Rapidly evolving treatment standards 7. Inability to adhere to therapy or medical appointments 8. Unstable or uncontrolled medical comorbidities	1. Train and expand scope of practice for nurse practitioners, clinical pharmacists, and physician assistants; enlist primary care providers; reserve hepatologists for most complex cases 2. Site or VISN-level coordination, with system redesign to increase efficiency; same-day services for evaluation, laboratory tests, and treatment initiation; integrate care 3. Telehealth or remote video teleconferencing, e-consults, expanded ECHO models, system redesign to increase clinic space, evening or weekend clinics, mobile van clinics 4. Site or VISN-level coordination, centralized reference laboratories for HCV RNA testing 5. Mapping of HCV patient locations and resources, expand ECHO and telehealth 6. Regularly updated policies, treatment guidelines, Web site or SharePoint, educational webinars 7. Careful patient selection and education, adherence support (phone calls, pill boxes, anticipation of specific problems), group clinics, peer support, integrated care and case management, patient navigators 8. Ensure the necessary care coordination, case management, mental health, and substance use services are in place to reach and continue to reassess treatment candidacy; use of electronic data tools for patient tracking and outreach

achieved among veterans with alcohol, substance use, and mental health disorders (89%–91%) to be similar to those without these conditions (91%–92%).[18,33]

In collaboration with the National Academic Detailing Office, the National Viral Hepatitis Program has also supported academic detailing of HCV and primary care providers to increase the use of alcohol pharmacotherapy among heavy and problematic drinkers with HCV infection. Liver and HCV clinics provide an opportune setting to increase access to initiation of pharmacotherapy for alcohol use disorder in preparation for HCV treatment initiation in this population.

Another successful strategy has been contingency management programs that reward veterans for completed successful behaviors or contact with HCV care providers. For each completed target behavior (eg, laboratory blood draw, medication refills, or completed appointments) veterans are rewarded with a prize ticket drawing ranging in value from complimentary phrases (ie, "great job") to vouchers for products or monetary denominations. Each completed consecutive contact escalates the number of tickets that can be drawn.

Integrated care has been particularly important for vulnerable populations and increases treatment initiation and SVR rates.[34] To maximize treatment among a difficult to reach and engage population, a comprehensive approach is needed that manages overall health, including comorbid psychiatric, substance abuse, and medical comorbidities, and that addresses factors that pose significant impediments to care, such as homelessness, rurality, and transportation. Mental health professionals, addiction specialists, care coordinators, case managers, and social workers are necessary resources to meet the individualized needs of this population. In collaboration with the Office of Academic Affiliations, the National Hepatitis Program supports a Human Immunodeficiency Virus (HIV) and Liver Disease Psychology Postdoctoral Residency Program at 10 VA sites. This fellowship emphasizes the behavioral, mental health, and substance use treatment of veterans with either HIV or HCV, and trains psychologists in this critical area to support Veterans Health Administration efforts to successfully treat veterans with HCV and care for veterans with HIV.

HITs have developed many innovative practices in response to the needs of their patients. Several VA facilities have embedded clinical pharmacists to manage and dispense HCV medications directly in the homeless clinic or have trained primary care providers who work exclusively with homeless veterans to treat HCV. Others have created small teams of multidisciplinary providers to bring HCV care to the veterans in their environment. These teams combine the use of mobile outreach vans and mobile technology to identify homeless veterans in the community, connect them to social work services, and initiate treatment. This has included going to railroad tracks and underpasses to find veterans, offer screening, and treat their HCV by delivering medication in fanny packs.

For veterans who have struggled with mental health challenges or substance use, VA clinicians have engaged Peer Support Specialists. Peers are veterans who have received training and certification and are in recovery from a mental health condition. Peer Support Specialist communication with fellow veterans about pursuing HCV treatment can have a substantial impact, particularly among those with doubts about treatment.

Although the VA continues to aggressively conduct outreach to these veterans and address modifiable factors that may result in eventual HCV treatment in the future, this will be a longer and more challenging process than in the past.

MOVING FORWARD

Challenges remain in engaging patients in HCV care, and providers will need to be flexible and responsive in their approach to care. Continued reassessment of how care is provided, strategizing to minimize gaps in care, and dissemination of best practices to improve access and quality of care will remain integral components of future success.

ACKNOWLEDGMENTS

The authors would like to acknowledge and thank all of the VA HCV health care providers and staff whose dedicated efforts and innovations have contributed to the VA's progress in eliminating HCV among veterans.

REFERENCES

1. Backus LI, Belperio PS, Loomis TP, et al. Hepatitis C virus screening and prevalence among US veterans in Department of Veterans Affairs care. JAMA Intern Med 2013;173:1549–52.

2. Dominitz JA, Boyko EJ, Koepsell TD, et al. Elevated prevalence of hepatitis C infection in users of United States veterans medical centers. Hepatology 2005; 41:88–96.
3. Beste LA, Ioannou GN. Prevalence and treatment of chronic hepatitis C virus infection in the US Department of Veterans Affairs. Epidemiol Rev 2015;37: 131–43.
4. Denniston MM, Jiles RB, Drobeniuc J, et al. Chronic hepatitis C virus infection in the United States, National Health and Nutrition Examination Survey 2003 to 2010. Ann Intern Med 2014;160:293–300.
5. Noska AJ, Belperio PS, Loomis TP, et al. Engagement in the hepatitis C care cascade among Homeless veterans, 2015. Public Health Rep 2017;132:136–9.
6. US Department of Veterans Affairs, Veterans Health Administration Web site. Available at: https://www.va.gov/health/aboutVHA.asp. Accessed August 24, 2017.
7. US Department of Veterans Affairs, National Center for Veterans Analysis and Statistics, Utilization. Available at: https://www.va.gov/vetdata/Utilization.asp. Accessed August 24, 2017.
8. Brown SH, Lincoln MJ, Groen PJ, et al. VistA—US Department of Veterans Affairs national-scale HIS. Int J Med Inform 2003;69:135–56.
9. Perlin JB, Kolodner RM, Roswell RH. The Veterans Health Administration: quality, value, accountability, and information as transforming strategies for patient-centered care. Healthc Pap 2005;5:10–24.
10. Backus LI, Gavrilov S, Loomis TP, et al. Clinical case registries: simultaneous local and national disease registries for population quality management. J Am Med Inform Assoc 2009;16:775–83.
11. US Department of Veterans Affairs, Viral Hepatitis Web site. Available at: https://www.hepatitis.va.gov/. Accessed August 24, 2017.
12. Toussaint JS, Berry LL. The promise of Lean in health care. Mayo Clin Proc 2013; 88:74–82.
13. Rogal SS, Yakovchenko V, Waltz TJ, et al. The association between implementation strategy use and the uptake of hepatitis C treatment in a national sample. Implement Sci 2017;12:60–73.
14. Backus LI, Belperio PS, Shahoumian TA, et al. Comparative effectiveness of the hepatitis C virus protease inhibitors boceprevir and telaprevir in a large U.S. cohort. Aliment Pharmacol Ther 2014;39:93–103.
15. Maier MM, Ross DB, Chartier M, et al. Cascade of care for hepatitis C virus infection within the US Veterans Health Administration. Am J Public Health 2016;106: 353–8.
16. Moon AM, Green PK, Berry K, et al. Transformation of hepatitis C antiviral treatment in a national healthcare system following the introduction of direct antiviral agents. Aliment Pharmacol Ther 2017;45:1201–12.
17. Belperio PS, Chartier M, Ross DB, et al. Curing hepatitis C virus infection: best practices from the U.S. Department of Veterans Affairs. Ann Intern Med 2017; 167(7):499–504.
18. Backus LI, Belperio PS, Shahoumian TA, et al. Real-world effectiveness and predictors of sustained virological response with all-oral therapy in 21,242 hepatitis C genotype-1 patients. Antivir Ther 2017;22(6):481–93.
19. Ioannou GN, Beste LA, Chang MF, et al. Effectiveness of sofosbuvir, ledipasvir/sofosbuvir, or paritaprevir/ritonavir/ombitasvir and dasabuvir regimens for treatment of patients with hepatitis C in the veterans affairs national health care system. Gastroenterology 2016;151:457–71.

20. Yehia BR, Schranz AJ, Umscheid CA, et al. The treatment cascade for chronic hepatitis C virus infection in the United States: a systematic review and meta-analysis. PLoS One 2014;9:e101554.

21. Arora S, Kalishman S, Thornton K, et al. Expanding access to hepatitis C virus treatment–Extension for Community Healthcare Outcomes (ECHO) project: disruptive innovation in specialty care. Hepatology 2010;52:1124–33.

22. Beste LA, Glorioso TJ, Ho PM, et al. Telemedicine specialty support promotes hepatitis C treatment by primary care providers in the Department of Veterans Affairs. Am J Med 2017;130:432–8.

23. Ourth H, Groppi J, Morreale AP, et al. Clinical pharmacist prescribing activities in the Veterans Health Administration. Am J Health Syst Pharm 2016;73:1406–15.

24. Rongey C, Shen H, Hamilton N, et al. Impact of rural residence and health system structure on quality of liver care. PLoS One 2013;8:e84826.

25. Backus LI, Belperio PS, Shahoumian TA, et al. Impact of provider type on hepatitis C outcomes with boceprevir-based and telaprevir-based regimens. J Clin Gastroenterol 2015;49:329–35.

26. Centers for Disease Control and Prevention. Advancing team-based care through collaborative practice agreements: a resource and implementation guide for adding pharmacists to the care team. Atlanta (GA): Centers for Disease Control and Prevention, U.S. Department of Health and Human Services; 2017. Available at: https://www.cdc.gov/dhdsp/pubs/docs/CPA-Team-Based-Care.pdf. Accessed August 30, 2017.

27. Recommendations for prevention and control of hepatitis C virus (HCV) infection and HCV-related chronic disease. Centers for Disease Control and Prevention. MMWR Recomm Rep 1998;47(RR-19):1–39.

28. National Hepatitis C Program Office. Hepatitis C: military-related blood exposures, risk factors, VA care. Available at: http://www.hepatitis.va.gov/provider/policy/military-blood-exposures.asp. Accessed August 30, 2017.

29. Ross DB, Belperio PS, Chartier M, et al. Hepatitis C testing in U.S. veterans born 1945-1965: an update. J Hepatol 2017;66:237–8.

30. Moyer VA, U.S. Preventive Services Task Force. Screening for hepatitis C virus infection in adults: U.S. Preventive Services Task Force recommendation statement. Ann Intern Med 2013;159:349–57.

31. Akiyama MJ, Kaba F, Rosner Z, et al. Hepatitis C screening of the "birth cohort" (Born 1945-1965) and younger inmates of New York City jails. Am J Public Health 2016;106:1276–7.

32. Jonas MC, Rodriguez CV, Redd J, et al. Streamlining screening to treatment: the hepatitis C cascade of care at Kaiser Permanente mid-Atlantic states. Clin Infect Dis 2016;62:1290–6.

33. Tsui JI, Williams EC, Green PK, et al. Alcohol use and hepatitis C virus treatment outcomes among patients receiving direct antiviral agents. Drug Alcohol Depend 2016;169:101–9.

34. Ho SB, Bräu N, Cheung R, et al. Integrated care increases treatment and improves outcomes of patients with chronic hepatitis C virus infection and psychiatric illness or substance abuse. Clin Gastroenterol Hepatol 2015;13:2005–14.

Localized US Efforts to Eliminate Hepatitis C

Annette Gaudino[a], Bryn Gay[a], Clifton Garmon[b], Mike Selick, MSW[c],
Reed Vreeland[d], Katie Burk, MPH[e], Emalie Huriaux, MPH[f], Shelley N. Facente, MPH[g],
Annie Luetkemeyer, MD[h], Phil Waters, JD[i], Camilla S. Graham, MD, MPH[j],*

KEYWORDS

- Hepatitis C virus • Elimination • Coalition • Advocacy • Legal
- People who inject drugs • Continuum of care

KEY POINTS

- Local strategies must be developed to implement hepatitis C elimination programs.
- Coalitions of community advocates, health and social service providers, researchers, legal experts, and government representatives have come together in New York State, San Francisco, California, and Massachusetts to create hepatitis C virus elimination plans.
- Barriers to the hepatitis C care continuum can be addressed on a local level using new and existing resources.
- Funding remains a challenge and focus of advocacy.

Disclosure Statement: End Hep C SF has received a charitable donation from Abbvie Pharmaceuticals and a grant from the Gilead Foundation (K. Burk). Research grant support to UCSF related to HCV from AbbVie (32175), Gilead and Merck (A. Luetkemeyer). Nothing to disclose (A. Gaudino, B. Gay, C. Garmon, M. Selick, R. Vreeland, E. Huriaux, S.N. Facente, P. Waters, C.S. Graham).

[a] Treatment Action Group, 90 Broad Street, Suite 2503, New York, NY 10004, USA; [b] VOCAL-NY, 80-A Fourth Avenue, Brooklyn, NY 11217, USA; [c] Harm Reduction Coalition, 22 West 27th Street, 5th Floor, New York, NY 10001, USA; [d] Housing Works, 57 Willoughby Street, 2nd Floor, Brooklyn, NY 11201, USA; [e] San Francisco Department of Public Health, 25 Van Ness, Suite 500, San Francisco, CA 94102, USA; [f] Project Inform, 273 Ninth Street, San Francisco, CA 94103, USA; [g] Facente Consulting, 5601 Van Fleet Avenue, Richmond, CA 94804, USA; [h] Division of HIV, Infectious Diseases and Global Medicine, Zuckerberg San Francisco General, University of California San Francisco, Box 0874, 995 Potrero Avenue, San Francisco, CA 94110, USA; [i] Center for Health Law and Policy Innovation, Harvard Law School, 122 Boylston Street, Jamaica Plain, MA 02130, USA; [j] Division of Infectious Disease, Beth Israel Deaconess Medical Center, Harvard Medical School, 110 Francis Street LMOB Suite GB, Boston, MA 02215, USA
* Corresponding author.
E-mail address: cgraham@bidmc.harvard.edu

Infect Dis Clin N Am 32 (2018) 293–311
https://doi.org/10.1016/j.idc.2018.02.009
0891-5520/18/© 2018 Elsevier Inc. All rights reserved.

id.theclinics.com

INTRODUCTION

We have now reached a sentinel point in addressing the scourge of hepatitis C virus (HCV) infection. Interferon, with its difficult side effects, is no longer used in the United States for HCV infection, we have tests to determine liver damage that do not require liver biopsy, and previously "difficult-to-cure" patient groups have a greater than 95% cure rate with 8 to 12 weeks of well-tolerated all-oral medications. These advances have led the National Academies of Medicine, Engineering and Science to declare that hepatitis C can be eliminated in the United States.[1]

The National Viral Hepatitis Action Plan details actions that agencies within the federal government can take to facilitate improvements in diagnosing patients, linking them to care, and supporting their successful completion of curative treatments.[2] Many of the systemic challenges facing us as a nation benefit from large-scale coordination of policies and actions at the federal level. However, much of our health care is organized on a state level, including departments of public health-sponsored surveillance, health insurance, and certain policies. Coalitions are emerging to address city and state-level elimination strategies, and these have several initiatives in common. This review discusses examples of programs from 2 states—New York and Massachusetts—and 1 city-wide effort, in San Francisco. Our goal is to facilitate the creation of HCV elimination campaigns in every state.

BACKGROUND: HEPATITIS C VIRUS IN NEW YORK STATE

Since 2001, more than 254,200 chronic HCV cases have been reported in New York state. In 2014, there were 16,169 chronic HCV cases and 127 acute cases reported. The statewide HCV case rate in 2014 was 83.4 per 100,000. The rate was higher in New York City (94.1 per 100,000) than outside of New York City (75.7 per 100,000). Although New York City has historically been the epicenter of the state's HCV epidemic, in 2014 more than one-half (51.2%) of new chronic hepatitis C cases were diagnosed outside of New York City.[3]

Since 2004, in New York state there has been a shift in the age distribution of reported HCV cases from being primarily among persons aged 40 to 60 years to being reported among a growing cohort of persons aged 20 to 40 years. This shift is especially striking outside of New York City. Recent increases of HCV are occurring outside of New York City among young people who inject drugs (PWID), which parallels the growing epidemic of prescription opioid misuse seen in suburban and rural areas. There has also been a shift in the distribution of cases by sex. In 2005, females aged 15 to 44 accounted for 35.7% of HCV cases reported outside of New York City. This proportion increased to 56.5%% in 2015.[4]

Hepatitis C Virus Services in New York State

Although New York state faces concerning gaps in its HCV continuum of care caused by ongoing barriers to HCV prevention and treatment, the state has built a strong foundation for an HCV elimination plan. New York state has one of that largest concentrations of skilled medical providers, prevention and harm reduction specialists, researchers, hepatitis C-focused coalitions, such as the New York City Hepatitis C Task Force, and public health officials in the nation, combined with a vibrant network of community outreach workers and community-based health activists throughout the state. There are several initiatives that build HCV clinical capacity and expand access to HCV treatment. The New York State Department of Health's AIDS Institute Hepatitis C Care and Treatment Initiative aims to increase the number of people with HCV who get linked to care and initiate and complete treatment. Each funded program provides linkage to care activities and on-site HCV medical care, care coordination, treatment, and supportive services in a clinical setting (ie, community health centers, drug treatment programs, and hospital-based clinics). The New York City Department of Health and Mental Hygiene (DOHMH) Project INSPIRE adapted the evidenced-based New York City HIV Care Coordination Program for HCV patients, and built capacity at 2 major medical centers by funding a multidisciplinary team including care coordinators and peer navigators to provided services, as well as supported clinical telementoring to build primary care provider capacity to deliver HCV care and treatment. Project INSPIRE aimed to improve patient outcomes and quality of care while reducing costs and proposed a payment model for sustained funding for these services. The New York City DOHMH Check Hep C Patient Navigation Program builds community health organization capacity and trains navigators to conduct effective HCV outreach, prevention, linkage to care, and clinical care coordination services to support complete HCV treatment and reinfection prevention after cure. Check Hep C is a flexible low-cost and low-threshold model for delivering patient navigation services that has been implemented at more than 45 community health organizations, including syringe exchange programs, community health centers, and hospitals, and has trained more than 100 peer and patient navigators in HCV patient navigation. New York State's more than 20-year history of support for syringe exchange and harm reduction services, and its role in originating and expanding medication-assisted treatment for opioid dependence, have informed human immunodeficiency virus (HIV), hepatitis, and substance use services worldwide. New York State has also been on the vanguard of successful and ongoing Medicaid reform that provides further support for new efforts to fill the gaps in the HCV care continuum.

The Catalyst for the Elimination of Hepatitis C Virus in New York State: The Human Immunodeficiency Virus Elimination Initiative "Ending the Epidemic"

The call to eliminate HIV first came in May 2013, when New York-based advocacy organizations convened community leaders, advocates, health and social service providers, researchers, and government representatives to assess the adequacy of New York's response to the HIV/AIDS epidemic and to discuss developing an action plan that would bring about the end of the epidemic in New York State. Community leaders partnered with the AIDS Institute and the DOHMH to convene key stakeholders who were tasked to identify priorities through a statewide community engagement process. These stakeholders held various town halls, rallies, actions, public lectures, and social media campaigns to raise awareness and pinpoint statewide priorities. Priority areas included policy, prevention, biomedical interventions, surveillance, access to care, messaging, and resources.

This first effort was the foundation for the Ending the Epidemic (EtE) initiative and informed a historic June 29, 2014, announcement from then-Governor Cuomo about his 3-point plan to end AIDS in New York State by the end of 2020—the first pledge of its kind in the United States.[5] The goal is to reduce the number of new HIV infections from an estimated 3000 to 750 by 2020 to reduce the prevalence of HIV in New York State. That same year, the governor appointed an "Ending the Epidemic Task Force" to create a blueprint to implement this plan. New York state's pioneering plan to end its HIV/AIDS epidemic by the end of 2020, and the recommendations made by the Governor's EtE Task Force also provide an example of how state, city, county, and community experts can set long-term goals and work toward achieving elimination targets.

The EtE initiative has already improved health outcomes across the HIV continuum of care, and New York state has begun meeting its EtE goals. These include (1) changing the HIV testing law, (2) gaining insurance coverage for health care specifically for transgender people, (3) the legal prohibition of using condoms as evidence for the two lowest levels of misdemeanor criminal charges for sex work, (4) enabling medical providers to access surveillance data to retain patients in care and help them to achieve viral suppression, and (5) allowing pharmacists to dispense starter kits for preexposure prophylaxis to prevent HIV transmission, among other adopted recommendations.

Developing an Initiative to Eliminate Hepatitis C in New York State

In Spring 2015, after meetings with community advocates who were intimately involved in the EtE campaign that was so successful the year before, community leadership invited the New York State Department of Health's AIDS Institute and New York City DOHMH into initial discussions to support a parallel initiative to eliminate hepatitis C in New York City and New York state. Many of the same advocacy organizations that were involved with EtE were reconvened with the stewardship of the New York state Hep C Elimination Campaign, and asked to develop a strategy for New York state to end hepatitis C. The response was unanimous and by Fall 2015, formation of a statewide Campaign to Eliminate HCV had begun.

Before the first steering committee meeting in March of 2016, the coalition leadership was composed of community-based HIV organizations and multiservice providers, harm reduction and treatment advocacy organizations, and multi-issue membership organizations that represented PWID. Leaders from these organizations wrote a discussion paper that served as an initial call to action for the rest of the state's HCV advocates that outlined the committee's vision for the work that lay ahead. This paper was the foundation for the coalition-building work that took place throughout the rest of 2015 and culminated in a statewide Summit for HCV Elimination in New York State.

The March 2016 meeting of the steering committee saw the development of a process for pursuing the vision, and a structure was created to carry it out. A group of 94 stakeholders from across the state, including state and local government representatives, epidemiologists, physicians, harm reduction and social service providers, and community advocates, formed the core coalition. It was to be guided by an advisory board that included the leading government agencies and the original members of the coalition. However, the steering committee had the authority to act for the campaign.

The steering committee decided to follow a path similarly taken by the EtE leadership and created 5 working groups that developed recommendations to inform the overall elimination strategy that would be presented to the New York state Governor. The groups were called Prevention/Harm Reduction/Prevention of Reinfection, Testing and Linkage to Care, Clinical Care/Treatment Access/Supportive Services, Surveillance and Data Metrics, and Social Determinants (**Fig. 1**).

Work group members were recruited from various institutions and fields, representing different geographic areas, experiences, expertise, work and community settings, and genders, and included professionals and people living with HIV, HCV, those who have used harm reduction services, and others disproportionately affected by HCV. Throughout the process, members were requested to consult other people in their networks, particularly to ensure the inclusion of practitioners and community representatives in the areas most affected by HCV. Each group was given a directive along with a set of questions to answer that were specific to the purpose of their group, and they were given 6 weeks to report back to the steering committee with their findings in the form of draft recommendations.

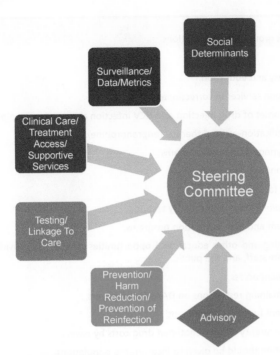

Fig. 1. New York work group structure.

Despite the extensive outreach to recruit a diverse membership, there were some limitations in the work groups' composition. This could be attributed to insufficient time and resources to announce the HCV elimination process or a lack of strong relationships within the more remote communities. There were gaps in participation by key impacted populations, especially people who inject or use drugs, Native and homeless populations, and those who were formerly incarcerated or who worked with people reintegrating into society. Ongoing efforts to engage the upstate, rural communities most impacted by the HCV and opioid epidemics in the statewide elimination campaign are needed. Stronger community voices and active participation would ensure a balance among the researchers, social service providers, and physicians.

The work group chairs reported their findings to the steering committee at a meeting held on November 28, 2016. Their analysis included gaps in services related to their area of focus, populations at risk, best practices, potential policy changes, and a list of their recommendations prioritized in order of need to achieve elimination (**Box 1**).

Establishing Elimination Targets

An important discussion arose around the establishment of elimination targets and the accompanying metrics with which to measure progress toward achievement. This work was done within the Data, Surveillance and Metrics work group, but the actual targets could not be determined until better estimates of the prevalence of people infected with chronic HCV are calculated, which the New York State Department of Health and the New York City DOHMH are coordinating efforts to complete in the near future. This work group has been trying to set elimination targets based on a prevalence estimate and consistent with the World Health Organization and National

---

Box 1
New York work group recommendations

Prevention

1. Health literacy and education.
2. HCV prevention services in correctional settings.
3. Prevent the onset of drug injection and HCV infection among young opioid users.
4. Access to medication-assisted therapy (buprenorphine).
5. Enhancing syringe exchange programs.
6. Safer injection/consumption facilities.

Testing/linkage to care

1. Facilitate and/or ensure confirmatory testing.
2. Expand patient and peer navigation programs.
3. Expand training and other educational opportunities for medical providers, testing and linkage to care staff, and the public.

Care and treatment access

1. Eliminate remaining restrictions on DAAs for all payers.
2. Address patient barriers to treatment.
3. Increase transparency about negotiated drug costs by payers.
4. Special attention should be given to incarcerated populations.

Data and metrics

1. Set realistic but ambitious targets for elimination.
2. Systematically track and disseminate information on progress toward achieving the goals of the initiative.
3. Strengthen surveillance systems.

Social determinants

1. Eliminate legal barriers for people who inject drugs.
2. Increase funding for discharge planning and care coordination services after release from correctional settings.
3. Implement culturally appropriate messaging to the multiple populations with higher HCV risk or prevalence.

Abbreviations: DAA, direct-acting antivirals; HCV, hepatitis C virus.

Academies of Sciences, Engineering, and Medicine targets. However, setting elimination targets tends to be a political decision, and depends on which stakeholders have the leverage to determine the appropriate target, the dynamics of the decision-making process, which stakeholder is responsible to monitor progress, and how accountability is implemented during the process.

In contrast, the elimination target of a decrease of new HIV infections to 750 by 2020 was easier to determine for EtE owing to the decades of surveillance systems in place for HIV, which could be attributed to greater resources and funding. For HCV, once a statewide prevalence estimate for New York state is in place, the 2 health departments will work with a consultant to model an elimination scenario and metrics.

New York State Hepatitis C Elimination Summit

After the Joint Steering Committee/Work Group Meeting in November 2016, plans were underway for the next major milestone: the statewide Hepatitis C Elimination Summit. This followed similar tactics of the EtE leadership, which were successful in engaging stakeholders, building consensus recommendations, developing a shared knowledge base, and creating a transparent process for going forward. It was held in Albany on February 7, 2017, and in the time leading up to that culminating event, the steering committee was tasked with reviewing the work group recommendations and refining and abridging them into a concise set of core positions that would be presented to those at the summit, agreed upon by consensus, and then advanced for gubernatorial support.

The New York State Summit was the first statewide elimination effort in the United States, drawing national attention. There were 252 state and local officials, elected representatives, medical and social service providers, and community stakeholders, including people living with HIV, HCV, who have used harm reduction services or others disproportionately affected by HCV, who participated in the meeting in person or online. Presentations described the impact of HCV on people across the state, their most urgent needs, and the pathway to elimination. Participants had the opportunity to respond to and endorse the community consensus statement. This was presented as a call to action for New York state elected officials, the goal for whom was the establishment of a formal Task Force to support the Five Pillars into which the work group recommendations had been adapted (**Box 2**).

The Consensus Statement was ratified unanimously, and following the meeting, the steering committee gathered endorsements from community organizations, medical providers and facilities, policymakers, and local governments. In all, 134 organizations have endorsed the statement and, in May of 2017, the document was sent the New York state governor with a request to advance the recommendations.

Stakeholder Listening Sessions

Ratification by the 252 people who attended or viewed the summit, followed by the written endorsement of the community organizations, was only the first step toward

---

Box 2
Five pillars for New York statewide HCV elimination

1. Enhance HCV prevention, testing, and linkage to care services for people who inject drugs, people who are incarcerated, men who have sex with men, and other populations disproportionately impacted by HCV infection.

2. Expand HCV screening and testing to identify people living with HCV who are unaware of their status and link them to care.

3. Provide access to clinically appropriate medical care and affordable HCV treatment without restrictions and ensure the availability of necessary supportive services for all New Yorkers living with HCV infection.

4. Enhance New York state HCV surveillance, set and track HCV elimination targets and make this information available to the public.

5. Commit New York state government and elected officials, public health professionals, HCV experts, and industry partners to leadership and ownership of the New York State Plan to Eliminate HCV alongside community members living with and affected by HCV.

Abbreviation: HCV, hepatitis C virus.

statewide consensus. The steering committee spent the next 6 months (February to August 2017) holding listening sessions in every part of New York state to ensure that stakeholders who had not been able to attend the summit could review the recommendations and provide feedback to the organizers that would further inform the document. From Buffalo to Staten Island, 20 sessions have been held so far, with more than 228 total attendees.

Conclusions from the New York State Elimination Program

New York State is the first state in the United States to create a set of recommendations to eliminate HCV, which can inform the gubernatorial task force's statewide strategy. New York state can be a model for other states because many of the same problems addressed during New York State's HCV Elimination Summit are being felt across the country: rural and suburban regions of the state face an epidemic of young opioid users; urban populations face poverty and limited access to services; the insurance industry faces ever-rising drug prices; patients face rising drug costs that outpace inflation; and no generic competition of the direct-acting antivirals (DAAs) exists in the United States.

We are now on firm ground to call for eliminating HCV in New York by treating as many patients as possible and curbing new transmissions, given the effectiveness and tolerability of current DAA regimens. We need to increase the number of people who know they have HCV by increasing public and health provider education, strengthening our testing law, and encouraging routine testing in clinical settings and increased targeted testing in drug treatment programs, syringe programs, and other places likely to serve people who may have been exposed to HCV. We can build a robust hepatitis C treatment infrastructure in New York state to care for all those previously and newly diagnosed by repurposing the very successful HIV treatment infrastructure and expanding hepatitis C treatment capacity within primary care, licensed drug treatments programs, and corrections facilities. Drug manufacturers and government must find a solution for high HCV drug prices that addresses the inherent budgetary strain of treating a high volume of patients. In the call to action emphasized in the consensus statement that was endorsed by community advocates across the state, the coalition requested a joint commitment by the Governor, the New York state Legislature and industry partners to find a viable, cost-effective solution that will expedite people's access to HCV testing, treatment, and care. On March 16, 2018, Governor Cuomo announced the State's commitment to eliminate HCV. Community leaders cheered, then set to work to make his pledge a reality.

SAN FRANCISCO HEPATITIS C VIRUS ELIMINATION INITIATIVE: *END HEP C SF*

San Francisco is profoundly impacted by HCV. An estimated 22,000 San Franciscans have HCV antibodies, and of those, approximately 12,000 are estimated to have current HCV infection.[6] As in many other communities, in San Francisco, HCV disproportionately impacts Baby Boomers (people born between 1945 and 1965) and some of our most vulnerable and stigmatized people, including PWID and men who have sex with men (**Fig. 2**).[7] In addition, San Francisco has the highest rate of hepatocellular carcinoma of any city in the United States, driven by both hepatitis B virus and HCV.[8]

Recognizing that San Francisco had been hit hard by the HCV epidemic, in 2008 representatives of public health organizations, research institutions, and civic groups convened to discuss and craft a local response. In May 2009, Mayor Gavin Newsom appointed a panel to serve on the Mayor's San Francisco Hepatitis C Task Force and charged the group with developing a comprehensive set of recommendations to

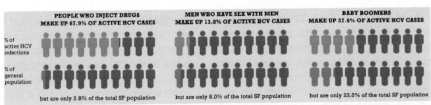

Fig. 2. Disproportionate burden of hepatitis C virus (HCV) in San Francisco, 2015. Although transgender women make up a small percentage of the total population of San Francisco (0.1%), End Hep C SF estimates that more than 1 of every 6 transgender women is currently living with HCV. Note that the above groups do not add up to 100%; it is possible for a person to be in more than one group.

address the HCV epidemic. The task force's initial recommendations were published in 2010 and are updated annually (available: http://sfhepc.org/recommendations/). The Hepatitis C Task Force successfully advocated for the creation of a viral hepatitis prevention coordinator position with the San Francisco Department of Public Health (SFDPH), as well as for allocation of local funds to broaden HCV testing and linkage to care efforts. With this proactive public health engagement on HCV and the advent of highly effective oral DAA therapy, San Francisco now has the tools necessary to greatly reduce HCV related morbidity and mortality, break the cycle of forward transmission, and ultimately eliminate HCV. To that end, in 2016 SFDPH, University of California, San Francisco, and other community partners established the *End Hep C SF* initiative to lay the groundwork for HCV elimination (available: www.EndHepCSF.org).

Several conditions make San Francisco an ideal place for a groundbreaking HCV elimination effort. Access to HCV prevention, testing, and treatment in San Francisco is strong compared with much of the greater United States, and San Francisco has a history of implementing cutting-edge, evidence-based public health interventions such as syringe access, opiate agonist therapy, health coverage for uninsured individuals, overdose prevention programs, rapid initiation of HIV treatment immediately after diagnosis, and early adoption of universal HIV treatment regardless of CD4 cell count.[9] In 2015, San Francisco became one of the first cities in the world to commit to achieving the UNAIDS vision of "Getting to Zero" for HIV (zero new HIV infections, zero HIV deaths, and zero HIV stigma by 2020).[10] San Francisco's Getting to Zero initiative provided inspiration for a similar elimination initiative focused on HCV.

End Hep C SF is a multisector independent consortium operating under the principles of collective impact. Collective impact involves people working together on a complex issue under 5 conditions: common agenda, shared measurement, mutually reinforcing activities, continuous communications, and backbone support.[11] The *End Hep C SF* founders recruited members for what was initially called the Steering Committee. This group met biweekly in the first quarter of 2016, learning about collective impact while laying the foundation for the initiative. After deliberation as to the best structure for the initiative, the Steering Committee formed 4 workgroups—(1)Research and Surveillance, (2)Prevention and Education, (3)Testing and Linkage, and (4)Treatment Access, then reached out to those working in HCV across the city in a variety settings and requested their participation in the initiative. Since its inception, *End Hep C SF* has strived to uphold the principles of collective impact and align with the framework's 5 conditions (available: http://www.fsg.org/approach-areas/collective-impact). To this end, we emphasize collective decision making, data sharing, and evaluation as key components of the initiative's process and diffused leadership model; we have also conducted structured evaluations to assess adherence to collective impact principles and will continue to do so at regular intervals.

As of the end of 2017, 32 organizations and more than 100 individuals had signed on as *End Hep C SF* partners, with representation from sectors including academia, local government, drug treatment programs, syringe access programs, homeless service organizations, pharmacies, private medical systems, HIV/AIDS service organizations, and advocacy groups. *End Hep C SF*'s organizational representatives participate in various ways, including membership on the Coordinating Committee or the 4 work-groups, guidance through the Executive Advisory Committee, or participation in semi-annual community-wide meetings. Many of our most actively involved stakeholders are staff of community-based organizations, committed to one or more key aspects of HCV elimination: diagnosis, treatment, prevention, and education. *End Hep C SF* has explicitly created opportunities for participation at varied levels of commitment to encourage broad-based representation in the initiative across San Francisco.

Vision and Priority Setting

End Hep C SF envisions a San Francisco where HCV is no longer a public health threat, and HCV-related health inequities have been eliminated. The initiative's mission is to support all San Franciscans living with and at risk for HCV to maximize their health and wellness. The initiative defined this vision, mission, corresponding values, and short-term goals in its first 3-year strategic plan published in March of 2017.[12] These priorities were established over a period of 4 months with the help of an external consultant who led workgroup members through a series of discussions related to available risk data, analysis of the existing landscape of interventions, and stakeholder wisdom about gaps and areas of potential high impact. Initial priority interventions were refined into measurable, achievable, time-based priorities for action both in 2017 and in 2018/2019 to move closer to elimination. A corresponding list of budget requests was simultaneously developed by the workgroups, identifying which priorities could not be achieved without additional funding and how much would be required. This list of funding needs was used to inform the San Francisco Hepatitis C Task Force's official request for the mayor's budget in 2017, as well as requests for funding from research institutions, private foundations, and corporate giving programs.

Core Strategies

In our first 2 years, *End Hep C SF* has focused on several keys strategies: addressing data gaps, reaching people living with HCV "where they are," developing models of HCV care and treatment outside of specialty care, and seeking innovative partnerships with insurers to support elimination.

Strategy: addressing data gaps

One of *End Hep C SF*'s core strategies is a focus on data, improving and aligning research and surveillance of HCV, and making better use of existing data to guide programs and policies. To understand the potential effect of *End Hep C SF* interventions, it is critical to have a strong estimate of citywide HCV prevalence, including in key populations with programmatic significance. However, despite the implementation of HCV surveillance systems and the inclusion of HCV measures in national health surveys, accurate estimates of total active HCV infections at the local level, including breakdown by key populations, are lacking. To address this data need, epidemiologists in the Research and Surveillance workgroup developed a process to triangulate surveillance, research, and local health systems data to produce a baseline estimate of the number of people in San Francisco with anti-HCV antibodies, as well as active HCV infection (detectable HCV RNA), with findings released in June 2017.[6] San Francisco's prevalence estimate is the result of an innovative, collaborative process made possible by the existence of *End Hep C SF*. Data regarding disparities among certain key populations will guide future efforts of the other workgroups, which will prioritize these populations for prevention, testing, linkage, and treatment interventions. Annual assessment of citywide HCV treatment starts as well as revised estimates of active HCV prevalence will be conducted to track progress toward HCV elimination.

Strategy: reaching people living with hepatitis C virus where they are
Education and outreach for key populations *End Hep C SF* maintains an explicit commitment to prioritizing marginalized populations for HCV interventions. In 2016, *End Hep C SF* launched the "New Treatments Have Changed the Game" HCV education initiative based on feedback from PWID during focus groups conducted by *End Hep C SF* partner GLIDE. GLIDE provides HCV testing, syringe access, and naloxone distribution services primarily to people who are homeless in San Francisco's Tenderloin neighborhood. Focus groups had the dual purpose of assessing clients' baseline knowledge of new developments in HCV treatment, and testing messages about HCV prevention, testing, and treatment. Three overarching messages for and by PWID resulted from the process: (1) "Sharing equipment spreads hep C. Come get sterile stuff." (2) "We can't treat hep C if we don't know we have it." (3) "Living with hep C? New treatments have changed the game." These messages were featured on posters with pictures of HCV service providers from 7 different *End Hep C SF* partner agencies (**Fig. 3**), viewable at http://www.endhepcsf.org/campaigns/.

Increased community-based testing *End Hep C SF*'s Testing and Linkage workgroup meets regularly to discuss community-based HCV testing practices and develop standards and protocols for testing in nonclinical settings. In the first year of *End Hep C SF*, this workgroup examined SFDPH surveillance data alongside community-based testing data and literature estimating the number of PWID citywide. The group set a target to increase community-based testing rates 4-fold over 3 years and have already increased testing rates by 18%, despite no significant increase in resources. This was done by programs integrating point-of-care rapid HCV testing with existing HIV testing services and reaching PWID and other key populations at syringe access programs, drug treatment programs, in residential hotels, on the street, in shelters, and other relevant settings.

Hepatitis C virus navigation services In 2016, *End Hep C SF* partners SFDPH, GLIDE, HealthRIGHT360, and the San Francisco AIDS Foundation launched HCV navigation services. These services support linkages to an HCV treatment provider for community members newly diagnosed with HCV, or those who have been living with HCV but are disconnected from care. The programs are specifically designed for people who are actively using drugs, homeless or marginally housed, and/or have cooccurring mental illness. The navigators educate clients about HCV, ensure their insurance status is up to date, connect them with appropriate providers, facilitate support groups, and help them to track appointments and medications. In the first year, 252 people connected to primary care, the majority of which included HCV treatment capability and at least 89 people achieved sustained virologic response at 12 weeks. These numbers have continually improved in the second year of programming as linkage strategies and data collection processes evolve.

Community engagement *End Hep C SF* is committed to hosting evening meetings twice annually for members of the larger community to learn more about local

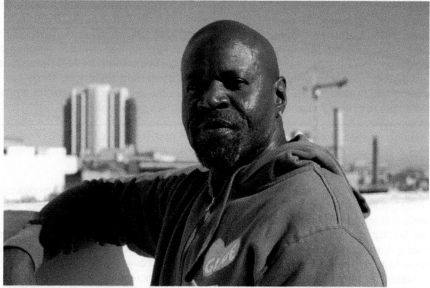

Living with Hep C?
New treatments have changed the game

There is new hope for people with Hep C
Come visit us to talk about the new cure

Fig. 3. Sample poster from the "New Treatments Have Changed the Game" campaign, a social marketing effort to boost hepatitis C virus testing and treatment rates among San Francisco people who inject drugs. (*Courtesy of* Glide Harm Reduction Program, San Francisco, CA; with permission.)

HCV services, and provide feedback to *End Hep C SF* about potential gaps in services and/or what should be scaled up. In August 2017, *End Hep C SF* hosted the first consumer advisory meeting entitled "Tales from the Cured." This meeting featured an explanation of *End Hep C SF*, a discussion of the HCV prevalence estimate, and an "Ask the Doctor" segment about new HCV treatments and interventions. A panel of 4 former clients of the HCV navigation programs discussed their experience being cured of HCV and the wide-reaching positive impact being cured has had on their lives. Meeting participants offered feedback on potential service locations and suggestions for peer-driven HCV linkage services.

Strategy: Developing Models of Hepatitis C Virus Care and Treatment Outside of Specialty Care

Primary care-based hepatitis C virus treatment
Providing HCV treatment in primary care is crucial given high need and the limited number of hepatology, gastroenterology, and infectious disease specialists treating HCV; the fact that many specialists lack experience working with PWID, people who are homeless, and others disproportionately impacted by HCV may also affect their ability to provide culturally competent care.[13] Further, referring a primary care patient to specialty care for treatment is an additional step that may hinder treatment initiation. In 2015, before the genesis of *End Hep C SF*, efforts began within the SFDPH's network of 19 clinical locations largely serving low-income San Franciscans, to train primary care providers to manage and treat HCV. Concurrently, efforts were underway at a local federally qualified health center (Tenderloin Health Services, part of Health-RIGHT360) to provide HCV treatment as part of primary care in a community clinic serving largely homeless and marginally housed patients. Through these efforts, dozens of primary care providers are newly treating HCV, and hundreds of patients have been cured in the primary care setting as a direct result (see Shelley N. Facente and collegaues' article, "New Treatments Have Changed the Game: Hepatitis C Treatment in Primary Care," in this issue).

Hepatitis C virus treatment outside of primary care
To further enhance access to HCV care and treatment, *End Hep C SF* has also focused on establishing innovative models for care in nonclinical settings frequented by many of the most stigmatized people living with HCV. These settings include residential drug treatment programs, methadone clinics, the street (via medical outreach to people who are homeless), the San Francisco jail, a sexual health clinic for men who have sex with men, and syringe access programs. Within opiate agonist therapy settings, 2 innovative HCV care and treatment programs launched by *End Hep C SF* partners are at the Opioid Treatment Outpatient Program (OTOP) at Zuckerberg San Francisco General Hospital and the Bayview Hunters Point Foundation. Both organizations are outpatient medication-assisted treatment clinics serving people with opioid use disorders, and both now provide DAAs via directly observed therapy for individuals who come in daily for methadone. OTOP has a history of serving people living with HIV who access methadone and other medication-assisted treatment for opioid dependence, and OTOP staff have years of experience providing HIV treatment and adherence support. Given this, OTOP clinicians, nurses, and counselors were well-positioned to start prescribing HCV DAAs and to support patient adherence to DAA regimens. OTOP implemented this model by hiring a full-time nurse through a grant from the California Department of Public Health. In the first year of OTOP's HCV treatment program, they have treated 68 patients. Bayview Hunters Point Foundation's methadone clinic does not have a history of treating HIV and worked closely with a primary care clinician and HCV treatment champion located at a neighboring SFDPH clinic to build capacity for HCV directly observed therapy and adherence support. To reach others who may not access health services in a primary care setting, the San Francisco AIDS Foundation is beginning to provide HCV treatment at its gay men's sexual health clinic and at one of its syringe access locations. Additionally, the SFDPH has begun treating people who are homeless through its Street Medicine team, and treating individuals incarcerated in the county jail through the SFDPH-run Jail Health Services. Funding the HCV treatment effort in the county jail is a unique challenge given the suspension of Medicaid and private

insurance benefits when people are incarcerated; there is a critical need for sustainable funding mechanisms for treatment in this highly impacted population.

Strategy: Seeking Innovative Partnerships with Insurers to Support Elimination

A unique partnership between *End Hep C SF* and the San Francisco Health Plan—the managed care plan for 87% of Medicaid enrollees in San Francisco—has helped facilitate many of these innovative approaches to HCV treatment. The San Francisco Health Plan participates regularly in *End Hep C SF*'s Treatment Access workgroup meetings and provides data about monthly HCV treatment uptake among Plan members. These data help the workgroup to monitor trends (ie, treatment compliance and completion rates, retreatment rates, prescriber trends) and strategize about ways to improve treatment uptake. The plan's workgroup participation has also offered clinicians the opportunity to understand the plan's process for determining preferred DAA regimens, alleviating clinicians' frustrations during the prior authorization process and motivating them to use preferred regimens when appropriate. The workgroup meetings have provided a forum for clinicians to give input into the plan formulary decisions, share the testing or treatment challenges with each medication, and work collaboratively to address barriers to effective care. For example, clinician feedback on treatment challenges introduced by a remote specialty pharmacy facilitated quality improvement efforts to simplify the ordering, refill, and delivery processes. The plan has been able to advocate effectively for funding support from the state with this detailed provider input. Additionally, the plan has provided technical assistance to clinics regarding prior authorizations and use of specialty pharmacies, and has provided financial support for innovative efforts, such as HealthRIGHT360's project to initiate HCV treatment in residential drug treatment facilities.

Future Directions

Data gaps

We still do not have comprehensive data on the number of individuals successfully treated for HCV in San Francisco. Instead, we have relied on available survey and surveillance data, modeling, and shared data on treatment from health systems. The Research and Surveillance workgroup continues to build on their initial prevalence estimation work, gathering data to create a cascade of HCV care in San Francisco. This will provide a better picture of HCV diagnosis, confirmation, and treatment rates. It will also inform forecast modeling, to determine the optimal combination of HCV treatment and prevention interventions within subpopulations to shorten HCV elimination timelines and improve cost feasibility.

Building capacity for hepatitis C virus interventions

The Prevention and Education workgroup is planning to use a widely distributed survey to measure the capacity of San Francisco organizations to integrate HCV interventions into their work, so targeted capacity-building efforts can begin. This group also plans to expand on the "New Treatments Have Changed the Game" campaign by creating a video featuring the stories of clients who have been cured of HCV. The Testing and Linkage workgroup continually works on scaling up HCV testing, and aims to develop peer-based HCV linkage services.

Expanding hepatitis C virus treatment access

The Treatment Access workgroup plans to continue to expand HCV treatment in nontraditional settings and seek funding to support HCV-dedicated nursing, as well as creating an academic detailing program. Academic detailing is an outreach education technique that helps clinicians provide evidence-based care to their patients through 1-on-1 conversations.[14] We plan to use academic detailing to improve screening and linkage to care in primary care settings, particularly in private health care settings outside the SFDPH. We are in the process of developing detailing materials and plan to begin the academic detailing program in 2018. Further, we plan to build on the success of the staff-based navigator program by building a cadre of peer navigators, training those with lived HCV treatment experience to support those living in their communities to be tested, linked to care, and treated for HCV.

Through our collective efforts to treat people living with HCV in both primary care and community-based settings, it has become evident that dedicated resources for HCV care and treatment are vital to their success. For example, SFDPH's efforts to treat people in the homeless shelter system were successful, with 6 people treated over 6 months of the program; however, the shelter treatment program has been paused because the provision of HCV treatment in this setting pulled limited nursing resources from the acute care services nursing staff must provide in the shelters. *End Hep C SF* will be working on strategies to overcome this barrier, which will likely include advocating for funds to support dedicated nursing staff.

Taken together, these planned initiatives will significantly scale up testing and treatment in San Francisco and move the needle closer to HCV elimination. *End Hep C SF* remains committed to broad representation of community members, service providers, and organizations disproportionately impacted by HCV, and to continually refining strategies through formal evaluation to maximize efficiency and effectiveness.

COALITION TO ELIMINATE HEPATITIS C VIRUS IN MASSACHUSETTS

The Massachusetts End Hep C-MA coalition grew out of a long-standing organization called the Massachusetts Viral Hepatitis Coalition. With the recognition that challenges facing people living with HCV infection and strategies for elimination were quite different from those needed to control or eliminate hepatitis B virus infection, it was decided to reorganize and create an organization that explicitly focused on the mission of HCV elimination. End Hep C MA was adopted from the San Francisco coalition's name, *End Hep C SF*. Activities described herein included work from both groups (termed the MA Coalition).

The MA Coalition has a similar structure to the New York State and San Francisco initiatives. It consists of a large coalition including health advocates from the fields of health access and health disparities, substance use services, housing, mental health, legal advocacy, poverty programs, health professionals including hepatitis C treaters from academic and community health centers, and people living with HCV. Members of the Massachusetts Department of Public Health provide information and advice but do not vote on decisions. Industry partners participate in open forums but do not vote on decisions. Subcommittees are where the bulk of the work is done, and include (1) awareness, engagement, and empowerment, (2) screening, services and case management, (3) insurance access, (4) corrections, and (5) harm reduction and prevention. The steering committee ensures that subcommittee work is on track, endorses other organizations' work, and provides input into state and national policies.

The MA Coalition is primarily an advocacy group that works to increase awareness about barriers to HCV care and treatment and identify and execute on strategies to reduce those barriers. Work done to remove restrictions on reimbursement of HCV treatment by Massachusetts Medicaid, which had national implications, and addressing the increased rate of HCV cases in younger people in Massachusetts is described.

Removing Insurance Restrictions

When the first all-oral DAA regimens were approved in 2013, there were wide variations in restrictions on access to these treatments by the various public and private insurance plans in Massachusetts. The fee-for-service (FFS) program of the Massachusetts Medicaid program, called MassHealth, approved coverage for the (at that time) off-label combination of sofosbuvir plus simeprevir for genotype 1 infection, or sofosbuvir plus ribavirin for other genotypes, without any patient restrictions. Prescribers had to seek prior authorization to ensure the appropriate selection of treatment based on patient characteristics. MassHealth collected data on which patients were receiving treatment and health outcomes including completion of treatment and sustained viral response rates. Despite the lack of restrictions, in the first year after DAAs were approved, less than 15% of eligible patients in FFS Medicaid had been treated.

In contrast, all 6 of the Medicaid managed care organizations (MCOs) in Massachusetts, which covered more than one-half of MassHealth recipients, had policies that restricted treatment to patients with advanced liver fibrosis (F3 to F4 stage liver disease), who had at least 6 months sobriety from substance use, and were receiving care or consultation from a specialist. The MA Coalition, led by members of the Center for Health Law and Policy Innovation of Harvard Law School, determined that the treatment restrictions being imposed by MCOs were contrary to Medicaid law.

Regulations set forth by the Centers for Medicare and Medicaid Services seek to ensure that Medicaid beneficiaries served by MCOs receive a comparable level of benefits and services as beneficiaries participating in the FFS system. These regulations state that MCOs must offer services "in an amount, duration, and scope that is no less than the amount, duration, and scope for the same services furnished to beneficiaries under FFS Medicaid."[15] Owing to the treatment restrictions being imposed by MassHealth MCOs where the FFS program offered open access, MCOs were not meeting their obligations under the law to provide the same level of coverage.

Acting on this knowledge, the MA Coalition pressured MassHealth officials to eliminate this treatment access disparity within MassHealth. This effort was bolstered when the Centers for Medicare and Medicaid Services, because of persistent efforts of advocates nationwide, released guidance to state Medicaid programs that explicitly called out these practices as inconsistent with the law.[16] Despite multiple meetings with MassHealth officials, MassHealth officials continued to identify contractual and financial barriers to implementing this change. The MA Coalition wrote to Massachusetts Attorney General Maura Healey outlining these concerns and threatening legal action to hold the Commonwealth accountable should the situation remain unchanged.

This effort did not prove directly successful, although it did serve to bring more attention to the issue, brought drug manufacturers to the discussion, and ultimately was a stepping stone for the MA Coalition's success. In January 2016, Attorney General Healey wrote to the leading manufacturer of HCV medications at the time, Gilead Sciences, warning the company that it could face legal action unless it acted to lower the price of its treatments. This threat received Gilead's attention, and they requested a meeting with Healey's office to discuss the issue. However, no action was taken by MassHealth. The MA Coalition continued to press MassHealth officials to solve the disparate treatment access issues between the FFS and MCO programs. This continued pressure, in combination with the public attention drawn to the problem as a result of Attorney General Healey's action, culminated in MassHealth finally taking action to hold its MCOs accountable. In July 2016, Daniel Tsai, Assistant Secretary for MassHealth, issued a bulletin to all MCOs providing services to MassHealth beneficiaries. The bulletin directed MCOs to cover HCV medications for all MassHealth members with no restrictions related to fibrosis score, substance use abstinence, or prescriber specialty, effective August 1, 2016.[17] As a result, all restrictions were lifted by all MCOs and MassHealth beneficiaries now enjoy the same open access policy, regardless of if they are enrolled in the FFS program or receive their services from an MCO. Commercial insurance plans operating in Massachusetts followed the lead of MassHealth and most plans have lifted restrictions on reimbursing DAAs, although there are formulary restrictions. The MA Coalition is working to ensure that all restrictions are removed for all plans.

Identifying Previously Undiagnosed Patients with Hepatitis C Virus Infection

The MA Coalition had supported legislation requiring that primary care centers offer HCV antibody testing to all patients born from 1945 through 1965, although there were no penalties attached to noncompliance with the law, nor additional funds to survey for compliance with the law. An informal survey conducted in the spring of 2017 showed that several major health systems still had no programs in place to facilitate testing of this birth cohort. Most of the health systems that did have programs in place relied on electronic medical record prompts. However, recent data in Massachusetts also demonstrate that nearly two-thirds of new cases of hepatitis C are in people born after 1965.[18] Cases of hepatitis C in this younger cohort are likely being driven by the youth opioid epidemic. The MA Coalition is now advocating that all adults age 18 and older in Massachusetts be offered an HCV test as a statewide pilot program.

SUMMARY

These 3 examples of US state and local HCV elimination initiatives have common elements. All have diverse coalitions composed of community-based organizations, academic and community health centers, and public health officials. In each model, relationships with public health officials are handled similarly; the public health officials provide data and assistance, but are also the recipients of policy initiatives. Each has created working groups to define and execute on coalition goals. There are also common challenges, including ensuring that the many diverse groups of people impacted by HCV are fairly represented in the coalition. A lack of funding for HCV-specific programs and insufficient access to HCV medications are both a challenge and a focus of advocacy for all 3 coalitions.

We are proposing that each state create an End Hep C *XX* coalition to facilitate joint advocacy on national level initiatives and Federal policy. An annual day of educating congress and other government agencies on the personal and economic impact of HCV could be tied to state-level efforts. Our nation has all the tools needed to eliminate HCV and now requires the focus and funding to make this a reality.

ACKNOWLEDGMENTS

The authors thank all members of the HCV elimination coalitions in New York, San Francisco, and Massachusetts for the work they do to make eliminating HCV a reality.

REFERENCES

1. National Academies of Sciences, Engineering, and Medicine. A national strategy for the elimination of hepatitis B and C: phase two report. Washington, DC: The National Academies Press; 2017.

2. The U.S. National Viral Hepatitis Action Plan for 2017-2020. Office of HIV/AIDS and Infectious disease policy of the U.S. Department of Health and Human Services. 2017. Available at: https://www.hhs.gov/sites/default/files/National%20Viral%20Hepatitis%20Action%20Plan%202017-2020.pdf. Accessed November 17, 2017.

3. New York State HIV Epidemiological Profile September 2016. Available at: https://www.health.ny.gov/diseases/aids/general/statistics/epi/docs/epi_profile2016.pdf. Accessed February 15, 2018.

4. New York State Department of Health. The changing face of the hepatitis C epidemic New York State (Excluding NYC) - new HCV case reports increased for young IDUs & females. Presentation. 2017. Available at: http://www.natap.org/2016/HCV/101216_01.htm. Accessed February 15, 2018.

5. New York State Department of Health. 2015 Blueprint for achieving the goal set forth by Governor Cuomo to end the epidemic in New York State by the end of 2020. Availbale at: https://www.health.ny.gov/diseases/aids/ending_the_epidemic/docs/blueprint.pdf. Accessed March 30, 2015.

6. Facente SN, Grebe E, Burk K, et al. Estimated hepatitis C prevalence and key population sizes in San Francisco: a foundation for elimination, in press.

7. End Hep C SF. Hepatitis C in San Francisco. San Francisco, CA. 2017. Available at: https://tinyurl.com/SF-HCVprevalence2017. Accessed August 1, 2017.

8. U.S. Cancer Statistics Working Group. United States cancer statistics: 1999-2014 incidence and mortality web-based report. Atlanta (GA): U.S. Department of Health and Human Services, Centers for Disease Control and Prevention and National Cancer Institute; 2017. Available at: http://www.cdc.gov/uscs.

9. Campbell CA, Canary L, Smith N, et al. State HCV incidence and policies related to HCV preventive and treatment services for persons who inject drugs — United States, 2015–2016. MMWR Morb Mortal Wkly Rep 2017;66:465–9.

10. UNAIDS. Countdown to zero: global plan for the elimination of new HIV infections among children by 2015 and keeping their mothers alive, 2011–2015. Geneva (Switzerland): UNAIDS; 2011. Available at: http://www.unaids.org/sites/default/files/sub_landing/files/JC2034_UNAIDS_Strategy_en.pdf.

11. Kania J, Kramer M. Collective impact: creating large-scale social change. Stanford social innovation review; 2011. Available at: http://www.fsg.org/sites/default/files/tools-and-resources/Collective_Impact_Webinar_presentation.pdf. Accessed August 10, 2017.

12. End Hep C SF. End Hep C SF strategic plan, 2017-2019. San Francisco, CA. 2017. Available at: https://tinyurl.com/EndHepCSFstrategicplan. Accessed August 10, 2017.

13. Kattakuzhy S, Gross C, Emmanuel B, et al. Expansion of treatment for Hepatitis C virus infection by task shifting to community-based nonspecialist providers: a nonrandomized clinical trial. Ann Intern Med 2017;167(5):311–8.

14. National Resource Center for Academic Detailing (NaRCAD). Introductory guide to academic detailing; 2017. Available at: https://www.narcad.org/uploads/5/7/9/5/57955981/introductory_guide_to_ad.pdf. Accessed August 15, 2017.

15. Code of Federal Regulations. 42 C.F.R. § 438.210: Coverage and authorization of services. 2002. Available at: https://www.gpo.gov/. Accessed September 20, 2017.
16. Assuring Medicaid beneficiaries access to hepatitis C (HCV) drugs. CMS Medicaid drug rebate program notice, release no. 172 (Nov. 5, 2015) Available at: https://www.medicaid.gov/medicaid-chip-program-information/by-topics/prescription-drugs/downloads/rx-releases/state-releases/state-rel-172.pdf. Accessed September 20, 2017.
17. MassHealth-Contracted Managed Care Organization (MCO) coverage of Hepatitis C virus (HCV) drugs and other drugs subject to MassHealth supplemental rebate agreements. MassHealth Managed Care Organization Bulletin 6, Daniel Tsai, Assistant Secretary for MassHealth. 2016. Available at: http://www.mass.gov/eohhs/docs/masshealth/bull-2016/mco-6.pdf. Accessed September 20, 2017.
18. Massachusetts Department of Public Health, Bureau of Infectious Disease and Laboratory Sciences. Hepatitis C virus infection surveillance report, 2007-2015; 2017. Available at: http://www.mass.gov/eohhs/gov/departments/dph/programs/id/. Accessed November 17, 2017.

New Treatments Have Changed the Game

Hepatitis C Treatment in Primary Care

Shelley N. Facente, MPH[a], Katie Burk, MPH[b], Kelly Eagen, MD[c,d,e],
Elise S. Mara, MPH[f], Aaron A. Smith, BS[b],
Colleen S. Lynch, MD, MPH[g,h],*

KEYWORDS

- Hepatitis C virus • HCV • Treatment • Primary care • Provider training
- Clinician training • Primary care provider

KEY POINTS

- Although direct-acting antiviral regimens have driven up demand for hepatitis C virus (HCV) treatment, only a fraction of HCV-infected individuals are offered treatment within specialty settings.
- In 2016 to 2017, the San Francisco Health Network (SFHN) worked to improve treatment access and better understand barriers still inhibiting SFHN primary care providers from prescribing HCV treatment.

Continued

Disclosure Statement: S.N. Facente has received consulting fees from Gilead Pharmaceuticals, Inc for projects other than those described in this article. The other authors have nothing to disclose.
[a] Facente Consulting, 5601 Van Fleet Avenue, Richmond, CA 94804, USA; [b] Community Health Equity and Promotion Branch, San Francisco Department of Public Health, 25 Van Ness Suite 500, San Francisco, CA 94102, USA; [c] San Francisco Department of Public Health, Medical Respite and Sobering Center, 101 Grove Street, Room 118, San Francisco, CA 94102, USA; [d] Tom Waddell Integrated Medical Services, San Francisco Health Network, San Francisco Department of Public Health, 101 Grove Street, Room 118, San Francisco, CA 94102, USA; [e] Department of Family and Community Medicine, University of California, San Francisco (UCSF), Zuckerberg, San Francisco General Hospital, 1001 Potrero Avenue, San Francisco, CA 94110, USA; [f] ARCHES Branch, San Francisco Department of Public Health, 25 Van Ness Avenue, Suite 500, San Francisco, CA 94102, USA; [g] Clinical Practice, Southeast Health Center, San Francisco Health Network, San Francisco Department of Public Health, ZSFG Office at Ward 82 Room 246, 2401 Keith Street, San Francisco, CA 94124, USA; [h] University of California, San Francisco (UCSF), Zuckerberg, San Francisco General Hospital, ZSFG Office at Ward 82 Room 246, 995 Potrero Ave San Francisco, CA 94110, USA
* Corresponding author. Clinical Practice, Southeast Health Center, San Francisco Health Network, San Francisco Department of Public Health, University of California, San Francisco (UCSF), ZSFG Office at Ward 82 Room 246, 2401 Keith Street, San Francisco, CA 94124.
E-mail addresses: colleen.lynch@sfdph.org; colleen.lynch@uscf.edu

Infect Dis Clin N Am 32 (2018) 313–322
https://doi.org/10.1016/j.idc.2018.02.012
0891-5520/18/© 2018 The Authors. Published by Elsevier Inc. This is an open access article under the CC BY-NC-ND license (http://creativecommons.org/licenses/by-nc-nd/4.0/).

Continued

- Through SFHN's HCV treatment expansion intervention, primary care providers were offered a 4-hour overview training about HCV treatment, an electronic referral system, and a team of HCV champions providing technical assistance within each clinic.
- Among SVHN patients tested for HCV over 3 years, 13.0% were found chronically infected; 578 patients were treated (19.9%), with no statistically significant differences between age, gender, or race/ethnicity of those treated and untreated.
- With minimal financial and time commitments, the SFHN primary care–based HCV treatment initiative resulted in a 3-fold increase in the number of patients treated for HCV in primary care.

INTRODUCTION

San Francisco residents are profoundly impacted by the hepatitis C virus (HCV), with approximately 2.5% of the general population seropositive for HCV as of 2015[1] compared with a national seroprevalence estimate of 1.4% (95% CI, 0.9%–2.0%).[2] HCV is a significant driver of morbidity, liver cancer, and death[3] and disproportionately has an impact on marginalized populations, including people of color, homeless individuals, people with a history of incarceration, and people who inject drugs.[4–8] The availability of highly effective oral HCV treatment with few side effects, known as direct-acting antivirals (DAAs), makes HCV cure possible in nearly all infected patients.[8]

In the pre-DAA era, HCV treatments were complex and largely managed by hepatologists, gastroenterologists, and infectious disease physicians. As tolerable and highly effective DAA regimens have driven up demand for treatment, the relative scarcity of these specialists to the large number of infected individuals has created a bottleneck effect, resulting in only a fraction of HCV-infected individuals offered treatment in any given year.[9] Even with reasonable capacity in the specialty setting, travel to specialty clinics or even the idea of attending appointments in unfamiliar settings with unfamiliar providers can be a barrier for marginalized populations disproportionately impacted by HCV.[10] As treatment courses in the DAA era have become shorter, simplified, and remarkably well tolerated, recent studies have demonstrated the efficacy of treating HCV in high-prevalence primary care settings.[11,12]

The San Francisco Health Network (SFHN) is San Francisco's safety net system of care, and serves the majority of the low-income and homeless populations of San Francisco. The percentage of all active adult SFHN primary care patients who have been diagnosed with HCV is 5.5%. Part of the San Francisco Department of Public Health, the SFHN includes primary care in 10 community-based and 4 hospital-based clinics throughout the city. In 2016, in an effort to increase HCV treatment access for all patients, SFHN leadership committed to training its primary care providers to treat uncomplicated cases of HCV in the primary care setting using a team-based model of care.

In 2017, the primary care–based HCV treatment initiative team at SFHN undertook an analysis to measure the impact of these efforts to improve treatment access within the SFHN primary care system and to better understand barriers still inhibiting SFHN primary care providers from providing HCV treatment to their patients.

METHODS

Through SFHN's HCV treatment expansion intervention, primary care providers within the SFHN were invited to participate in a 4-hour overview training about

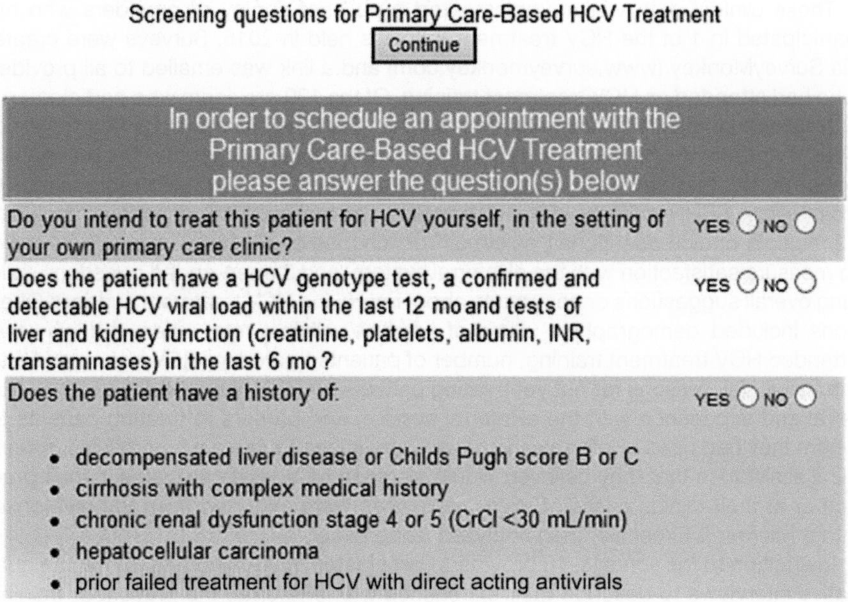

Screening questions for Primary Care-Based HCV Treatment

| Continue |

In order to schedule an appointment with the
Primary Care-Based HCV Treatment
please answer the question(s) below

Do you intend to treat this patient for HCV yourself, in the setting of your own primary care clinic?	YES ○ NO ○
Does the patient have a HCV genotype test, a confirmed and detectable HCV viral load within the last 12 mo and tests of liver and kidney function (creatinine, platelets, albumin, INR, transaminases) in the last 6 mo?	YES ○ NO ○
Does the patient have a history of:	YES ○ NO ○

- decompensated liver disease or Childs Pugh score B or C
- cirrhosis with complex medical history
- chronic renal dysfunction stage 4 or 5 (CrCl <30 mL/min)
- hepatocellular carcinoma
- prior failed treatment for HCV with direct acting antivirals

Fig. 1. Screenshot from the SFHN primary care–based HCV treatment eReferral system.

primary care–based HCV treatment and best practice models for team-based HCV care. A secure electronic referral system (eReferral) to support primary care–based HCV treatment was created to give providers individualized treatment consultations for their patients (**Fig. 1**). Finally, primary care clinics were supported by a team of HCV champions providing technical assistance to help design individualized treatment workflows within each clinic. The intervention was designed to be sustainable and scalable, requiring limited additional investment of resources. A grant from the California Department of Public Health supported 0.15 full-time equivalent of clinician and pharmacist time to staff the eReferral system and 0.4 full-time equivalent of an analyst to manage treatment data, and all other support for the initiative was provided in-kind from the SFHN (see **Fig. 1**).

For the authors' analysis, data from the SFHN's electronic medical record (EMR) from October 1, 2014, through December 31, 2017, were reviewed. Data were collected on patients with at least 1 primary care visit in the previous 2 years (n = 53,039), including age, gender, and race/ethnicity; the number of patients tested for HCV (n = 22,447); the number with positive HCV RNA results (ie, confirmed to be chronically infected) (n = 2910); and the number initiating DAA treatment (n = 578). Patients receiving treatment during and after the primary care–based HCV treatment intervention were compared with those who had yet to receive treatment. These EMR data were supplemented with data from the primary care–based HCV treatment eReferral metrics to determine the number of primary care patients treated preintervention versus postintervention and the number and quantity of prescriptions written by each provider. Data were analyzed using SAS software SAS version 9.4 (SAS Institute, Cary, North Carolina) Version 9.4 (SAS Institute, Cary, North Carolina) and STATA version 15.0 (StataCorp, College Station, Texas) for summary statistics and Pearson chi-square tests.

These clinical data were supplemented by a brief survey of providers who had participated in 1 of the HCV treatment trainings held in 2016. Surveys were created via SurveyMonkey (www.surveymonkey.com) and a link was emailed to all providers who had attended an HCV treatment training. Of the 120 providers who participated in 1 of these trainings, 111 were still employed by the SFHN and were asked to participate. Two reminder emails were sent during the 4-week period that the survey was open; during that time 39.6% (n = 44) completed the survey, with representatives from every SFHN primary care clinic. Surveys included 16 questions, including 12 multiple-choice questions ("select all" or "choose one"), two 5-point Likert scales to measure satisfaction with the eReferral system, and 2 open-ended questions soliciting overall suggestions or comments about improving HCV treatment support. Questions included demographics (clinic of practice, clinical role, when and why they attended HCV treatment training, number of patients treated for HCV before and after the training[s], reasons for not yet treating patients for HCV [if applicable], use of eReferral and experience with the eReferral system, and barriers to treating patients for whom they had used eReferral) and other suggestions for learning modalities or technical assistance that they believed would increase HCV treatment rates in their practice or at their clinics overall. Survey responses were exported from SurveyMonkey into a Microsoft Excel file, then analyzed using Excel.

In addition to the surveys, 15 providers participated in 20-minute to 60-minute qualitative interviews to describe their experience with eReferral, the prescriber training, and HCV treatment in primary care overall. Interviews were conducted via phone, using a 10-question, semistructured interview guide. Interviews were thematically analyzed with open coding to allow themes to emerge from the data.[13] Findings were merged into a final summary that was shared with HCV clinical champions for verification prior to dissemination.

RESULTS
Treatment and Prescribing Data

Analysis of SFHN data demonstrates that of the total 22,447 adults tested for HCV between October 1, 2014, and December 31, 2017, 2910 were found chronically HCV infected (13.0%). During the period of the analysis, 578 patients were treated (19.9%). Importantly, there were no statistically significant differences overall between the age, gender, or racial/ethnic demographics of those who had been treated by the SFHN (n = 578) and those who were chronically HCV infected but not yet been treated (n = 2332) (Table 1).

The number of patients treated in primary care tripled from the period during which DAAs were available but HCV primary care treatment trainings had not been conducted (10/1/2014–1/31/2016), referred to as the "pre-intervention period," compared with the 23 month "post-intervention period" (2/1/2016–12/31/2017), with 143 patients treated preintervention (8.9 patients per month) compared with 435 treated postintervention (18.9 patients per month). The number of SFHN clinics providing primary care–based treatment also increased from 5 preintervention to 12 postintervention. These data indicate substantial increases in HCV treatment access in the SFHN primary care setting (Table 2).

Use of Capacity-Building Services in Relation to Prescribing Practices

From March 1, 2016, through November 30, 2017, 280 prescriptions for HCV treatment were written by 68 providers trained during 1 of the HCV treatment trainings. This was an average of 4.1 prescriptions per trained provider; however, when

Table 1
Demographics of all active San Francisco Health Network patients tested for HCV from October 1, 2014, to December 31, 2017, by HCV status and treatment status as of December 31, 2017[e]

	Tested[a] for Hepatitis C Virus	Infected[b] with Hepatitis C Virus	Untreated[c] for Hepatitis C Virus		Treated for Hepatitis C Virus		Odds of Being Treated if Hepatitis C Virus Infected
			No.	%	No.	%	
Total	22,447	2910	2332	80.1	578	19.9	—
Male[d]	12,702	2065	1637	79.3	428	20.7	1.2 (P = .07)
Female	9745	845	695	82.2	150	17.8	ref[f]
Baby boomer (born 1945–1965)	10,188	2031	1615	79.5	416	20.5	1.1 (P = .20)
Not baby boomer	12,259	879	717	81.6	162	18.4	ref[f]
Asian	4977	153	131	85.6	22	14.4	.65 (P = .07)
Black/African American	4040	1005	811	80.7	194	19.3	.92 (P = .45)
American Indian/Alaskan Native	200	58	43	74.1	15	25.9	1.3 (P = .34)
Native Hawaiian/Pacific Islander	223	13	8	61.5	5	38.5	2.4 (P = .12)
Hispanic	6116	379	299	78.9	80	21.1	1.02 (P = .84)
White	5041	1081	858	79.4	223	20.6	ref[f]
Unknown/missing	1850	221	182	82.4	39	17.6	.82 (P = .31)

[a] "Tested" denotes having record of an HCV antibody, genotype, and/or viral load test between October 1, 2014, and December 31, 2017.
[b] "Infected" specifies adult individuals with an active clinical record (ie, seen in the last 2 years of pull date, 1/25/2018), an SFHN clinic as a primary care clinic, and evidence of HCV infection (a positive antibody test, detectable viral load, HCV genotype, and/or documented HCV treatment initiation) between October 1, 2014, and December 31, 2017.
[c] "Untreated" is defined as having HCV infection, as defined previously, but with no HCV treatment initiation documented in the EMR.
[d] Nonbinary gender (ie, transgender) is not routinely captured in the SFHN EMR so is not reported here.
[e] No statistically significant differences were found between the proportion of patients treated or untreated for their HCV by gender, age, or ethnicity.
[f] ref, denotes to the reference in an odds ratio table.

Table 2
San Francisco Health Network primary care hepatitis C virus treatment numbers preintervention (10/1/2014–1/31/2016) and postintervention (2/1/2016–12/31/2017)

	Preintervention (16 mo)		Postintervention (23 mo)		
	Total No.	No./mo	Total No.	No./mo	Increase (%)
Total patients treated[a]	143	8.9	435	18.9	112
Total clinics represented among treated	5	N/A	12	N/A	140

[a] Five treated cases had no listed primary care provider.

excluding 3 "superprescribers" who fell more than 2 SDs from the mean, the total number of prescriptions dropped to 168, with an average of 2.6 per provider.

From February 1, 2016, through December 31, 2017, 63 providers used the eReferral system for a total of 261 individual patient cases (an average of 4.14 patient cases per provider). At the same time, 63 prescriptions were written by providers using eReferral, and another 330 prescriptions were written by providers who did not use eReferral (although 112, or 34%, of those were written by the 3 superprescribers [discussed previously]). See **Table 3** for more details on the use of eReferral for HCV prescriptions in the SFHN.

Provider Survey Data

Survey and interview results provided additional insight into the effectiveness of the multimodal capacity-building intervention. Almost 2 of 3 survey respondents (28/44) were primary care providers licensed to prescribe HCV treatment directly. The remaining respondents were registered nurses (18%), pharmacists (4%), in an administrative roles (eg, program manager or nurse manager), 1 medical evaluation assistant, and 1 urgent care provider.

Of the respondents who were prescribing providers and participated in 1 of the 2 HCV treatment trainings (n = 31), more than 85% had never treated a patient for HCV prior to the training session. At the time of the survey (6–16 months post-training, depending on which training they had attended), that number dropped below 50%, with 15 of the 27 people who said they had treated no patients before the training reporting treating at least 1 patient post-training. The distribution of the number of patients treated pretraining and post-training is seen in **Fig. 2**.

For those clinicians who said they still had not treated any patients for HCV post-training (n = 20), 8 reported having no patients in need of HCV treatment (eg, patients

Table 3
San Francisco Health Network hepatitis C virus treatment data with and without eReferral (2/1/2016–12/31/2017)

	N
Number of eReferrals made[a]	261
Number of eReferrals that started treatment	105
Number of treatment starts with no eReferral on record	330
Number of providers using eReferral system	63
Number of unique providers with at least 1 treatment start	37

[a] Four patients were referred twice during the period.

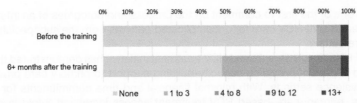

Fig. 2. Provider self-report of the number of patients treated for HCV before the treatment trainings versus at the time the provider survey was sent out. Depending on the date of the treatment training the provider completed, the post-training time interval ranged from 6 months to 16 months.

with HCV were already being treated in another setting) or being unable to prescribe (eg, none of their patients had HCV or their patients' HCV was being treated in another setting). Of the remaining 12, 8 said they did not have any patients they thought could adhere to treatment, and/or their patients had too many competing priorities to allow for HCV treatment at the current time. The other 4 said they did not know how to navigate the prior authorization process to obtain medications (2 people), did not feel comfortable prescribing treatments to their patients yet (3 people), or they knew how to do it but there was no one at the clinic to assist and they believed they could not do it themselves (2 people).

Interview feedback regarding the technical assistance component for clinics was generally positive, although some respondents acknowledged it was not sufficient in and of itself, thereby validating the importance of the multimodal intervention design. Although technical assistance was beneficial for clinic workflow and reminders to use the eReferral system, the most successful clinics were those with at least 1 clinician HCV champion in-house. "Having dedicated people who are helping with this topic makes it easier," a provider explained. "They can be the expert…we have providers who are experts on HIV medicine, or experts on trans medicine, and that makes it easier for me to help with prescribing those things." Numerous providers noted that sometimes inexperienced providers needed more than education to begin treating; consistent support was needed until they could "build muscle memory." More information about the types of additional clinic-specific support providers requested is in **Fig. 3**.

DISCUSSION

The tolerability and efficacy of HCV DAAs present an opportunity for care systems to provide curative treatment of patients living with HCV in new and innovative ways. This

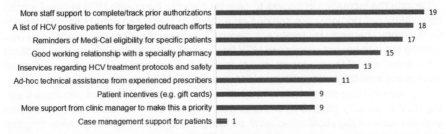

Fig. 3. Provider survey responses (n = 44) to a multiple choice ("select all") question about what more could be offered at their clinic to increase the number of patients treated for HCV.

article is one of the first to comment on the process and outcomes of an intervention that aimed to shift HCV care for uncomplicated patients from the subspecialty to primary care setting.

The SFHN primary care–based HCV treatment initiative has demonstrated the feasibility and impact of providing capacity-building support to primary care providers in high-prevalence settings. With minimal financial and time commitments for training providers, primary care–based HCV treatment access increased 3-fold in a period of just over 3 years as a result of this initiative. Providers within the authors' system showed rapid learning and deployment of the skills of HCV treatment.

A strength of the authors' eReferral model is that the primary skill required of providers to treat HCV is the ability to assess treatment readiness. The central eReferral team provides case consultation, including treatment recommendations. As a result, trainings do not require providers to become individually competent to understand the nuances of regimen selection or follow ongoing changes in DAA options. By shifting the responsibility of regimen selection to the eReferral consultation team, providers more readily become able to treat HCV in the primary care setting. The authors suspect that the providers who began treating HCV during this period were a group already interested in and motivated to offer HCV treatment within their practices; the additional supports offered through the treatment initiative merely provided a catalyst for action. The results of the provider survey reveal that even after the trainings, providers felt supported by both the eReferral system and other colleagues in their own clinics with a breadth of experience in treating HCV.

One of the treatment initiative's major goals was to ensure that treatment access was equitable across population groups. The authors' data show that primary care providers are treating a representative population of those infected with HCV within the SFHN; the demographics of patients treated for HCV in primary care were statistically similar to those HCV-infected patients who had not yet been treated. The authors are currently undertaking a formal analysis of patients who have been treated for HCV in primary care to ensure effective and high-quality treatment through this initiative and to ensure that patients marginalized by social factors not explored in this article are able to obtain HCV treatment in primary care.

The authors' analysis is limited by a fairly small sample size from the provider survey; it is also true that providers may have been more likely to respond to the survey invitation if they were enthusiastic about HCV treatment or about the training intervention. Primary care providers, however, indicated a willingness to take on the task of HCV treatment with the support of experienced providers and clinic teams. Taken together, introductory trainings, eReferral, and clinic technical assistance provided a variety of options to support prescriber knowledge and confidence. Providers reported appreciation of the support provided.

Despite the increases in access to care for patients living with HCV in San Francisco's safety net primary care settings as a result of these capacity-building interventions, many barriers to treatment persist for patients. Providers who received training but had not yet prescribed HCV treatment highlighted concerns about patient adherence, lack of team support, and burdensome treatment authorization processes as reasons why they were still unable to initiate HCV treatment.

The authors have several plans to continue to scale up numbers of providers treating HCV in primary care. One of the largest ongoing barriers identified by providers was the lack of logistical clinic level support; the authors plan to provide ongoing training to nursing and clinical pharmacy staff to assist with the necessary tasks associated with HCV treatment (ie, procuring medication, supporting adherence, and monitoring laboratory test results). The impact of having a trained nursing or pharmacy staff member is that that 1 of these team members can support multiple clinical providers, thereby increasing the number of providers treating and total number of patients treated. The authors also aim to organize more provider trainings for providers who missed the first trainings or have subsequently joined the network. These trainings will highlight community-based patient navigation programs that can support more challenging patients through treatment. The authors will continue to offer individualized support through eReferral. Resident teaching is a final piece of the efforts to scale up overall numbers of providers treating in primary care.

PUBLIC HEALTH IMPLICATIONS

Many of the patients treated in SFHN primary care settings were unlikely to have been successfully treated in specialty clinics. As an example, in 1 study in Zuckerberg San Francisco General Hospital's liver specialty clinic, 42% of patients living with HCV were determined by providers to be treatment ineligible, with substance use and housing instability a major reason for provider-determined treatment ineligibility among African American patients. For those determined appropriate for treatment, approximately 1 of every 3 patients were lost to follow-up before treatment was completed.[14]

Although the data related to primary care–based treatment are encouraging, an even broader spectrum of patients likely could be treated with the offer of additional support within the primary care setting, such as patient navigators, social workers, and nurses or pharmacists onsite to support directly observed therapy for HCV medications. Large-scale improvements in HCV treatment rates for patients in primary care settings could substantially contribute to local,[7] regional,[15] and national efforts[16] to eliminate HCV as a public health threat.

REFERENCES

1. Facente SN, Grebe E, Burk K, et al. Estimated hepatitis C prevalence and key population sizes in San Francisco: a foundation for elimination. PLOS ONE, in press.
2. National Center for Health Statistics CfDCaPC. National Health and Nutrition Examination Survey Data (NHANES) 2011-2012. Hyattsville (MD): Services USDoHaH, trans; 2012.
3. Ly KN, Hughes EM, Jiles RB, et al. Rising mortality associated with Hepatitis C virus in the United States, 2003-2013. Clin Infect Dis 2016;62(10):1287–8.
4. Centers for Disease Control and Prevention. Surveillance for viral hepatitis - United States, 2014. Viral hepatitis - statistics & surveillance 2016. Available at: http://www.cdc.gov/hepatitis/statistics/2014surveillance/commentary.htm. Accessed February 22, 2018.
5. Rodrigo C, Eltahla AA, Bull RA, et al. Historical trends in the Hepatitis C virus epidemics in North America and Australia. J Infect Dis 2016;214(9):1383–9.
6. Rustgi VK. The epidemiology of hepatitis C infection in the United States. J Gastroenterol 2007;42(7):513–21.
7. End Hep C SF. End Hep C SF strategic plan, 2017-2019. San Francisco (CA). 2017.
8. Burstow NJ, Mohamed Z, Gomaa AI, et al. Hepatitis C treatment: where are we now? Int J Gen Med 2017;10:39–52.
9. McGowan CE, Fried MW. Barriers to hepatitis C treatment. Liver Int 2012; 32(Suppl 1):151–6.

10. Bruggmann P, Litwin AH. Models of care for the management of hepatitis C virus among people who inject drugs: one size does not fit all. Clin Infect Dis 2013; 57(Suppl 2):S56–61.

11. Kattakuzhy S, Gross C, Emmanuel B, et al. Expansion of treatment for Hepatitis C virus infection by task shifting to community-based nonspecialist providers: a nonrandomized clinical trial. Ann Intern Med 2017;167(5):311–8.

12. Norton BL, Fleming J, Bachhuber MA, et al. High HCV cure rates for people who use drugs treated with direct acting antiviral therapy at an urban primary care clinic. Int J Drug Pol 2017;47:196–201.

13. Strauss A, Corbin J. Basics of qualitative research: grounded theory procedures and techniques. Newbury Park (CA): Sage; 1990.

14. Schaeffer S, Khalili M. Reasons for HCV non-treatment in underserved African Americans: Implications for treatment with new therapeutics. Ann Hepatol 2015;14(2):234–42.

15. New York State Hepatitis C elimination campaign. End Hep C NY. 2017. Available at: https://www.endhepcny.org/. Accessed February 22, 2018.

16. Buckley GL, Strom BL, editors. A national strategy for the elimination of Hepatitis B and C. Washington, DC: The National Academicies of Sciences, Engineering, and Medicine; 2017.

Five Questions Concerning Managing Hepatitis C in the Justice System

Finding Practical Solutions for Hepatitis C Virus Elimination

Anne C. Spaulding, MD, MPH[a,b,]*, Madeline G. Adee, cMPH[a],
Robert T. Lawrence, MD, MEd[c], Jagpreet Chhatwal, PhD[d],
William von Oehsen, JD[e]

KEYWORDS

• HCV elimination • Prison • Jail • Incarceration • Hepatitis C • Medicaid

KEY POINTS

- Most hepatitis C virus (HCV) in the United States is transmitted by injection drug use and most Americans who inject drugs are incarcerated at some point.
- HCV is concentrated in corrections; framework of population health compared with a focus on the individual may be necessary to address the epidemic.
- Surveillance data on HCV in correctional facilities is inconsistent and there are barriers to screening, but opt-out testing can work.
- Current direct-acting antiviral prices are prohibitively high for prison health care budgets; very few incarcerated persons receive treatment.
- There are options available for prison systems to overcome the gap between demand for and availability of treatment.

Disclosure/Potential Conflicts of Interest: Dr A. Spaulding has received funding through her institution from Gilead Sciences. She has consulted for Ogilvy CommonHealth, which received a grant from Gilead Sciences. Dr J. Chhatwal has received funding through his institution from Gilead Sciences and Merck. He has consulted for Gilead Sciences and Merck. External funding: NSF grants numbers 1722906 (A. Spaulding) and 1722665 (J. Chhatwal). All other authors have nothing to disclose (M. Adee, R. Lawrence, W. von Oehsen).
[a] Department of Epidemiology, Rollins School of Public Health, Emory University, 1518 Clifton Road Room 3033, Atlanta, GA 30322, USA; [b] Department of Medicine, Morehouse School of Medicine, 720 Westview Dr SW, Atlanta, GA 30310, USA; [c] Alaska Department of Corrections, 550 West 7th Avenue, Suite 1860, Anchorage, AK 99501, USA; [d] Institute for Technology Assessment, Massachusetts General Hospital, Harvard University, 101 Merrimac Street, Floor 10, Boston, MA 02114, USA; [e] Powers Pyles Sutter & Verville PC, 1501 M Street Northwest, Seventh Floor, Washington, DC 20005-1700, USA
* Corresponding author. Department of Epidemiology, Rollins School of Public Health, Emory University, 1518 Clifton Road, Room 3033, Atlanta, GA 30322.
E-mail address: aspauld@emory.edu

Infect Dis Clin N Am 32 (2018) 323–345
https://doi.org/10.1016/j.idc.2018.02.014
0891-5520/18/© 2018 Elsevier Inc. All rights reserved.

id.theclinics.com

INTRODUCTION

Ignoring the portion of the United States' hepatitis C epidemic made up of persons with a history of incarceration leads to serious underestimations of hepatitis C virus (HCV) prevalence. At present in the United States, even among persons living in households, injection drug use is the most common route of infection with HCV.[1] As an illicit activity, parenteral drug use commonly results in incarceration; almost all people who inject drugs have a history of incarceration.[2,3] To eliminate HCV, the United States must engage the criminal justice system by increasing routine screening and making treatment with the new direct-acting antivirals (DAAs) against HCV accessible to persons who are imprisoned.[4]

The United States leads the world in the rate of incarceration.[5] In the United States, prisons house persons convicted of a crime and serving a sentence of a year or more. Jails detain persons awaiting trial or sentenced to shorter stays. The median length of a jail stay is 2 to 5 days.[6] Six states have unified jail/prison systems. All US correctional facilities have a high concentration of people who inject drugs (PWID) and thus a high prevalence of HCV. Recidivism is common in the US justice system and many persons, once incarcerated, tend to cycle in and out of facilities repeatedly[7] (**Fig. 1**). A 2014 article combined estimates of persons living with HCV who were homeless or institutionalized with those dwelling in households (NHANES [National Health and Nutrition Examination Survey] data). It estimated that 10 million Americans spent at least part of last year incarcerated and likely 30% of all Americans with hepatitis C pass through a prison or jail annually.[8] Among the 1.5 million Americans who are in prison at any given timepoint,[9] the authors estimate that 18%,[9] or 270,000, have antibodies to HCV. State prisons responding to a 2015 survey reported they are aware of about 106,000 (39%) persons so diagnosed.[10] Three-quarters of the 18% (13.5% or 1 in 7) are viremic[1] and thus candidates for HCV treatment once diagnosed.

Prisons, as opposed to jails, serve as particularly important sites to expand access to DAAs, because of the longer duration of sentences, which permits completion of a full course of treatment.[11] Directly observed medication administration helps ensure adherence. Those leaving prison typically have fewer connections to community health resources and so treatment while imprisoned is strategic. Rarely is a person in jail a candidate for starting DAAs, but jails occasionally initiate treatment of persons with advanced disease. Although prison can be a more strategic venue for treatment, few prisons aggressively seek to identify more persons to treat. Two-thirds of state prisons either offer no screening or only offer targeted testing of inmates reporting high-risk behavior, which significantly limits detection and potential treatment in this high-prevalence population.[8,12,13]

Beginning in 2012, more people died of HCV-related infections than of 60 other nationally notifiable infectious conditions, including human immunodeficiency virus (HIV), hepatitis B, and tuberculosis.[14] Nonetheless, hepatitis C has not generated the sense of urgency or diversion of funds associated with other infectious disease epidemics, perhaps because of its slow course, low prevalence in the general population, high cost of treatment, or spread outside the public's eye, primarily within groups that reside in the social shadows of poverty and drug use. As a result, a recent survey showed that the median proportion of people in state prisons with known HCV infection receiving treatment is only 0.49% (range, 0%–5.9%).[10] More and more prisons are being sued for denying treatment to those with hepatitis C, and at least 1 federal judge has declared that withholding medical treatment from a person incarcerated in a state prison constitutes cruel and unusual punishment.[15]

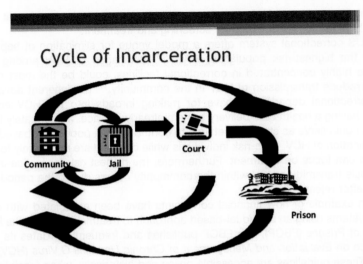

Fig. 1. Trajectories of persons caught in the criminal justice system. In the United States, after an alleged offense is committed, the individual may go to jail while awaiting trial. Those found guilty of a felony with a sentence greater than 1 year may be sent to prison. The arrows in this diagram illustrate the recurrent nature of confinement for those who have ever passed through a jail or prison; recidivism rates are high. (*Courtesy of* B. Zack, The Bridging Group, Oakland, CA; with permission.)

This article poses 5 questions to illustrate dilemmas faced by correctional and public health administrators in the screening and treatment of hepatitis C in correctional populations. It explores how some strategies for reducing medication costs can be pursued by individual states and some by federal policy change alone, and discusses how treating persons who are incarcerated will be essential to bring the hepatitis C epidemic under control.[4]

QUESTION 1: IS HEPATITIS C VIRUS IN CORRECTIONS MORE EFFECTIVELY ADDRESSED USING THE FRAMEWORK OF POPULATION HEALTH COMPARED WITH A FOCUS ON THE INDIVIDUAL?

A paradigm shift, from an individual to population focus, usually occurs in the evaluation and management of infectious disease when a pathogen becomes widespread. When a disease threatens to affect wide portions of a population, the will and resources to address the epidemic must come from the broader society, often governing agencies. Under a population health–based paradigm, health planners use mechanisms for detection, contact investigation, and treatment of a widespread disease with the end goal of eradicating the disease. In the United States, the evaluation and management of HCV is currently in the transition between an individual-based and population-based approach.

Under an individual-based health care model, curative DAAs reach individuals who have meaningful access to health care and adequate resources to cover the cost of medications. This approach lowers HCV-related mortalities for some. Reaching most infected individuals, rectifying the current uneven access to treatment in the United States, and arresting the spread of HCV requires a shift toward a population-based process of evaluation and treatment. Like HIV or infectious tuberculosis, treatment of HCV becomes prevention when communities target individuals at high risk for transmission for screening and treatment.

The US correctional system offers a model venue for elimination of hepatitis C among the highest-risk population, PWID.[16] Elimination of HCV among PWID, who are highly concentrated in correctional facilities, could be the most efficient way to reduce transmission of HCV in the community.[17] The inherent advantages that correctional departments have for making inroads into the HCV epidemic include having a health care delivery system already in place. If adequately funded, prisons could serve as strategic settings to contribute to a population-based model for elimination of HCV. High-risk individuals while confined are more likely to be sober and can focus on treatment. Furthermore, the highest risk for justice-involved individuals transmitting HCV within the community occurs during the period immediately after release.[18]

As an example of how financial constraints have been associated with correctional systems using an individual-based approach to treatment, there is the Federal Bureau of Prisons (FBOP). The FBOP publishes and frequently updates its clinical guidance on *Evaluation and Management of Chronic Hepatitis C Virus (HCV) Infection*.[19] These guidelines are accessible online and historically, when feasible, many states' prison systems have based their protocols on these guidelines. Whether following these guidelines will withstand legal and ethical scrutiny is being tested in federal courts. Access to treatment is not universal in the FBOP; patients with advanced stages of fibrosis are prioritized (**Box 1**). In 2015, this led to treating

---

Box 1
The Federal Bureau of Prisons aspartate transaminase to platelet ratio index method of prioritizing patients for treatment

- FBOP guidelines recommend universal anti-HCV antibody screening of all sentenced inmates, and for those who are anti-HCV positive, reflex HCV RNA viral load testing and reflex testing for HCV genotype.

- Certain comorbid medical conditions that are associated with HCV, or the necessity of immunosuppressant medication for a comorbid medical condition, may prioritize individuals for treatment.

- Treatment priority is usually based on degree of severity.[19] After diagnosis, the health providers look for signs of hepatic cirrhosis, with or without decompensation. Advanced disease prioritizes persons for treatment.

- As a predictor for advanced disease, an aspartate transaminase (AST) to platelet ratio index (APRI; [(AST/AST upper limit) $\times$ 100]/platelet count [10^9/L]) is calculated if no obvious cirrhosis is assessed. The APRI has been recommended as a screening tool where prevalence of HCV is high but resources for screening for fibrosis and cirrhosis are sparse.[24]

- Individuals with an increased APRI score are referred for liver imaging to confirm signs of cirrhosis or fibrosis, which, if present, qualify the patient for the highest priorities for treatment. For all patients with an APRI of 2.0 or greater, treatment is highest priority.

- If the APRI is greater than 1.0, fibrosis stage 2 or greater was found on a liver biopsy in the past, or certain comorbid conditions (eg, HIV, diabetes) are present, hepatitis treatment can still be prescribed, but priority is intermediate.

- The provider provides a pretreatment assessment. If priority criteria for treatment are met, a DAA can then be prescribed.

- Continuity of care for individuals who have already started DAAs before incarceration also creates a priority for treatment.

just 2.4% of infected persons.[20] Although the FBOP has recently relaxed its criteria of which stage of fibrosis will be prioritized for treatment, and lifestyle factors such as alcohol or illicit drug use are not categorically disqualifying, treatment of all incarcerated persons infected with HCV is far from available. A correctional health system usually examines the return on investment, both during the time frame of incarceration and over the lifetime of the individual, that an intervention will bring.[11] If HCV treatment costs decreased precipitously, the return on investing in DAAs for HCV would compare favorably with other health interventions in correctional medicine. Treatment of HCV would then decrease in line with the public health approach to other infectious disease epidemics.

Consider the population health–based approach taken by the US Department of Veterans' Affairs (VA). In 2016, supported by congressional funding and (an unpublished) negotiated reduction in pharmaceutical prices to approximately $15,000 (personal communication, Jules Levin, NATAP, 2018), the VA expanded treatment to all veterans with chronic HCV who do not have medical contraindications. The Veterans Health Administration follows screening guidelines endorsed by the US Centers for Disease Control and Prevention (CDC) and the US Preventive Services Task Force that recommend 1-time screening for all persons born between 1945 and 1965, and risk-factor screening for all those born outside this time frame.[21,22] The VA system follows joint treatment guidelines established by the American Association for the Study of Liver Diseases and the Infectious Disease Society of America (HCVguidelines.org). Treatment is no longer reserved for those with advanced liver disease or cirrhosis. Veterans with a chronic infection, even with no evidence of liver disease, qualify for treatment unless, ironically, the veteran happens to be incarcerated. Per VA policy, benefits for veterans infected with HCV are suspended when a veteran is in jail or prison under the assumption that the veteran's health care is covered by the corrections system.

Political will and, perhaps more important, favorable economics have allowed the VA to adopt population-based screening and treatment. Circumstances are not as favorable for correctional departments. Compounding the problems is the relative concentration of individuals infected with HCV within correctional institutions with rates more than 4-fold higher than the estimated 4% prevalence in the US veteran population[8,12,23] **(Table 1)**.

The responsibility for funding prison health care depends on the jurisdiction. The federal government funds the FBOP; they can acquire drugs at a steep discount off a federal supply schedule (see Appendix 1). State governments alone are responsible for underwriting all state prison health care. Federal funds, including Medicaid and

Table 1
Comparison of population dynamics in the Veterans' Affairs Health System and in correctional systems

	VA Health System	Prison/Jails
HCV seroprevalence (%)	4	18
Point prevalence: number of patients with HCV in 1 d	170,000	386,000
Period prevalence: number of individual patients with HCV over 1 y	170,000	~2 million

The Veterans' Affairs Health System does not continuously add or subtract its population. Most incarcerated persons pass through only jail, and jails turn over their populations repeatedly over the course of 1 year.

Medicare; private insurance; and pharmaceutical manufacturers' patient assistance programs do not cover state prison health care costs. The carve-out of correctional health care budgets from the rest of the US medical system poses the first challenge in treating persons in this sector of the epidemic.

QUESTION 2: WHAT ARE SOME ISSUES WITH TESTING FOR HEPATITIS C VIRUS IN PRISONS? DOES THE BENEFIT FOR POPULATION HEALTH OUTWEIGH THE INCREASING DEMAND FOR INDIVIDUAL HEALTH SERVICES?

Looking for Problems Whose Solutions Are Unfunded

The unaffordability of HCV treatment creates a disincentive for prisons to screen for HCV. Prisons have no legal mandate to screen for disease. However, once a disease such as hepatitis is diagnosed, deliberate indifference to health needs has been determined by the US Supreme Court to be a violation of the eighth amendment of the Constitution prohibiting cruel and unusual punishment.[11,15] Thus with screening, states may be obliged to incur greater medical costs for care and treatment.

National Survey on Surveillance in State Prisons Shows Reluctance to Screen

Routine, universal screening, without regard to purported risk factors, has occurred in either jails, prisons, or both in at least 28 of the 50 states. **Fig. 2** shows data collected in a recent survey of state prison medical directors, published literature on screening in jails, and an earlier survey of which state prison systems had conducted surveillance.[8,12] To these estimates, the authors have added data from recent surveillance

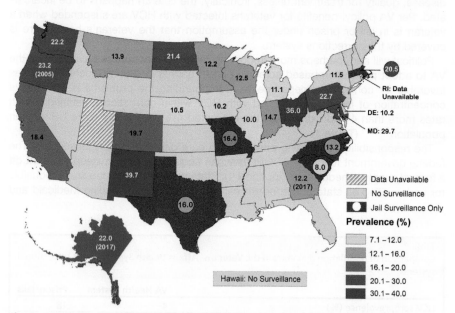

Fig. 2. Prevalence of antibodies to HCV in US state prison systems: estimates from 2016 National Survey of State Prison Systems unless date otherwise specified; with local jail data added. States that did not respond to survey, but where local jail data were available, are shaded in gray. The jail prevalence is provided in the circle within the state. (*Adapted from* Spaulding AC, Anderson EJ, Khan MA, et al. HIV and HCV in U.S. prisons and jails: the correctional facility as a bellwether over time for the community's infections. AIDS Rev 2017;19(3):142; with permission.)

in the Alaska and Georgia departments of corrections by this article's authors. The US Preventive Services Task Force's recommendations on whom to screen for HCV lists incarceration as a risk factor.[22] Studies show that limiting correctional screening to those with other risk factors excludes many persons infected with HCV.[25-27] Unlike screening for HCV, screening for HIV in prisons at intake is the norm, which shows that prison systems can systematically offer testing for blood-borne infections.[12] Screening reveals an HIV infection in an average of 1.3% of the prison population.[28] Many jails in areas of high HIV prevalence also perform routine screening for HIV.[6] Budgets are sufficient to treat the small proportion of persons with HIV.

Challenges with Comparing Data from the Reports of Multiple States' Hepatitis C Virus Screening Programs

Prison-provided surveillance data are not directly comparable because of inconsistencies in how data on HCV prevalence are collected; current data on HCV prevalence in prisons come from surveillance of entry, stock, and exit populations. Uncertainties that come from screening programs also arise when persons with unknown status and known positives are not addressed in a prespecified manner, as shown by a recent review[29] of HCV screening in the unified jail/prison system of Rhode Island (**Fig. 3**). Promotion by a professional society or government agency of a standard method to report prison prevalence of HCV would help states compare their data. Standardization would have a second effect: it would facilitate surveillance efforts for the United States as a whole, because the data could be added to nationwide estimates of HCV prevalence and geographic distribution.

First Case Study: Public Health Administrator Outside, Looking in on the Georgia Department of Corrections

Imagine yourself as a public health administrator in the state of Georgia. Historically, the Georgia State Department of Corrections (GDC) did not systematically perform HCV screening in its population of approximately 45,000, with 17,000 entrants and exits yearly. Beginning in 2016, a project team from Rollins School of Public Health, Emory University, sought to address hepatitis C case finding. With the backing of the Georgia Department of Public Health, the Emory team began a demonstration project of voluntary exit testing for antibodies to HCV with reflex testing for RNA. Funding came from industry. The offer of screening did not depend on prior testing, high

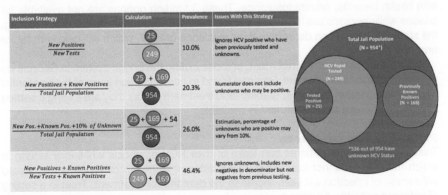

Fig. 3. Uncertainty over HCV prevalence, based on choice of numerator and denominator. (*Data from* Beckwith, et al. Journal of Public Health 2016, from modified analysis published in AIDS Review 2017.)

risk for HCV exposure, or HIV status. Emory staff provided periodic in-person information sessions on hepatitis for about-to-be-released persons; afterward, each attendee was given a chance to sign a testing consent form. Georgia has legally mandated screening for HIV on exit and HCV screening was added to this blood draw for those wanting testing. An Emory-employed social worker was engaged to provide help with discharge planning and linkage to community care for those diagnosed with HCV infection.

The project began in 1 prison, but as of January 2018, exit testing is occurring in 5 of 33 state prison facilities. To date, just 12.5% of persons who have undergone the full information session have opted out of exit testing. A total of 299 persons have been tested for anti-HCV antibodies; reflex polymerase chain reaction (PCR) testing is performed when antibodies are found. Seroprevalence was 10.7% and 56% of those who were anti-HCV positive (6.0% of all tested persons) were viremic. About 6.3% of tests were done in patients in the 1945 to 1965 birth cohort, and 26.3% of persons tested were anti-HCV positive; among those younger than the baby boomer generation, 6% were HCV seropositive. Two patients with viremia volunteered that they already knew about their infection; questions about prior diagnosis were not systematically asked.

After the demonstration project period, there are 3 possible options for HCV screening:

Cease testing
This option would not promote access to cure for infected people. However, without continued allocation of resources, and support from the Department of Public Health, correctional administrators may consider this the only feasible strategy going forward.

Continue opt-in exit testing
The benefits are that non-targeted HCV screening at exit situates testing in an existing infrastructure for health care. For Georgia, testing occurs at a time when phlebotomy is already mandated, so no additional health workers are needed. Persons found to be viremic on exit can access treatment in the community, where patients may qualify for federally funded programs (eg, Medicaid/Medicare/Veterans' Health Administration/Indian Health Service); patient assistance programs established by pharmaceutical companies; and, for a minority of persons leaving the prison who secure employment with health benefits, private insurance. These 3 funding options are not available for prisons while persons are incarcerated. Furthermore, by routine, nontargeted testing, the state of Georgia can determine the prevalence of HCV, which will help with future program planning.

The risks are that many, if not most, of those exiting the prison system in Georgia do not have access to health care. Persons found to have infection learn of their potential need for vaccination, cancer screening, and treatment just as they are exiting a setting in which comprehensive treatment is available.

Shift testing from exit to entry
The benefits are that patients can learn of their HCV diagnosis while in a setting in which the prison cannot be deliberately indifferent to health care needs. Increased awareness of infection will likely increase the demand for treatment. Treat in a setting of enforced sobriety. Additional care, such as vaccinations and cancer screening, can be provided. The prevalence of HCV viremia is lower in Georgia than in many other states. If the number of cases found is less than the number originally perceived to

exist, setting up a screening and treatment program may be feasible, especially if the cost of medications is decreasing.

The risk is that persons may not finish treatment before release. Although prisons may commence treatment only for those with greater than 3 months left on their sentence, some may leave early; treatment models for continuity of care after release would be required.[30] The heart of a treatment program is identifying persons to treat, but finding cases may be perceived as obligating a system to underfunded programs.

QUESTION 3: WHAT ARE OPPORTUNITIES AND CHALLENGES FACING HEALTH ADMINISTRATORS FOR TREATING HEPATITIS C IN A STATE PRISON SYSTEM?

In managing hepatitis C once diagnosed, when funds are insufficient to cure all, US prison systems, in addition to low commitment to screening, have adopted a combined approach of prioritizing the most urgent cases and negotiating lower prices for medications.

Second Case Study: Alaska, Navigating the Complexities of Screening for and Treating Hepatitis C Virus from the Inside

Imagine yourself as a medical director for the Department of Corrections in Alaska, one of 6 states whose justice system combines both jail and prison services. Alaska has 12 correctional facilities spread over a geographic area more than twice the size of Texas. Although Alaska averages 30,000 criminal remands (pretrial commitments) per year, because of recidivism these intakes do not represent unique individuals. For example, in 2017 a total of 17,565 individuals were remanded to an Alaskan facility. Approximately 45% of these entrants stay in the system greater than 1 year.

Alaska makes treatment decisions without reference to sentence, but, for the sake of determining the feasibility of a population-health approach, consider a hypothetical scenario in which a state such as Alaska treats the population of individuals with a sentence greater than 1 year. Because about 45% of entrants remain in the system beyond 1 year, the authors estimate that 17,565 × 0.45, or 7900 individuals, would be screened and considered for treatment if infected.

Case finding

Routine testing for HCV antibody is performed by the Alaska State Virology Laboratory for any person in the system as part of an opt-in testing model (on request by the patient or initiated by the provider). Beginning in 2016, seropositive results were reflexively tested for genotype. Although PCR is not performed by the state virology laboratory for screening purposes, a positive genotype is considered a surrogate for the presence of virus. The patient is presumed to be virus free when genotype cannot be determined. A quantitative test for viral load is drawn for individuals being considered for treatment.

Prevalence

A chart audit at 2 facilities, Spring Creek Correctional Center in Seward, Alaska, a male facility housing up to 551 sentenced persons, and the Highland Mountain Correctional Center in Eagle River, Alaska, a female facility housing up to 404 sentenced and unsentenced women, revealed that approximately 22% of persons in the correctional population are anti-HCV antibody positive.

Applying these findings to the entire system, if 22% of 7900 entrants whose stay exceeds 1 year are infected, then 1738 persons may be antibody positive, and 1300 are HCV viremic.

Budget

Not including behavioral health, the Alaska Department of Corrections Division of Health and Rehabilitation Services spends approximately $30 million per year on its health care services for all confined persons. At the initial prices for DAAs, the cost of treating all viremic persons would have been greater than this entire budget.

Converting to a population-health approach is feasible, but only if the cost of treatment is proportionate to the prevalence of a disease in the population being treated (**Fig. 4**). Consider a comparison between the proportionate costs of HCV treatment and HIV treatment. HIV prevalence is approximately 1%; each treated patient costs $40,000 per year, or $4 million if 100 are treated a year. With discounts, the cost of treating each patient with HCV is $40,000, the same price as a year's worth of HIV treatment, but more than 20 times more persons in prisons and jails are infected than with HIV.

There are several options a state prison system can pursue to maximize the number of cures:

Note that these are not mutually exclusive options. The more persons discovered to have infection, the greater the need for a way to pay for more treatment. If the overall budget for health care does not increase, the price per cure must decrease.

1. Increase in-prison HCV screening: with such high prevalence of hepatitis C, if testing were more aggressive (eg, opt-out rather than opt-in), more persons would know their antibody status. This approach is promoted by the FBOP.

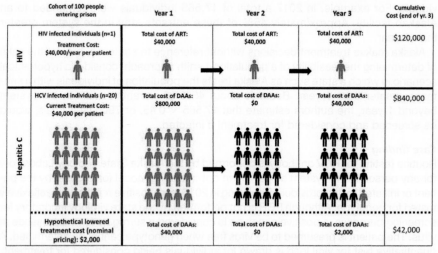

Fig. 4. Hypothetical treatment cost for a cohort of 100 people, entering the Alaska Department of Corrections, incarcerated for 3 years (upper limit of typical length of stay for persons with felony conviction), with HIV treatment cost for comparison. Assuming HIV prevalence of 1% and HCV prevalence of 20%, this shows that, with such a high prevalence of HCV in correctional populations, the burden of drug costs is incurred up-front when cases are identified, then annual expenditures decline for these entrants as individuals are cured. This expenditure is compared with the cost of HIV treatment, which is spread over the length of time an individual is incarcerated. The initial cost is $40,000 per treatment course. At a reduced price of $2,000, an estimated nominal price per regimen (explained later), the Alaska Department of Corrections could much more easily afford treatment of individuals with hepatitis C. ART, antiretroviral therapy.

Benefits: More persons will learn whether they are infected. Recommendations for persons with viremia could be followed: immunize against hepatitis A, hepatitis B, and pneumococcus. For those with advanced liver disease, perform upper endoscopy to rule out esophageal varices and image the liver to rule out masses suggestive of hepatocellular carcinoma. Refer persons for treatment.

Risks: If opt-out testing is offered too aggressively, those with inadequate understanding of a right to refuse may feel coerced to undergo testing. With more testing, demand for medical services, including treatment of hepatitis C, could outstrip the budget.

2. Negotiate acquisition cost for treatment: state prison systems and local jails have a limited number of options to reduce the price of treatment. Although they are scarce, vehicles do exist to obtain lower-priced medications to treat their correctional populations. The Medicaid drug rebate provisions require that the manufacturers give their best price to the Medicaid program, but there are ways for state prison systems to work around this best-price requirement, as outlined in question 5.

Benefits: Prices for DAAs can be reduced and more patients can therefore be treated.

Risks: Most options require cooperation on the part of at least 1 pharmaceutical company, and careful navigation of federal drug pricing laws.

3. Prioritize persons for treatment based on severity or comorbid conditions. See response to question 1 for the approach recommended by the FBOP guidelines.

Benefits: Patients are assessed system wide in an equitable way. Resources are used to treat persons for whom treatment is most urgent. Patients who will experience little disease progression if treatment is postponed for a year or two may be treated later, when the price of treatment decreases.

Risks: Although the APRI (aspartate transaminase to platelet ratio index) score has a high specificity for detecting cirrhosis, it has a low sensitivity (**Box 2, Table 2**). Reliance

---

Box 2
Applying the Federal Bureau of Prisons guidelines to state systems: Georgia and Alaska

Adapting the HCV management guidelines of the FBOP to a state program could be a feasible first step toward the eventual goal of having hepatitis C treatment follow the American Association for the Study of Liver Diseases guidelines. The number of cases of HCV needing treatment that the Georgia prison system would find if opt-out testing were initiated for entrants could be estimated, in keeping with the FBOP guidelines. The number of cases found could then be compared with the number the system has the capacity to treat per year. In GDC in financial year 2017, 219 persons were treated.

Parameters: it was necessary to determine what percentage of patients with HCV viremia would have an APRI more than 1.0. In the Alaska Department of Corrections, 13% had APRI greater than 1.0. Evaluation, management, and follow-up may be difficult to conduct if the time the individual is the correctional system is less than 1 year, so only patients with an expected length of stay greater than 1 year are considered for treatment in this example. In addition, experience shows that about 91% of patients offered treatment in prison accept it.[32] Approximately 23% of persons with HCV viremia were treated in GDC. This percentage is strikingly similar to the percentage of persons with HCV viremia in the Washington Department of Corrections: they estimated that 23% of their population with HCV viremia had an APRI greater than 1.0.[33]

Summary: note that testing entrants to the Georgia prisons system would identify roughly the number of new patients that the prison infrastructure has the capacity to treat. The number treated in Alaska would be about 155 patients a year.

Table 2
Comparing treatment projections: Alaska and Georgia prison systems, 2018

	Alaska Department of Corrections	Georgia DC
Number of unique entrants per year	17,565	17,000
Number viremic if prevalence similar to pilot study	2900	1020
Number with stay (jail + prison) >1 y	1305	1020
Number with APRI>1.0	170 (13%)	240 (23.5%)
Number consenting to treatment (91%)	155	219

on the APRI score may be misleading. One systematic review found that more than 50% of negative APRI results, using a cutoff of 2.0 as recommended by the FBOP, could be falsely negative, thereby providing a false sense of reassurance regarding the patient's liver status.[31]

QUESTION 4: WHAT ARE CURRENT DIRECT-ACTING ANTIVIRAL PRICES, AND WHAT BARRIERS EXIST FOR PRISONS TO REDUCE THESE PRICES?

State prisons typically buy medications on the open market through wholesalers at prices that represent the highest markups in the US drug market.[10,34] As of the start of 2018, the listed price, or average wholesale price (AWP), of new DAA regimens ranges between $26,400 and $96,000 per treatment course in the United States. Although several studies have shown that these drugs are cost-effective in the general population at the given price,[35,36] they remain unaffordable for many payers, especially prison health services, even after accounting for existing discounts.[10] Because of budget constraints, state corrections cannot purchase the amount of medication needed to meet the demand.

How Price Is Derived

A good benchmark for comparing drug prices is the average manufacturer price (AMP), which is defined in federal law and generally represents the manufacturer's average price nationwide for a drug within the retail class of trade.[37,38] Not all prices, such as AMP, are published, but, because they are derivatives of other prices, these unpublished numbers can be estimated. Using financial year 2018 pricing data supplied by the GDC for their AWP for DAAs ($69,773) and the 340B price when their patients with hepatitis C use a safety-net hospital ($38,186), the authors estimated AMP for an 84-day course of treatment.

The AWP represents a markup of approximately 17% over wholesale acquisition cost (WAC). Hence, WAC is $57,912. If the 340B price represents 23.1% less than the AMP, then AMP is $49,657 (ie, 38,186/0.769). If Medicaid pricing represents a 24% discount off AMP, then the Medicaid rebate price is $37,399. Although the VA price is unpublished, multiple providers have informally disclosed that it is in the $10,000 to $11,000 range. The nominal price must be less than 10% of the AMP. An 84-day course of treatment costs $400 or less to manufacture[39,40] (Fig. 5, Table 3). Additional details on pricing and calculations are in Appendix 1.

Barriers to Reducing Price

Because of the market impact of certain federal laws, pharmaceutical companies cannot simply discount their medications to a level that would permit prisons to purchase sufficient supplies of drug to meet correctional population demands. In particular, the

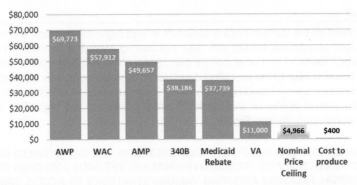

Fig. 5. Estimated price per course of treatment, for most commonly used DAAs. Length of treatment used in this calculation is a 12-week, or an 84-day, supply of drugs. See appendix for an expanded explanation of each pricing level. (*Data from* Georgia Department of Corrections, November 2017. Cascade format introduced at online site for "340B University." Available at: www.HRSA.gov. Accessed March 19, 2018.)

manufacturers cite the adverse financial consequences of discounting their medications as a result of the federal laws underlying (1) the Medicaid drug rebate program (MDRP), (2) the 340B drug pricing program (340B program), (3) the federal ceiling price (FCP) to which the federal government's 4 largest drug purchasers (the VA, Department of Defense, Public Health Service, and Coast Guard) are entitled, and (4) the average sales price (ASP) formula used by the Medicare Part B program to reimburse hospitals and clinicians for physician-administered drugs[41–44] (see Appendix 1 for more details.) The most significant threat to manufacturer pricing arises out of a unique requirement in the MDRP that a manufacturer extend its best price on brand-name drugs to the entire Medicaid and 340B programs, with only a few exceptions.[45] The result is that if a correctional facility were successful in negotiating deep discounts, those discounts would likely reduce the prices at which manufacturers could legally sell their drugs within federal programs. Industry clearly has an incentive to overstate the impact of these federal programs when negotiating with potential purchasers, but the barriers are nonetheless real.

Table 3
Summary of prices in the hepatitis C therapeutics market

Term	Abbreviation	Meaning	Georgia Price ($)
Average wholesale price	AWP	Sticker price	69,773
Wholesale acquisition price	WAC	What wholesalers pay	57,912
Average manufacturer's price	AMP	What it costs the manufacturer	49, 657
Price paid by a 340B covered entity	340B	Maximum price that can be paid by a safety-net entity (340B program of HRSA)	38,186
Nominal price	—	≤10% of AMP (see response to question 5)	4000 (hypothetical)

Abbreviation: HRSA, Health Resource and Service Administration.
  All prices are authors' estimates of actual prices, unless otherwise stated.

Net Result

The net result of the current pricing structure is that high-risk persons are not being treated, and companies cannot sell their product to meet the demand. There is a gap between demand and what can be purchased under existing market conditions. Of note, this is similar to the so-called deadweight-loss concept: why existing regulations and patent law surrounding DAA pricing leads to a market situation "enjoyed by neither the patent holder or the public"[46] when prices are too high. This situation leaves an untapped market (**Fig. 6**).

QUESTION 5: HOW CAN PRISON SYSTEMS OVERCOME THE GAP BETWEEN DEMAND FOR AND AVAILABILITY OF TREATMENT? WHAT ARE THE PROS AND CONS OF CORRECTIONAL FACILITIES ADOPTING VARIOUS STRATEGIES TO ACCESS DIRECT-ACTING ANTIVIRALS AND MANAGE HEPATITIS C?

Given the complex web of federal drug pricing laws and the financial pressures they exert on manufacturers not to discount their prices in the nonfederal market, state and local correctional systems currently have limited options for reducing the prices they pay for DAAs (see Appendix 1). It is therefore essential that state or local correctional departments pursue a purchasing strategy that is exempt from best price. After that, they can consider more refined methods for reducing their DAA acquisition costs.

State or Local Departments of Corrections Can Potentially Use the Following Strategies to Purchase Drugs at a Lower Price than they Currently Pay, Without Violating the Best-price Rule

1. Contracts with entities eligible for discounts under the 340B Drug Pricing Program: the 340B program enables safety-net providers to qualify for reduced prescription drug prices. Pharmaceutical companies participating in Medicaid must offer drug discounts to 340B-covered entities, which include disproportionate share hospitals and federally qualified health centers serving lower-income communities. State prisons are not eligible for coverage under 340B, but they may enter a contract with a covered entity to treat an incarcerated person as a patient of the covered facility.[11]

  Benefits: Moderate discounts are possible with these mechanisms.
  Risks: Discounts are inadequate to substantially increase the number of persons infected with HCV that the justice system can treat.

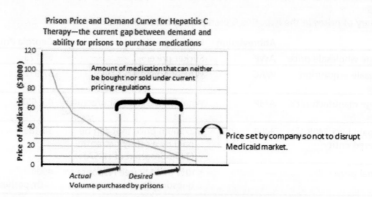

Fig. 6. The untapped DAA market. The lower horizontal line represents a price that permits prisons to purchase the volume needed to adequately address hepatitis C.

2. Pooled procurement: another potential strategy is known as pooled procurement, by which states, counties, and municipalities band together and buy medications in bulk from the manufacturer. By purchasing in bulk, states may obtain lower prices for medications. Some states also participate in the Minnesota Multistate Contracting Alliance for Pharmacy (www.mmcap.org), a group-purchasing organization for government facilities to negotiate reduced prices. The depth of the discounts that states are able to obtain are unknown because the contracts are kept confidential. The drug prices that state prison systems reported to a *Wall Street Journal* reporter in 2016 showed that discounts are often just slightly less than full list price.[47] In order to obtain more substantial discounts with pooled procurement, that are less than best price, this strategy would need to be combined with a Section 1115 waiver (detailed later).

Benefits: Moderate discounts are possible with these mechanisms.

Risks: Discounts are inadequate to increase the number the system can treat substantially.

3. Nominal pricing: state correctional systems, or group purchasing organizations of which they are a part, could request nominal pricing from the manufacturer. A nominal price is defined as a price less than 10% of AMP[48] and paid by any facility identified in Section 1927(c) (1) (D) (i) of the Social Security Act, or any determined to be a safety-net provider by the Secretary of Department of Health and Human Services (DHHS).[49] The DHHS Secretary can approve of nominal pricing based on the type of facility, services provided, population served, and the number of other nominal price eligible facilities in the same service area.[50] Although the exact AMP is confidential, this would make the price substantially less.

Benefits: Prisons and jails are clearly within the realm of public institutions deemed appropriate for nominal pricing consideration. Given that a complete course of DAAs costs between $200 and $400 to produce, this would still be more than the production cost for the pharmaceutical company. Importantly, using nominal pricing would not affect the manufacturers' Medicaid market or best price. Transactions could be proposed to Centers for Medicare & Medicaid Services (CMS) in advance to confirm that the manufacturer is not incurring any risk by extending nominal pricing to correctional facilities. Nominal pricing would create the most substantial discount.

Risks: Agreement to nominal pricing is entirely at the discretion of the pharmaceutical company.

State Departments of Corrections Can Also Team with the State Medicaid Program in Order to Use the Following Strategy

A. Section 1115 waiver: states may act individually to request exemption from the best-price rule via a waiver permitted under Section 1115 of the Social Security Act. If approved by the federal government, the waiver could allow the state Medicaid agency to negotiate supplemental rebates from manufacturers on behalf of itself and other state agencies (eg, the Department of Corrections) that were exempt from best-price calculations. By negotiating on behalf of other state agencies that are willing to use the state Medicaid's preferred drug list, the Medicaid agency would presumably have greater leverage in negotiating supplemental rebates from manufacturers. This strategy would require state agencies to collaborate to win approval of the waiver from the federal government. The companies could then pursue either a new lower price or charge a fee by month for whatever amount of drug would be demanded by state entities, a sort of subscription plan.

As summarized earlier, vehicles do exist for states to obtain lower-priced medications to treat their prison populations. Because these options require states to invest significant resources for limited benefits, some stakeholders have questioned whether legislative change may be necessary to empower states to negotiate lower prices.

Legislative Change That Would Allow Departments of Corrections to Purchase Drugs at a Lower Price Without Violating the Best-Price Rule

1. Change the best price rule statutorily: one proposal is to amend federal regulations that stipulate which entities are excluded from Medicaid's best-price rule. There are currently 19 exceptions to the best-price rule, and through legislation a 20th exception could be created. If state prisons were added as an excluded or exempt entity, they could negotiate prices lower than Medicaid and receive discounts like those available to the VA and Indian Health Service. This possibility has the benefit of applying to state prisons in all states if changed.

Other Solutions Require Examining Patent Law for the New Direct-Acting Agents

1. Purchasing a patent: The National Academies of Medicine in their phase II report on the elimination of hepatitis B and C recommended that the DHHS should purchase the patent or licensing rights to a DAA that could then be used to treat patients left uncovered at present. This recommendation would require voluntary cooperation from at least 1 pharmaceutical company. Furthermore, the company willing to grant patent rights to a drug may be selling a product that would not do well under current marketplace conditions, such as a DAA with activity against only a limited number of genotypes or associated with a cure rate less than the 99% seen with the most recently developed agents. To the best of our knowledge, since the report was published in April 2017, no company has volunteered to sell their patent.
2. Evoking eminent domain: in April of 2017, a group of experts in law, economics, and public health met at Johns Hopkins University to provide advice, specifically to the state of Louisiana, on purchasing treatment of Medicaid beneficiaries and prisons. The group then wrote an open letter to Louisiana's Secretary of Health, which advocated the state invoke a little-used provision in the US Code: 28 U.S.C §1498, which authorizes the government to make use of patented inventions, including medication.[51] This strategy would essentially evoke eminent domain over use of the patented medication. The company holding the patent can obtain compensation for use of the patented invention but cannot prevent the government from the action.[46] This power was used particularly frequently in the 1960s for procuring drugs, such as antibiotics, by the Department of Defense and the Veterans Health Administration.[46] In more recent times, the US government threatened to invoke §1498 to obtain ciprofloxacin in bulk at the time of the anthrax attacks in 2001. This threat was never carried out because, in response, Bayer reduced the cost of the medication by more than 70% during negotiations with the federal government.[46]

DISCUSSION

Society benefits by more aggressively screening for and treating hepatitis C in incarcerated populations. Screening and treatment of incarcerated persons is cost-effective for society as a whole, and would reduce hepatitis C burden in the overall US population. Several modeling studies have evaluated the long-term benefits and costs of providing HCV screening and treatment in corrections. He and colleagues[16] showed that universal opt-out screening of inmates for HCV in United States prisons would reduce ongoing HCV transmission, the incidence of advanced liver diseases, and liver-related deaths. Universal HCV screening followed by treatment with DAAs had an incremental cost-effectiveness ratio (ICER) of $19,800 per additional quality-adjusted life year (QALY), which is lower than that of the birth-cohort screening in the general population ($35,700–$65,700 per QALY).[52–55]

An interesting finding of the modeling study by He and colleagues[16] was that most of the benefits of interventions in prisons would accrue in the community, because a larger proportion of releasees to the community would have been cured of the disease. Compared with no screening, universal screening for up to 10 years would diagnose 123,000 new HCV cases, and 71,000 of those would be diagnosed among inmates currently incarcerated. Furthermore, such interventions would prevent 12,500 new HCV infections in the next 30 years. Of the averted infections (ie, incidence), around 90% of them would have occurred in the general population; that is, outside the prisons. Furthermore, HCV screening in prisons would prevent a total of 12,500 liver-related deaths, 1200 liver transplants, 9000 cases of hepatocellular carcinoma, and 7500 cases of decompensated cirrhosis, and most of them would be prevented outside prisons.

A study by Martin and colleagues[56] showed that doubling prison testing rates (such as through opt-out testing) with oral DAAs would be cost-effective in United Kingdom prisons (ICER £15,090 [approximately US$20,059] per QALY gained). In addition, if greater than 10% of referred PWID are treated in prison (2.5% base case), HCV treatment would be highly cost-effective (ICER<£13,000 [approximately US$17,280]). Another study by Martin and colleagues[57] showed that increasing case finding can be cost-effective in prisons if continuity of treatment and care is ensured after release.

Evidence for the value of HCV screening and treatment in corrections available from modeling studies can guide policy makers in establishing evidence-based guidelines that can restrict disease spread and improve outcomes in those already infected. The prioritization of cases in treating hepatitis C with curative DAAs has been called into question by data from a recent study that showed DAA treatment is important for reducing mortality at all stages of fibrosis.[58] HCV prevention efforts focusing on corrections not only will reduce HCV burden but will provide a good value for care. From a societal perspective, investing in prison health care to increase access to screening and treatment would be money well spent.

SUMMARY

- The opioid epidemic may be contributing to the plateau in prison HCV prevalence. The previously seen decline in prevalence has stalled. Greater access to HCV treatment in prison settings could help re-ignite a decline in prevalence of the disease.
- Access to prison-based treatment requires knowledge of whom to treat. At current levels of funding for HCV management, prisons are not aggressively seeking cases.
- In order to make screening acceptable in a system focused on avoiding deliberate indifference to known health problems, a policy to treat only the most urgent cases may be the lesser of 2 evils. The alternative is to continue not to screen, although the ideal solution is to reduce prices.
- Within current laws and regulations, use of nominal pricing seems to be the most viable option for substantially reducing prices. If this is not approved by the Secretary of Health and Human Services or if no pharmaceutical company is willing to sell medications at this price, other strategies are necessary. Some negotiating

power can be realized by individual corrections departments. However, changes in laws and policy at the federal level may be needed to help prisons contribute to efforts to make hepatitis C a rare disease for everyone.

ACKNOWLEDGMENTS

The authors are grateful for helpful comments from: Emeli Anderson MSPH, cPhD, and Chava Bowden, BS, Emory University; Elizabeth Paukstis JD Viral Hepatitis Round Table; James Cassell, PA-C, and Laura Brooks, Alaska Department of Corrections; and Newton Kendig MD, GW School of Medicine. The opinions expressed in this document do not necessarily reflect these advisors, or their current or past organizations and affiliations. The authors thank Georgia Department of Corrections for data on medication purchases, and Marsha Simon of Simon & Company, Washington DC, for information on nominal pricing for family planning clinics. The authors thank Carolyn Mackey and Junyu Chen of Emory University for background research and assistance in preparing the article for publication.

REFERENCES

1. Denniston MM, Jiles RB, Drobeniuc J, et al. Chronic hepatitis C virus infection in the United States, National Health and Nutrition Examination Survey 2003 to 2010. Ann Intern Med 2014;160(5):293–300.
2. Alcabes P, Vlahov D, Anthony JC. Characteristics of intravenous drug users by history of arrest and treatment for drug use. J Nerv Ment Dis 1992;180(1):48–54.
3. Genberg BL, Astemborski J, Vlahov D, et al. Incarceration and injection drug use in Baltimore, Maryland. Addiction 2015;110(7):1152–9.
4. National Academies of Sciences, Engineering, and Medicine. A national strategy for the elimination of hepatitis B and C: phase two report. Washington, DC: National Academies Press; 2017.
5. World prison brief, Webpage of the International Centre for Prison Studies, University of London. Available at: http://www.prisonstudies.org/world-prison-brief-data. Accessed February 3, 2018.
6. Spaulding AC, Perez SD, Seals RM, et al. The diversity of release patterns for jail detainees: implications for public health interventions. Am J Public Health 2011; 101(Suppl 1):S347–52.
7. Spaulding AC, Drobeniuc AM, Frew PM, et al. Jail, an unappreciated medical home: assessing the feasibility of a strengths-based case management intervention to improve the care retention of HIV-infected persons once released from jail. PLoSOne 2018;13(3):e0191643.
8. Varan AK, Mercer DW, Stein MS, et al. Hepatitis C seroprevalence among prison inmates since 2001: still high but declining. Public Health Rep 2014;129(2):187–95.
9. Carson EA, Anderson E. Prisoners in 2015. Washington, DC: US Department of Justice, Office of Justice Programs, Bureau of Justice Statistics; 2016. NCJ 250229. Available at: https://www.bjs.gov/index.cfm?ty=pbdetail&iid=5869. Accessed January 20, 2017.
10. Beckman AL, Bilinski A, Boyko R, et al. New hepatitis C drugs are very costly and unavailable to many state prisoners. Health Aff 2016;35(10):1893–901.
11. Spaulding A, Kim A, Harzke A, et al. Impact of new therapeutics for hepatitis C virus infection in incarcerated populations. Top Antivir Med 2012;21(1):27–35.

12. Spaulding AC, Anderson EJ, Khan MA, et al. HIV and HCV in U.S. prisons and jails: the correctional facility as a bellwether over time for the community's infections. AIDS Rev 2017;19(3):134–47.

13. Beck AJ, Maruschak LM. Hepatitis testing and treatment in state prisons. Washington, DC: US Department of Justice, Office of Justice Programs; 2004.

14. Ly KN, Hughes EM, Jiles RB, et al. Rising mortality associated with hepatitis C virus in the United States, 2003–2013. Clin Infect Dis 2016;62(10):1287–8.

15. Estelle v. Gamble 429 U.S. 97 (1976).

16. He T, Li K, Roberts M, et al. Prevention of hepatitis C by screening and treatment in US prisons. Ann Intern Med 2016;164(2):84–92.

17. Martin NK, Vickerman P, Grebely J, et al. Hepatitis C virus treatment for prevention among people who inject drugs: modeling treatment scale-up in the age of direct-acting antivirals. Hepatology 2013;58(5):1598–609.

18. Cepeda JA, Niccolai LM, Lyubimova A, et al. High-risk behaviors after release from incarceration among people who inject drugs in St. Petersburg, Russia. Drug Alcohol Depend 2015;147:196–202.

19. Federal Bureau of Prisons. Evaluation and management of chronic hepatitis C virus (HCV) infection. Clinical guidance. 2016. Available at: https://www.bop.gov/resources/pdfs/hepatitis_c.pdf. Accessed September 7, 2017.

20. Committee on Finance, United States Senate. The price of sovaldi and its impact on the U.S. health care system. 2015. Available at: https://www.finance.senate.gov/download/the-price-of-sovaldi-and-its-impact-on-the-us-health-care-system-full-report. Accessed February 24, 2017.

21. Smith BD, Morgan RL, Beckett GA, et al. Recommendations for the identification of chronic hepatitis C virus infection among persons born during 1945-1965. MMWR Recomm Rep 2012;61(RR-4):1–32.

22. Moyer VA. Screening for hepatitis C virus infection in adults: U.S. Preventive Services Task Force recommendation statement. Ann Intern Med 2013;159(5):349–57.

23. Dominitz JA, Boyko EJ, Koepsell TD, et al. Elevated prevalence of hepatitis C infection in users of United States veterans medical centers. Hepatology 2005;41(1):88–96.

24. Lin ZH, Xin YN, Dong QJ, et al. Performance of the aspartate aminotransferase-to-platelet ratio index for the staging of hepatitis C-related fibrosis: an updated meta-analysis. Hepatology 2011;53(3):726–36.

25. Kuncio DE, Newbern EC, Fernandez-Viña MH, et al. Comparison of risk-based hepatitis C screening and the true seroprevalence in an urban prison system. J Urban Health 2015;92(2):379–86.

26. Larney S, Mahowald MK, Scharff N, et al. Epidemiology of hepatitis C virus in Pennsylvania state prisons, 2004–2012: limitations of 1945–1965 birth cohort screening in correctional settings. Am J Public Health 2014;106(6):e69–74.

27. Stockman LJ, Greer J, Holzmacher R, et al. Performance of risk-based and birth-cohort strategies for identifying hepatitis C virus infection among people entering prison, Wisconsin, 2014. Public Health Rep 2016;131(4):544–51.

28. Maruschak LM, Bronson J. HIV in prison. Washington, DC: Bureau of Justice Statistics; 2017. NCJ 250641. Available at: https://www.bjs.gov/content/pub/pdf/hivp15st.pdf. Accessed October 10, 2017.

29. Beckwith CG, Kurth AE, Bazerman LB, et al. A pilot study of rapid hepatitis C virus testing in the Rhode Island Department of Corrections. J Public Health (Oxf) 2016;38(1):130–7.

30. Klein SJ, Wright LN, Birkhead GS, et al. Promoting HCV treatment completion for prison inmates: New York State's hepatitis C continuity program. Public Health Rep 2007;122(Suppl 2):83–8.

31. Chou R, Wasson N. Blood tests to diagnose fibrosis or cirrhosis in patients with chronic hepatitis C virus infection: a systematic review. Ann Intern Med 2013; 158(11):807–20.

32. Allen SA, Spaulding AC, Osei AM, et al. Treatment of chronic hepatitis C in a state correctional facility. Ann Intern Med 2003;138(3):187–90.

33. Assoumou SA, Wang J, Tsui J, et al. Characterization of a population with hepatitis C infection in a U.S. state prison. 6th International Symposium on hepatitis care in substance users. Jersey City, NJ, September 6–8, 2017.

34. Rosenthal ES, Graham CS. Price and affordability of direct-acting antiviral regimens for hepatitis C virus in the United States. Infect Agent Cancer 2016; 11(1):24.

35. He T, Lopez-Olivo MA, Hur C, et al. Systematic review: cost-effectiveness of direct-acting antivirals for treatment of hepatitis C genotypes 2-6. Aliment Pharmacol Ther 2017;46(8):711–21.

36. Chhatwal J, He T, Hur C, et al. Direct-acting antiviral agents for patients with hepatitis C virus genotype 1 infection are cost-saving. Clin Gastroenterol Hepatol 2017;15(6):827–37.e8.

37. 42 U.S.C. 1396r-8(k)(1).

38. 42 C.F.R. 447.504.

39. Hill A, Khoo S, Fortunak J, et al. Minimum costs for producing hepatitis C direct-acting antivirals for use in large-scale treatment access programs in developing countries. Clin Infect Dis 2014;58(7):928–36.

40. van de Ven N, Fortunak J, Simmons B, et al. Minimum target prices for production of direct-acting antivirals and associated diagnostics to combat hepatitis C virus. Hepatology 2015;61(4):1174–82.

41. 42 U.S.C. 1395 w-3a.

42. 38 U.S.C. 8126.

43. 42 U.S.C. 256b.

44. 42 U.S.C. 1396r-8.

45. 42 U.S.C. 1396r-8 (c)(1)(C)(i).

46. Brennan H, Kapczynski A, Monahan CH, et al. A prescription for excessive drug pricing: leveraging government patent use for health. Yale Journal of Law & Technology 2016;18(1):7. Available at: http://digitalcommons.law.yale.edu/yjolt/vol18/iss1/7.

47. Fields G, Lofuts P. High cost of new HCV drugs strains prison budgets, locks many out of care. Wall Street Journal 2016. Available at: https://www.wsj.com/articles/high-cost-of-new-hepatitis-c-drugs-strains-prison-budgets-locks-many-out-of-cure-1473701644. Accessed September 13, 2016.

48. 42 C.F.R. 447.502.

49. 42 U.S.C. 1396r-8(c)(1)(D)(i).

50. 42 U.S.C. 1396r-8(c)(1)(D)(ii).

51. Sharfstein JM, GA, JMB, et al. Letter to Rebekah E. Gee, Secretary of Health, State of Louisiana. 2017. Available at: http://ldh.la.gov/assets/docs/HepatitisC/ResponsememotoSecretaryGeeHCV.pdf. Accessed October 10, 2010.

52. Eckman MH, Talal AH, Gordon SC, et al. Cost-effectiveness of screening for chronic hepatitis C infection in the United States. Clin Infect Dis 2013;56(10): 1382–93.

53. Rein DB, Smith BD, Wittenborn JS, et al. The cost-effectiveness of birth-cohort screening for hepatitis C antibody in U.S. primary care settings. Ann Intern Med 2012;156(4):263–70.
54. McGarry LJ, Pawar VS, Panchmatia HR, et al. Economic model of a birth cohort screening program for hepatitis C virus. Hepatology 2012;55(5):1344–55.
55. Liu S, Cipriano LE, Holodniy M, et al. Cost-effectiveness analysis of risk-factor guided and birth-cohort screening for chronic hepatitis C infection in the United States. PLoS One 2013;8(3):e58975.
56. Martin NK, Vickerman P, Brew IF, et al. Is increased hepatitis C virus case-finding combined with current or 8-week to 12-week direct-acting antiviral therapy cost-effective in UK prisons? A prevention benefit analysis. Hepatology 2016;63(6):1796–808.
57. Martin NK, Hickman M, Miners A, et al. Cost-effectiveness of HCV case-finding for people who inject drugs via dried blood spot testing in specialist addiction services and prisons. BMJ Open 2013;3(8) [pii:e003153].
58. Cepeda JA, Thomas DL, Astemborski J, et al. Increased mortality among persons with chronic hepatitis C with moderate or severe liver disease: a cohort study. Clin Infect Dis 2017;65(2):235–43.
59. Available at: https://www.medicaid.gov/medicaid/prescription-drugs/medicaid-drug-rebate-program/index.html. Accessed March 19, 2018.
60. 42 C.F.R. 447.509 (a) (1).
61. 42 C.F.R. 447.509.
62. 42 C.F.R. 447.509 (a) (6).
63. 42 U.S.C. 1396r-8 (k)(3).
64. Veterans Health Care Act of 1992, Pub. L. No. 102-585 §602, 106 Stat. 4943, 4967–4971 (1992).
65. 42 U.S.C. 1396 r -8(c)(1)(C)(ii)(III).
66. von Oehsen WH, Ashe M Duke K. Pharmaceutical discounts under federal law: state program opportunities. Oakland (CA): Pharmaceuticals and Indigent Care Program, Public Health Institute; 2001.

APPENDIX 1: PRICING LEVELS OF DRUGS IN THE US MARKET

- AWP is a drug-specific published price that was originally intended to represent the average price paid to wholesalers by pharmacies, doctors, and other customers (including correctional pharmacies) but that is now considered more like a sticker or list price than an actual market price.[37,38]
- WAC is the estimated manufacturer's list price to wholesalers, before any rebates or discounts are applied.
- AMP is the average price paid to a manufacturer by wholesalers for the manufacturer's drugs distributed to retail community pharmacies and by retail community pharmacies that purchase the drug directly from the manufacturers, subject to certain exceptions.[37] Pharmaceutical companies are required to report this price quarterly to the federal government.
- MDRP.

Background and Additional Information on the Medicaid Drug Rebate Program

The Omnibus Budget Reconciliation Act of 1990 is the enabling legislation for the MDRP, which results in savings for the Medicaid program. The MDRP is administered by the CMS, an agency within the DHHS.[59] Congress's goal in creating the rebate program was to ensure that federal and state taxpayers, who fund the Medicaid program, are not paying more for pharmaceuticals than any other US purchaser. It achieves this goal by contractually obligating each pharmaceutical manufacturer to pay state Medicaid programs a quarterly rebate for each covered outpatient drug reimbursed by Medicaid. Although participation in the drug rebate program is optional for manufacturers, they have a strong incentive to enter into rebate agreements with the government because both Medicaid and Medicare are prohibited from reimbursing any drug manufactured by a company that refuses to execute a rebate agreement.[44]

For brand-name drugs, the rebate is based on the greater of either (1) a 23.1% discount off the drug's AMP or (2) the difference between the AMP and the manufacturer's best price for that drug.[60] In either case, an additional rebate is due if the drug's AMP increases more than the consumer price index, a measure of inflation.[59] The Medicaid rebate net price is the net price paid to a manufacturer after deducting the statutory rebate amount from the original price of the drug.[61] Because the Medicaid net price for a brand-name drug is at least as good as the best price for that drug, the Medicaid net price should generally be better than any price available in the private sector. With respect to generic and over-the-counter drugs, the rebate is 13% of the drug's AMP.[59,62]

The MDRP statute defines many of the key terms contained in the law's language. For example, based on the statute's definition of "manufacturer," the rebate obligations extend to not only traditional producers of pharmaceuticals but also to drug repackagers and relabelers.[63] Under the statute's definition of "covered outpatient drug," the class of drugs subject to rebates includes both prescription and nonprescription drugs and prescription biologic products, depending on the setting in which they are used.[63]

Could Prisons Qualify for Best Price?

Under 42 C.F.R. 447.505, which sets forth rules under Section 1927(c) (1) (C) of the Social Security Act, state prisons are not currently listed as exempt from the rule and are thus unable to buy medications at costs lower than the best price that drug companies offer to Medicaid, other than with certain exceptions listed earlier.

Some have advocated legislation to permit prisons to access drugs under the best-price agreement. One risk to proposing this strategy is that the Congressional Budget Office (CBO) may need to rate this proposal before congress votes on it. The CBO may assume that, if new discounts are proposed, the manufacturers would cut rebates elsewhere, including the price for medications purchased by the US government. With this assumption, the price for drugs purchased by Medicaid would increase. However, the assumption does not follow edicts encoded in federal law or regulation. Given that the state prison market is virtually untapped, industry would not need to increase prices elsewhere to offset the new discount; instead, their markets would be expanding. If Medicaid agencies lobby against extending an exception to prisons, prisons can ask their state Medicaid to cooperate with them to reduce prices.

- 340B: maximum price that can be charged to a 340B covered entity. The 340B ceiling price is calculated quarterly by the drug's manufacturer by subtracting the MDRP rebate amount from AMP. The minimum MDRP rebate for brand name drugs is AMP $\times$ 23.1%.[60]
- The Federal Supply Schedule. Under the Veterans Health Care Act of 1992,[64] the VA negotiates drug prices on behalf of many government agencies. Deepest discounts are for 4 entities (known as the Big 4) that are on the Federal Supply Schedule: the VA, Department of Defense, Public Health Service, and the US Coast Guard. Their price for medications is the FCP, which must represent at

least 24% off the AWP. Lesser discounts may be given to other federal agencies, such as the FBOP,[10] but the federal prison system still enjoys discounts not shared by state governments.[20]

The nominal price is the price that is less than 10% of AMP.[48] Five categories of purchasers and a sixth category of safety-net providers approved by the DHHS Secretary are allowed to negotiate and pay a nominal price, without establishing a new best price for purposes of the MDRP and 340B programs.[49,50,65]

- Cost to produce: $400 or less.[39,40]

Although the precise impact of the MDRP, 340B, FCP, and ASP laws on the prices paid by state and local correctional institutions can vary significantly by program,[66] they all disincentivize manufacturers from discounting their prices, including those charged for the new DAAs. That is because, if a state or local correctional facility is successful in negotiating deep discounts, those discounts would likely lower the prices at which the drugs' manufacturers could legally sell their drugs within those federal programs. All 4 programs rely on an averaging mechanism for calculating pricing so that, if a manufacturer agrees to sell 1 or more of its drugs at a low price within the nonfederal correctional market, those sales will have the effect of reducing the drugs' average price, which, in turn, will reduce program payment for those drugs. Sales to nonfederal correctional institutions are a small share of the total US pharmaceutical market so their impact on these average federal prices will be incremental and therefore modest. The more significant threat to manufacturer pricing arises out of a unique requirement in the MDRP that a manufacturer extend its best price on brand name drugs to the entire Medicaid and 340B programs. The impact of the Medicaid best-price requirement is more dramatic because, rather than reducing pricing incrementally, it can lead to a sharp decline in pricing that is sudden and triggered by a single transaction. In calculating best price, a manufacturer must, among other things, include cash discounts, volume discounts, rebates, and free goods (when contingent on any purchase requirement) but not take into account prices that are merely nominal in amount.[65]

Treatment of Chronic Hepatitis C in Patients Receiving Opioid Agonist Therapy: A Review of Best Practice

Brianna L. Norton, DO, MPH[a,*], Matthew J. Akiyama, MD[a],
Philippe J. Zamor, MD[b], Alain H. Litwin, MD, MS, MPH[a]

KEYWORDS

- Hepatitis C virus • Opioid agonist therapy • Drug-drug interactions
- Direct acting antivirals • Best practice

KEY POINTS

- Injection drug use is the most common route of transmission of the hepatitis C virus and high rates of infection are observed among individuals on opioid agonist therapy.
- Although people who inject drugs carry the highest burden of hepatitis C, few have initiated treatment.
- Cohort studies and subsets of large clinical trials have demonstrated comparable HCV treatment efficacy for individuals who are on opioid agonist therapy compared with those who are not.
- Significant barriers including screening, linkage to care, disease knowledge, perceptions of poor candidacy, concerns about adherence, and unsubstantiated beliefs about reinfection remain.
- Because many persons on opioid agonist therapy continue to use drugs, we propose a strategy of treatment and cure-as-prevention is imperative to curb the hepatitis C epidemic.

Disclosure: A.H. Litwin has served on the advisory board of Abbvie, BMS, Gilead Sciences, and Merck. P.J. Zamor has served on the speakers bureau for Gilead, AbbVie, Merck, and Bristol Myers Squibb, and on the advisory board for Gilead, AbbVie, and Bristol Myers Squibb. M.J. Akiyama has been the recipient of a Gilead Investigator Sponsored Research Grant. B.L. Norton has no conflicts of interest. This review was funded in part by NIDA K23DA039060, NIDA K24DA036955, and NIDA R01 DA034086.

[a] Division of General Internal Medicine, Albert Einstein College of Medicine, Montefiore Medical Center, 3300 Kossuth Avenue, Bronx, NY 10467, USA; [b] Division of Hepatology, Carolinas Healthcare Systems, 1025 Morehead Medical Drive, Suite 600, Charlotte, NC 28204, USA
* Corresponding author.
E-mail address: bnorton@montefiore.org

Infect Dis Clin N Am 32 (2018) 347–370
https://doi.org/10.1016/j.idc.2018.02.001
0891-5520/18/© 2018 Elsevier Inc. All rights reserved.

id.theclinics.com

INTRODUCTION

Mortality from hepatitis C virus (HCV) infection has increased over the past 15 years and HCV now exceeds human immunodeficiency virus (HIV) as a cause of death in the United States.[1] Up to 4 million people in the Unites States are thought to be infected with HCV[2,3] and the true prevalence is likely to be even higher.[4] The risk of morbidity and mortality related to HCV infection is markedly decreased in patients who achieve a cure with antiviral therapy.[5,6]

Injection drug use is the most common route of transmission of HCV, particularly among younger people, where the incidence of HCV is increasing.[2,7] The prevalence of HCV in the United States among persons who inject drugs (PWIDs), both former and current PWID, is 70% to 77% resulting in a population of approximately 1.5 million PWIDs with HCV in the United States alone.[8] Between 2007 and 2012, reports of new HCV infection increased 50% nationally and 17 US states reported a 200% increase.[9] At least 70% of those infections are related to injection drug use among older adolescents and young adults. Globally, approximately 10 million PWIDs are thought to be infected with HCV.[8]

Opioid treatment programs (OTPs), such as methadone maintenance programs, provide opioid agonist therapy (OAT) to more than 300,000 opioid-dependent patients in the United States.[10] Buprenorphine is also widely prescribed for OAT, primarily outside of OTPs and in the outpatient medical setting. More than twice as many people are prescribed buprenorphine than methadone nationwide[11,12] and 9.3 million buprenorphine prescriptions were filled in the United States in 2012 alone.[13] Approximately 70% of patients on OAT are HCV antibody positive,[14–16] and many continue to use and inject drugs while in drug treatment.[17,18]

Although PWIDs carry the highest burden of HCV disease, few initiate treatment. HCV providers often exclude PWIDs owing to perception of poor candidacy and disappointing treatment outcomes, concerns about treatment adherence, or unsubstantiated beliefs about reinfection.[19–22] Patient barriers include limited HCV knowledge, competing life priorities owing to other comorbidities or to drug use, low perceived vulnerability from a disease without early symptoms, and fears of HCV treatment side effects.[23,24] PWIDs also cite the stigma and discomfort encountered in the health care setting, leading to poor self-efficacy and inability to navigate the health care system.[19,25] Furthermore, the majority of US states and health insurance companies have recently required varying durations of abstinence ranging from 1 to 12 months to approve prior authorization for direct-acting antiviral (DAA) HCV medications.[26]

Multiple models suggest that even a moderate increase in HCV treatment uptake and cure in PWIDs will reduce overall HCV prevalence, with potential HCV disease eradication.[27–29] Treatment guidelines do not exclude PWIDs from HCV treatment and, in fact, guidelines from the American Association for the Study of Liver Diseases and the Infectious Diseases Society of America recommend that HCV therapy must be considered for each individual, whether they are current users of illicit drugs or are on OAT.[4,30] Furthermore, HCV treatment outcomes are no different in people who use drugs compared with people who do not use drugs.[31,32] With the advent of highly effective, all-oral treatments for HCV infection, we review the current evidence-based approaches to the treatment of HCV in PWID (both current and former) who are taking OAT, a population that is already engaged in medical care and may be readily available to initiate HCV treatment.

EFFICACY OF HEPATITIS C VIRUS TREATMENT IN PATIENTS ON OPIOID AGONIST THERAPY

Before 2011, HCV was treated with a 24- or 48- week course of pegylated interferon (PegIFN) and ribavirin (RBV). In 2011, 2 HCV NS3/4A protease inhibitors, telaprevir and boceprevir, were approved for the treatment of HCV genotype (GT) 1 in combination with PegIFN/RBV after studies showed they improved sustained virologic response (SVR) rates in patients with HCV GT1 compared with PegIFN/RBV alone.[33,34] Clinical registration trials of these new DAA therapies have generally excluded or minimized entry of patients who are either active PWIDs or on OAT. However, cohort studies have shown that similar results can be achieved in these patient populations when compared with clinical trial results, which we outline below and are summarized in **Table 1**.

Pegylated Interferon and Ribavirin

In large clinical trials of PegIFN/RBV, patients infected with HCV GT1 achieved an SVR rate of around 42% to 46%, whereas approximately 76% to 82% of patients with HCV GT2/GT3 achieved SVR.[35,36] Studies of PegIFN/RBV in patients receiving OAT have demonstrated SVR rates of 36% to 45% in GT1 and 57% to 88% in GT2/G3, demonstrating that SVR rates are broadly comparable with those in clinical trials.[16,37–45] A number of studies have directly compared the efficacy of PegIFN/RBV in patients who are receiving OAT compared with those not on OAT and have also shown similar SVR rates between the 2 populations.[37,46,47]

Direct-Acting Antivirals

Post hoc analyses of phase II and III clinic trials
In the SPRINT-1 (Safety and Efficacy of Boceprevir in Previously Untreated Subjects With Chronic Hepatitis C Genotype 1), SPRINT-2, and RESPOND-2 (Retreatment with HCV Serine Protease Inhibitor Boceprevir and PegIntron/Rebetol 2) trials of boceprevir, 20 patients on methadone received PegIFN/RBV plus boceprevir and 4 received PegIFN/RBV plus placebo. In the boceprevir group, SVR rates were 50% in the 20 patients on methadone versus 63% in the 1528 patients not on methadone. In the placebo group, SVR rates were 25% in the 4 patients on methadone versus 37% in the 543 patients not on methadone.[48] Given the limited number of patients involved, it is difficult to draw conclusions from these data, but SVR rates were broadly comparable.[49]

Of all the patients treated with fixed dose sofosbuvir/ledipasvir in the 3 phase III ION trials (Efficacy and Safety of Ledipasvir/Sofosbuvir Fixed-Dose Combination for 12 Weeks in Subjects With Chronic Genotype 1 or 4 HCV and HIV-1 Co-infection), 70 received opioid replacement therapy (40 on methadone, 30 on buprenorphine with or without naloxone). In retrospective analyses, the mean SVR rate in patients not on OAT was 96.8% (1822 of 1882) and the mean SVR rate for patients on OAT was 94.3% (66 of 70). The overall cure rates were similar.[50]

Six patients on OAT (5 methadone and 1 naltrexone) were enrolled in the phase III ALLY-2 trial (A Phase 3 Study to Evaluate Combination Therapy With Daclatasvir and Sofosbuvir in the Treatment of HIV and Hepatitis C Virus Coinfection), which studied the combination of daclatasvir and sofosbuvir in HIV and HCV coinfected patients. All 6 patients on OAT achieved SVR with 12 weeks of combination therapy and there were no adverse events related to OAT, nor dose adjustments in OAT.

Data from the ASTRAL-1, -2, and -3 (Sofosbuvir/Velpatasvir Fixed Dose Combination for 12 Weeks in Adults With Chronic HCV Infection) trials, demonstrated that

Table 1
Published clinical studies evaluating HCV treatment outcomes among patients on OAT

Treatment Setting	Treatment	Overall SVR	GT1 SVR	GT2 or 3 SVR	Reference
Direct-acting antivirals					
Phase III, randomized, placebo-controlled, double-blind trial of treatment-naïve patients with HCV GT1, GT4, and GT6 who were ≥80% adherent to visits for OAT. ITG received 12 wk; DTG received placebo for 12 wk, 4-wk wash-out, then open-label treatment for 12 wk.	Elbasvir, grazoprevir (n = 301)	ITG: 91.5% DTG: 89.5%	ITG: 93.5% (GT1): 91.7% (GT4): 60% DTG: 90.6% (GT1): 100% (GT4): 50%	NA	Dore et al,[54] 2016
Phase II trial HCV GT1 patients on chronic methadone (n = 19) or buprenorphine (n = 19)	Ombitasvir, paritaprevir, ritonavir, and dasabuvir + weight-based RBV (n = 37)	97.4%	97.4%	NA	Lalezari et al,[52] 2015
Retrospective cohort study of patients treated in a community-based primary care clinic.	SOF, PegIFN, RBV(n = 18) SOF, RBV (n = 4) SOF, SIM (n = 22) SOF, LDV (n = 23)	96% OAT, drug use: 95% OAT, no drug use: 100% No OAT, drug use: 90% No OAT, no drug use: 95%	95% n = 84	G2: 100% G3: 100% G4: 100%	Norton et al,[59] 2017
PegIFN and ribavirin					
Metaanalysis of 36 studies; studies must include ≥10 people who use drugs treated for HCV	PegIFN, RBV (n = 2866)	55.5%	45% (GT1, GT4)	70%	Dimova et al,[38] 2013

Description	Treatment				Reference
Retrospective review of patient charts from an office-based OAT program run by a GP in Zurich, Switzerland. HCV medication was administered in the GP practice. Specialized care was available from hepatologists and psychiatrists within 3 of referral.	PeglFN, RBV (n = 35)	71%	74%	76% (GT3)	Seidenberg et al,[44] 2013
Two US OAT clinics with a colocated hepatitis clinic. Internist-addiction medicine specialist was the primary care provider for most patients, and provided HCV care under the supervision of a hepatologist.	PeglFN, RBV (n = 24)	54%	44%	66% (GT2) 100% (GT3)	Martinez et al,[16] 2012
Retrospective cohort study of a concurrent group treatment program at an OTP in New York offering comprehensive, integrated substance abuse treatment, medical and psychiatric care.	PeglFN, RBV (n = 27)	42%	44%	NR	Stein et al,[45] 2012
Nonrandomized, open-label study at 4 tertiary hospital hepatitis clinics in Australia. Patients were all receiving OAT.	PeglFN, RBV (n = 53)	57%	36%	71% (non-GT1)	Sasadeusz et al,[42] 2011
Patients under observed heroin maintenance therapy at German treatment centers received HCV treatment.	PeglFN, RBV (n = 26)	69%	42%	100% (GT2) 90% (GT3)	Schulte et al,[43] 2010
Observational UK study at a hospital-based infectious disease unit. All patients had HCV GT2/GT3. The study included 60 former drug users, the majority of whom were on OAT.	PeglFN, RBV (n = 125)	Nondrug users: 73% Former drug users: 73% (44/60) Active drug users: 40% (4/10)	NA	Nondrug users: 73% (91/125) Former drug users: 73% (44/60) Active drug users: 40% (4/10)	Alvarez-Uria et al,[37] 2009
Retrospective analysis of treatment outcomes at multiple OAT clinics in New York providing onsite HCV treatment. Treatment was administered by physicians and physician assistants trained in HCV care and following a standardized procedure developed with a hepatologist.	PeglFN, RBV (n = 73)	45%	40% (GT1/GT4)	75% (GT2) 36% (GT3)	Litwin et al,[41] 2009

(continued on next page)

Table 1
(continued)

Treatment Setting	Treatment	Overall SVR	GT1 SVR	GT2 or 3 SVR	Reference
A multicenter, randomized, controlled, prospective study in Austria of patients with GT2/GT3 HCV and on stable OAT. HCV therapy administered by a multidisciplinary team at an addiction clinic.	PegIFN, RBV (n = 17)	88%	NA	88%	Ebner et al,[39] 2009
Two Canadian clinics offering addiction services including OAT, syringe exchange, counseling, and onsite consultation with infectious disease specialists. Addiction specialist performed the initial HCV medical evaluation. Nurses administered weekly PegIFN injection and monitored adherence to RBV, which was self-administered; 53% of patients were on methadone.	PegIFN, RBV (n = 28) IFN, RBV (n = 12)	55% (PegIFN, RBV = 61%; IFN, RBV = 42%)	44%	64%	Grebely et al,[84] 2007
Patients on stable OAT without illicit drug use for 6 mo were prospectively matched with patients not on OAT without drug use and treated for HCV at German medical centers.	PegIFN, RBV (n = 100)	OAT: 42% Non-OAT: 56% (*P* = .16)	GT1/4: OAT: 38% Non-OAT: 55% (*P* = .59)	OAT: 48% Non-OAT: 57% (*P* = .76)	Mauss et al,[96] 2004

Abbreviations: DTG, deferred treatment group; GP, general practitioner; GT, genotype; ITG, immediate treatment group; NA, not applicable; NR, not reported; OAT, opioid agonist therapy; PegIFN, pegylated interferon; RBV, ribavirin; SIM, simeprevir; SOF, sofosbuvir; SVR, sustained virologic response.

sofosbuvir/velpatasvir was well-tolerated among patients on OAT. SVR was achieved by 49 of 51 patients (96%) on OAT and 966 of 984 patients (98%) not on OAT with similar adherence and adverse event profiles in both groups.[51]

Phase II and III clinical trials

Data from a phase II, multicenter, open-label, single-arm study in HCV GT1-infected patients on methadone or buprenorphine with or without naloxone who received 12 weeks of coformulated ombitasvir/paritaprevir/ritonavir and dasabuvir plus weight-based RBV has been published. This study enrolled 38 treatment-naïve or PegIFN/RBV treatment-experienced noncirrhotic patients with HCV GT1 infection who were on stable OAT with methadone (n = 19) or buprenorphine with or without naloxone (n = 19). SVR was achieved by 97% of patients[52] (37 of 38), which was similar to non-OAT patients treated with the same regimen in the phase II trial.[53] No changes to the dose of methadone or buprenorphine were required during the study in any patient.[52]

The phase III C-EDGE CO-STAR trial (A Phase III Randomized Clinical Trial to Study the Efficacy and Safety of the Combination Regimen of MK-5172/MK-8742 in Treatment-Naïve Subjects With Chronic HCV GT1, GT4, and GT6 Infection Who Are on Opiate Substitution Therapy) evaluated the efficacy and safety of the investigational once-daily tablet elbasvir/grazoprevir in patients with HCV GT1, GT4, or GT6 infection who were receiving OAT, the majority of whom were also currently using drugs. Ninety-four percent of patients (189 of 201) treated with elbasvir/grazoprevir for 12 weeks achieved cure, similar to cure rates in other large trials of elbasvir/grazoprevir in patients not on OAT. The use of nonprescribed illicit drugs, such as cocaine, amphetamines, marijuana, and other opiates, was observed in 59.2% of patients at baseline and remained steady throughout the trial; however, adherence to treatment was high and 97% of patients took at least 95% of their study medication over the 12 weeks of therapy. There were no adverse events related to OAT, and no dose adjustments to OAT while on HCV treatment were required.[54]

Real-world clinical data

There are many recent unpublished data (abstracts presented) that have evaluated the efficacy of DAAs in persons on OAT in both prospective clinical trials and retrospective cohort studies. The PREVAIL study was one of the first clinical trials to evaluate various models of care for DAA treatment onsite at a methadone clinic.[17] Persons were randomized to either individual onsite treatment, weekly group treatment, or directly observed therapy (DOT). SVR rates were high in all groups, with a trend toward better outcomes in the more supportive models of care (SVR rates of 90% [46 of 51] for individual, 98% [50 of 51] for DOT, and 96% [46 of 48] for group; $P = .76$). All patients were on OAT, and nearly one-half were also currently using drugs (49.3% [74 of 150] had a positive urine toxicology screen at baseline). Urine toxicology results were not associated with SVR rates ($P = .99$). In multiple retrospective real-world cohorts studies, SVR rates for patients on OAT have been high, ranging from 95% to 100%.[55–58] In all of these studies patients were treated for HCV onsite at the OTP, and in many cases, the clinicians used this unique setting to offer DOT. Another study treated patients for HCV onsite at a community-based primary care clinic. SVR rates were high for patients on OAT, and cure rates were similar to patients not on OAT (SVR rates of 97% [35 of 36] for patients on OAT, 95% [41 of 43] for those not on OAT; $P = .99$). The majority of patients (56%) on OAT were also currently using drugs.[59]

Addressing barriers to hepatitis C virus treatment in patients on opioid agonist therapy

Although SVR rates have been comparable for patients on OAT versus nondrug users, a low proportion of PWIDs ever initiate HCV treatment.[14,16] In 1 study comparing current opioid users with those without opioid dependence, 8.8% of patients with opioid use disorder initiated treatment compared with 18% of those without an opioid use disorder.[60] In general, studies show that linkage to HCV care and evaluation for PWIDs is poor, and that less than 10% of PWIDs who are evaluated for their HCV infection ever initiate antiviral therapy.[23,32] Furthermore, only 60% to 70% of patients at OTPs are offered screening for HCV.[41,61] Between 2003 and 2011, there was no significant change in the proportion of OTPs offering HCV screening, although the proportion of for-profit OTPs offering screening decreased and the proportion of nonprofit OTPs offering screening increased.[61] Factors associated with HCV screening for patients in substance abuse treatment were the provision of primary care at the OTP center (odds ratio, 3.18; 95% confidence interval [CI], 1.99–5.38), a hospital-affiliated setting (odds ratio, 2.56; 95% CI, 1.5–4.37), and a nonprofit/public setting (odds ratio, 1.79; 95% CI, 1.08–3.03).[62] Based on recommendations from the US Preventive Services Task Force, the Centers for Medicare & Medicaid Services covers a single HCV test for patients at high risk of infection (history of illicit injection drug use or blood transfusion before 1992) and for adults born between 1945 and 1965 who do not fall into the high-risk category. Annual testing for individuals who continue to inject drugs after a negative HCV test is also covered.[63] Given the nearly universal history of injection drug use at OTPs, HCV screening rates should reach nearly 100% in these setting, especially given the fact that the majority of patients accessing OTPs have insurance.

Another barrier to treatment lies in the fact that significant gaps in HCV knowledge have been identified among high-risk populations, including PWIDs. This lack of knowledge and misinformation hinders the ability of HCV-positive persons to appropriately interpret their disease and decreases their interest in care, potentially contributing to the persistently low uptake of HCV treatment in this population.[64] Therefore, patient education on HCV is critical to the success of implementing HCV screening and treatment at OTPs.[65] Studies have shown that improved HCV knowledge leads to an increased interest in HCV care, as well as adherence to an HCV specialty clinic appointment (64% adherence for patients who received education vs 39% adherence for patients without education; $P<.0001$).[66] Furthermore, education on HCV infection, treatment, side effects, and coping strategies was shown to improve SVR rates in patients on OAT infected with HCV GT1/GT4 who received PegIFN alfa-2a and ribavirin therapy (SVR of 76% vs 55% of patients without the education program; $P = .038$).[67] Recommendations for the management of HCV in PWIDs include pretherapeutic education on HCV transmission, risk factors for progression of fibrosis, HCV treatment regimens and side effects, reinfection, and harm reduction strategies.[68]

Failure to complete the evaluation process once linked to care, and physician-perceived patient risk factors as contraindications to therapy (such as drug use) have been among the most common reasons patients are not considered for HCV treatment.[69–71] Historically, liver biopsy has often been the greatest barrier to completing the evaluation process for HCV treatment owing to fear, payer complications, lack of transportation, and subspecialist reluctance to perform a liver biopsy on patients undergoing OAT.[15,16] It is vital that the extent and progression of liver fibrosis and cirrhosis be monitored and managed because the population of patients on OAT is aging and higher rates of cirrhosis can be expected. Guidelines published by American Association for the Study of Liver Diseases and the Infectious Diseases Society of

America support the noninvasive evaluation of liver fibrosis. Liver biopsies are now rare, which should further reduce the barrier to pretreatment staging among PWIDs and patients on OAT. Transient elastography or panels of fibrosis biomarkers (Aspartate Aminotransferase Platelet Ratio Index score, Fibrosis-4, or Fibrosure) are well-established for the assessment of liver fibrosis and should be used to increase the number of patients who can complete an assessment for treatment,[30,68] and patients should be specifically educated regarding the fact that biopsies are unnecessary for treatment initiation.

Fears that patients on OAT or active PWIDs may have low adherence to HCV therapy may also result in low HCV treatment rates. However, studies in the IFN era showed similar adherence in patients with and without a history of drug use.[42,47,72] In 1 study of 71 patients maintained on methadone and treated with PegIFN/RBV, intermittent drug users were similarly adherent to those strictly abstinent from illicit drugs.[73] In the era of DAAs, 1 study of 61 methadone maintained patients on sofosbuvir-based regimens showed that the mean weekly adherence by electronic monitors was 88% and mean adherence by visual analogue scale was 95%. SVR rates were similar to registration trials with sofosbuvir-based regimens.[74] Finally, the CO-EDGE C-STAR phase III trial of fixed-dose once daily grazoprevir/elbasvir enrolled only patients on OAT, of whom nearly 60% continued illicit drug use while on HCV treatment. All participants within that trial achieved greater than 80% adherence and 96.5% achieved greater than 95% adherence.[75]

Furthermore, current drug use is not a contraindication for HCV treatment.[76] In a metaanalysis of 36 studies of people who use drugs treated for HCV with PegIFN/RBV, 13 studies reported the number of patients who were current drug users and found that current drug use was not associated with treatment failure ($P = .76$).[38] In 1 study of PegIFN/RBV, persons with frequent drug use (n = 9) had a decreased SVR (22%) when compared with occasional drug use (n = 10 [80%]; $P = .12$), although this was not significant owing to the very low number of patients. This finding was mainly due to a higher rate of discontinuation in patients with frequent drug use (56%) than in those who did not use drugs or had occasional drug use (29%).[40] Discontinuations will likely be less, even for people with current drug use, in the in the era of DAAs where side effects are tremendously reduced and adherence to therapy is easier given once daily regimens. In the recent phase III trial of a grazoprevir/elbasvir coformulation, current illicit drug use during HCV treatment was common (59%), and the proportion of people who had positive urine drug screens remained consistent during the 12 weeks of therapy. The SVR rate was the same for people who had positive urine drug screens compared with those with consistently negative urine drug screens (95.5% and 95.4%, respectively).[18]

Another perceived barrier to treating former or active PWIDs is the fear of HCV reinfection after successful treatment if a patient returns to or continues active drug use. A thorough review focusing on reinfection in the era of interferon found that, although approximately one-half of patients return to active drug use after successful HCV treatment, reinfection rates among patients were low (1%–5%); this finding may be due to the development of partial protective immunity as well as use of harm reduction measures.[77] In the recent phase III trial of grazoprevir/elbasvir in patients on OAT, there were 6 probable reinfections out of the 301 patients after treatment completion (4.6 reinfections per 100 person-years). One-half of these patients (3 of 6) had spontaneous clearance of their reinfection. A study conducted in Norway specifically evaluated patients who continued to inject drugs after DAA treatment completion; reinfections rates were 4.9 per 100 person-years. Long-term follow-up studies are needed to improve our understanding of the impact of reinfection in the era of

DAAs. Even when considering a consistent rate of reinfection, models suggest that HCV treatment among people who are actively injecting drugs can still substantially decrease the prevalence of HCV.[28] Although we may initially see reinfection rates increase after treatment among PWID (owing to the increase in the number of people susceptible to infection), studies suggest that even a moderate scale-up of treatment among PWID will eventually reduce the pool of the infected, leading to a decrease in transmission and overall HCV prevalence.[78,79] Therefore, if we are to achieve HCV elimination, we must actively treat people who use drugs and expect to see some occurrence of reinfections. Patient care after successful treatment for HCV should take into account the possibility of a return to drug use and take measures to limit the risk of reinfection, such as education around harm reduction, referral to syringe exchange services, and cotreatment of drug-using partners and friends. Patients with continued risk factors should be screened with HCV RNA testing annually and, if reinfection occurs, patients should be tested for the possibility of a new HCV GT and baseline resistance. The limited risk of reinfection should not exclude PWIDs from receiving treatment for HCV,[68] especially because decreasing transmission and the overall prevalence of HCV requires specific attention to the treatment of people who are actively injecting drugs.

Models of care for hepatitis C virus therapy in patients on opioid agonist therapy

As reviewed recently by Bruggmann and Litwin,[80] the administration of HCV therapy to patients with a history of drug use can be managed under a number of different settings, including OAT clinics, primary care centers, or in specialty clinics. Management of therapy may also include delivery by DOT[71] or in conjunction with peer-based treatment support.[81] The key to successful HCV treatment in PWIDs is the availability of a multidisciplinary team, including substance abuse services, psychiatric treatment, and primary medical care.[68,80] A metaanalysis of 19 studies of PWIDs treated with PegIFN/RBV considered the effect of HCV GT, HIV coinfection, and the involvement of a multidisciplinary team on SVR. In a multivariate analysis, these investigators showed that involvement of a multidisciplinary team improved SVR rates ($P<.0001$) independent of any other factors.[38]

Provision of HCV screening, assessment, and therapy onsite at OTPs or in a primary care setting has many advantages. Screening of patients on OAT and people who are actively injecting drugs ensures that HCV infection is diagnosed quickly and targeted education programs can be initiated. Staff at OAT clinics are familiar with the needs of their patients, many of whom will have psychosocial needs not regularly encountered by HCV specialists at hospital-based HCV clinics. Furthermore, adherence to HCV therapy can be monitored if HCV therapies are administered with OAT in a DOT setting. Providing HCV-specific training to existing staff, teaching primary care providers how to deliver HCV treatment onsite in OTPs,[15,41] inviting outside specialists to administer HCV care at the OTP, or facilitating regular review of OTP patients by consultant hepatologists[80] are all methods in which to provide HCV care within OTP settings. Community-based primary care clinics can also be an ideal setting in which to provide HCV evaluation and care. A US-based study used telehealth technology to train primary care staff at 21 community-based or prison clinics to provide interferon-based HCV treatment, and ongoing support was delivered via weekly teleconferences with a multidisciplinary team of providers. The community-based and prison clinics achieved the same SVR rates as the hospital-based university HCV clinic (58%; $P = .9$).[82] In 1 study of patients receiving onsite HCV treatment at an urban primary care clinic, with support from an HCV care coordinator, there were no differences in cure rates for persons who use drugs (96%) compared with persons who do not use drugs (95%).[59] These methods could also be replicated for HCV treatment in OTP settings.

Group Treatment

Group treatment may also improve adherence and thereby SVR rates. In an OTP-based study of concurrent group treatment with PegIFN/RBV, during weekly meetings patients discussed adherence to medication and adverse events, received their PegIFN injection, and provided mutual support. More than one-half (15 of 27) of the patients had positive urine drug tests during treatment for opiates, cocaine, or both. The majority of patients (26 of the 27) opted to continue concurrent group treatment after the first 12 weeks of treatment, demonstrating the acceptability of this intervention.[45] In the PREVAIL study, persons on OAT were randomized to individual onsite treatment versus weekly group treatment versus or DOT. SVR rates were high in all groups, but there was a trend toward better outcomes in the more supportive models of care (SVR rates of 90% [46 of 51] for individual, 98% [50 of 51] for DOT, and 96% [46 of 48] for group; $P = .76$). In the OTP setting, there exists a unique opportunity to address HCV education, lack of support, and adherence concerns by conducting groups, a modality in which many PWID are familiar.

Directly Observed Therapy

In the IFN era, DOT demonstrated promising results in several models of care among drug users and individuals on OAT. Comparable rates of SVR were seen among active drug users using PegIFN given through DOT with self-administered RBV to those seen in clinical trials of nondrug users.[83,84] The administration of DOT by nursing and medical staff in a methadone maintenance clinic aided in addressing concurrent substance use and mental illness, and facilitated access to and completion of treatment.[85] Specialized outpatient drug treatment centers have also been used successfully to deliver DOT among methadone- and buprenorphine-maintained PWID receiving PegIFN through DOT.[86] Data on DOT in the era of DAAs are limited; however, in a prospective study of 61 PWID with chronic HCV treated with sofosbuvir-based regimens, pill count adherence was higher among those patients receiving DOT (77%) versus those treated in a group (70.7%) versus those treated by an individual provider (73.2%), but these differences were not statistically significant. SVR rates for the participants that received DOT was 100% (13 of 13); the overall SVR rates were 98% (60 of 61).[74] Again, in the PREVAIL study, persons SVR rates were high in all treatment arms, but there was a trend toward better outcomes in the more supportive models of care (SVR rates of 90% [46 of 51] for individual, 98% [50 of 51] for DOT, and 96% [46 of 48] for group; $P = .76$), particularly DOT. Given the unique setting of OTPs, where many patients are coming to the program multiple times a week, DOT for HCV treatment may be a viable and easy to implement treatment strategy.

Side Effect Management

Side effect management in the IFN era was complicated by nausea, insomnia, myalgia, irritability, and depression,[35,36] all similar to the symptoms of opioid withdrawal; however, the concern that these side effects could trigger resumption of drug use was not shown to be true.[87] Furthermore, a metaanalysis of 14 studies of PWIDs treated with PegIFN/RBV found no effect of psychiatric comorbidities on SVR ($P = .76$),[38] and the prescription of prophylactic or on-treatment antidepressants showed a decrease in IFN-related depression.[88] DAAs have much fewer side effects and are generally well-tolerated. Although there are few phase III studies specific to patients on OAT, the phase II trial with ombitasvir/paritaprevir/ritonavir and dasabuvir plus RBV in HCV GT1-infected patients on methadone or buprenorphine showed similar AE and discontinuation rates as patient not on OAT in phase II trials.[52] The most common adverse events were nausea, fatigue, and headache. Similarly, of the 70 patients on OAT in the ION-3 trial of sofosbuvir/ledipasvir treatment was safe and well-tolerated.[50] In the phase III trial of elbasvir/grazoprevir in patients on OAT using methadone or buprenorphine, adverse events were the same for patients on study drug versus placebo. The most common adverse events were fatigue (17%), headache (13%), nausea (10%), and diarrhea (9%).[54,75]

Pharmacokinetics Between Direct-Acting Antivirals and Opioid Agonist Therapy

Many DAAs have the potential to interact with methadone and buprenorphine through the metabolism, inhibition, and induction of the cytochrome P4503A enzyme.[89] Consequently, specific drug combinations have been noted to alter opioid drug levels. Despite common metabolic pathways, studies to date have shown no significant signs and symptoms of opioid withdrawal or toxicity that would preclude concurrent administration (**Table 2**).[90]

Patients on OAT or people who actively use drugs may also be receiving other medications for comorbid conditions such as HIV coinfection or depression. Careful attention must be given to both prescribed and nonprescribed drugs including antiretrovirals for HIV, antidepressants, antihypertensives, sedatives, statins, acid reducers, erectile dysfunction medications, anticonvulsants, and herbal remedies (especially St John's Wort and milk thistle). Interactions between these drugs and DAAs have been reviewed recently by Mauss and Klinker.[46]

Liver transplantation in patients on opioid agonist therapy

Once a patient with HCV-related cirrhosis develops decompensation (ascites, variceal bleeding, hepatic encephalopathy) and/or hepatocellular carcinoma, liver transplantation should be considered. Experience with liver transplantation in patients receiving OAT is extremely limited; however, liver transplantation is a therapeutic option for patients with a history of drug use and OAT is not a contraindication for transplantation.[68] Two case reports have demonstrated that the procedure can be successful in this population.[72,91] Of the 8 patients in these cases, all were former drug users (no active injection drug use for at least 5 years) and 2 received OAT.[72,91] Graft survival, patient survival, and rejection rates were similar in former injection drug users compared with non–injection drug users,[72] and of the 2 patients treated for HCV, 1 patient achieved SVR and remained infection-free at 4 years after transplant.[72,91] Although intraoperative anesthesia and postoperative analgesia can present a challenge in patients on OAT, collaboration with pain specialists can help to remove this as a barrier to care.[91]

Hepatitis C virus prevention and elimination

With the advent of new curative therapy, HCV elimination may be possible; however, this goal can only be achieved by focusing on HCV prevention and treatment among PWIDs, the key drivers of the HCV epidemic. Prevention of HCV requires appropriate screening among high-risk populations such as PWIDs, and the implementation of syringe exchange and OTPs, as well as an aggressive approach to HCV treatment as prevention. HCV testing to increase awareness of one's HCV status is crucial to educate persons about harm reduction measures, such as engaging in safer sex and reducing household sharing of razors and toothbrushes, as well as the abolition of sharing any drug paraphernalia (including needles, cookers, cotton, water, pipes, and nasal devices). One study in Australia estimated that syringe exchange programs directly averted 50% of new HCV infections (97,000) during 2000 to 2009.[14]

Table 2
Drug interactions between methadone or buprenorphine and DAAs

DAA	Methadone	Buprenorphine (Naloxone)	Symptoms of Withdrawal	Treatment Recommendation	Reference
Telaprevir	R-methadone C_{max}: 0.71 (0.66–0.76) AUC: 0.71 (0.66–0.76) S-methadone C_{max}: 0.65 (0.60–0.71) AUC: 0.64 (0.58–0.70)	Buprenorphine C_{max}: 0.80 (0.69, 0.93) AUC: 0.96 (0.84, 1.10) Norbuprenorphine C_{max}: 0.85 (0.66, 1.09) AUC: 0.91 (0.71, 1.16)	No difference in symptoms between opioid alone or opioid with telaprevir as measured by SOWS	No dose adjustment	Luo et al,[97] 2012; Van Heeswijk et al,[98] 2013
Boceprevir	R-methadone C_{max}: 0.90 (0.71–1.13) AUC: 0.85 (0.74–0.96) S-methadone C_{max}: 0.83 (0.64–1.09) AUC: 0.78 (0.66–0.93)	Buprenorphine C_{max}: 1.18 (0.93–1.50) AUC: 1.19 (0.91–1.57) Norbuprenorphine C_{max}: 0.54 (0.36–0.83) AUC: 0.55 (0.36–0.86)	No evidence of opioid withdrawal or opioid excess, measured by SOWS	No dose adjustment	Hulskotte et al,[99] 2015
Simeprevir	R-methadone C_{max}: 1.03 (0.97–1.09) AUC: 0.99 (0.91–1.09) S-methadone C_{max} AUC: unchanged, data not reported	No data	No data		Ouwerkerk-Mahadevan et al,[100] 2016
Sofosbuvir	R-Methadone C_{max}: 0.99 (0.85–1.16) AUC: 1.01 (0.85–1.22) S-Methadone C_{max}: 0.95 (0.79–1.13) AUC: 0.95 (0.77–1.17)	No data	None as measured by DDQ, SOWS, or pupil diameter	No dose adjustment	Denning et al,[101] 2011
Sofosbuvir, ledipasvir	No PK data	No PK data	No difference in pooled Phase 2/3 data for CNS adverse events for patients on methadone vs not on methadone	No dose adjustment	German et al,[102] 2014

(continued on next page)

Table 2
(continued)

DAA	Methadone	Buprenorphine (Naloxone)	Symptoms of Withdrawal	Treatment Recommendation	Reference
Ombitasvir, paritaprevir, ritonavir, and dasabuvir	R-Methadone C_{max}: 1.04 (0.98–1.11) AUC: 1.05 (0.98–1.11) S-Methadone C_{max}: 0.99 (0.91–1.08) AUC: 0.99 (0.89–1.09)	Buprenorphine C_{max}: 2.18 (1.78, 2.68) AUC: 2.07 (1.78, 2.40) Norbuprenorphine C_{max}: 2.07 (1.42, 3.01) AUC: 1.84 (1.30, 2.60)	No difference in pupil diameter, SOWS, or DDQ score between opioid alone or opioid with HCV regimen	No dose adjustment. Monitor for increased sedation for patients on buprenorphine given increase in C_{max} AUC	Menon et al,[103] 2015
Daclatasvir	R-Methadone C_{max}: 1.07(0.97–1.18) AUC: 1.08 (0.94–1.24) S-Methadone C_{max}: 0.95 (0.79–1.13) AUC: 0.95 (0.77–1.17)	Buprenorphine C_{max}: 1.30 (1.03–1.64) AUC: 1.37 (1.24–1.52) Norbuprenorphine C_{max}: 1.65 (1.38–1.99) AUC: 1.62 (1.30–2.02)	No effect on opioid withdrawal or toxicity scores measured by COW and OOA	No dose adjustment	Garimella et al,[104] 2015
Grazoprevir	R-Methadone C_{max}: 1.03 (0.96–1.11) AUC: 1.09 (1.02–1.17) S-Methadone C_{max}: 1.15 (1.07, 1.25) AUC: 1.23 (1.12–1.35)	Buprenorphine C_{max}: 0.90 (0.76–1.07) AUC: 0.98 (0.81–1.19) Norbuprenorphine C_{max}: 1.10 (0.97–1.25) AUC: 1.13 (0.97–1.32)	No symptoms or signs of toxicity or withdrawal in clinical trials	No dose adjustment	Fraser et al,[105] 2013
Elbasvir	R-Methadone C_{max}: 1.07 (0.95–1.20) AUC: 1.03 (0.92–1.15) S-Methadone C_{max}: 1.09 (0.95–1.25) AUC: 1.09 (0.94–1.26)	Buprenorphine C_{max}: 0.94 (0.82–1.08) AUC: 0.98 (0.89–1.08) Norbuprenorphine No data	No symptoms or signs of toxicity or withdrawal in clinical trials	No dose adjustment	Marshall et al,[106,107] 2013
Velpatasvir	No PK data	No PK data	No symptoms or signs of toxicity or withdrawal in clinical trials	No dose adjustment	Grebely et al,[51,108] 2016

Abbreviations: AUC, area under the curve; C_{max}, maximum concentration; CNS, central nervous system; DAA, direct-acting antiviral; DDQ, desire for drugs questionnaire; NA, not available; OOA, opioid overdose assessment; PK, pharmacokinetic; SOWS, subjective opiate withdrawal scale clinical opiate withdrawal scale.

Furthermore, participation in methadone maintenance has been shown to significantly lower the rate of risky injecting and sexual behavior among PWIDs. In 1 study, the estimated cumulative incidence of HCV per 100 PWIDs per year before methadone maintenance participation was 36.48 (95% CI, 25.84 - 47.11), compared with 13.84 (95% CI, 6.17–21.51) after methadone maintenance participation, potentially averting 22.64 (95% CI, 19.67–25.6) new HCV infections per 100 PWIDs per year.[92] There is much evidence to support the combination of both these harm reduction approaches, and modeling studies have shown that, in a setting where the HCV prevalence is 40%, scaling up opioid substitution therapy and needle exchange coverage can decrease the HCV prevalence over 10 years by up to one-third.[93] Making these programs available to the rapidly growing population of young PWIDs is of particular importance because this population has been shown to be a key driver of new infections in the United States. HCV cure as prevention will also be an important component to HCV prevention and eradication. Given the new highly effective and easy-to-use HCV regimens, reducing the prevalence of disease through aggressive treatment stands to reduce rates of new infections. This point is particularly important for populations a with high prevalence and incidence, such as PWIDs. For a PWID population that starts with an HCV prevalence of 65%, minimal scale-up of treatment to 98 per 1000 PWIDs annually could significantly reduce the HCV prevalence by 75% within 15 years.[79] Because the near majority of patients on OAT continue to use and inject drugs,[17,54,94] HCV care and treatment in OTPs where PWID are already engaged in medical care is crucial to HCV elimination efforts. Reducing the incidence and prevalence of HCV with potential for elimination is possible, but a strategy of seek, test, treat, and cure, particularly among PWIDs, must be adopted.

Scale-up to 22, 54, or 98 per 1000 PWID annually could reduce prevalence by three-quarters within 15 years.

SUMMARY

The majority of new HCV infections in the United States are transmitted via injection drug use and the prevalence of HCV in current and former PWID is high. The incidence of new infections is particularly high among young PWID.[95] However, data on HCV treatment in the era of DAAs are limited for patients on OAT and for active PWID, and more research is needed regarding the optimal models of care for increasing diagnosis, treatment uptake, adherence, and completion, and rates of SVR. Young suburban and rural PWIDs, a growing population, must have access to syringe exchange and OAT to prevent acquisition and transmission of HCV, and novel approaches are needed to engage them in HCV care and treatment.

Although new DAA medications promise high HCV cure rates, few PWIDs initiate treatment, even when they are engaged in OAT.[14,16] Despite a number of barriers to HCV treatment for this population, both real and perceived, HCV can be successfully cured in patients on OAT and active PWIDs, and data suggest that similar cure rates are achieved by patients on OAT compared with those not on OAT in the era of DAAs. Measures should be taken to improve the uptake and success of treatment in this population.

Universal HCV screening should be implemented at OAT programs, substance abuse clinics, and primary care clinics that treat patients with substance abuse disorders. HCV patient education can help to improve patients' understanding of the risk of HCV to their health, dispel myths about HCV medications, and encourage harm reduction to reduce risk of transmission. IFN-free and RBV-free regimens carry a lower burden of adverse events, and can be dosed as once-daily regimens. Such regimens are more amenable to prescription and monitoring by nonspecialists than PegIFN/RBV-based regimens, which allows the opportunity to treat PWIDs within their primary care medical homes, and where they receive OAT. Providing care to patients via multi-disciplinary teams of physicians, nurses, psychiatrists, and addiction counselors trained in HCV care, and with the close support of HCV providers, results in the best treatment outcomes and has been established at a number of OAT clinics and primary care centers treating some of the most underserved patients in the United States, Canada, Europe, and Australia. Successful implementation of new HCV therapy for a population that carries one of the highest burdens of infection should be a goal of all health care providers involved in the treatment of HCV and/or drug addiction. It is only through aggressive treatment of PWIDs that we will reduce the morbidity and mortality of this disease, with the potential for elimination.

HCV care recommendations for patients receiving opioid replacement therapy

Screening and prevention: Mandatory HCV antibody screening of all patients accessing OTPs and yearly screening of patients who currently use drugs.
- Onsite HCV RNA testing to confirm chronic HCV is best; reflex testing where possible.
- If confirmation with an HCV viral load cannot be performed, HCV antibody–positive patients should be referred to a clinic where HCV RNA measurement can be done.
  - Case managers, patient navigators, or peer escorts may facilitate adherence to follow-up visits.
- All HCV antibody–negative patients should be counseled to prevent future HCV infection. Patients should be advised not to share syringe, cooker, cotton, or rinse water.
- Patients should be referred to harm reduction and syringe exchange programs as necessary.
- Clinical registries should be created to ensure that case management is provided for patients with HCV who are not currently engaging in care.

Education: Provide patient education on HCV transmission, risk factors for progression of fibrosis, HCV medication, adherence, reinfection, and harm reduction strategies to HCV-positive patients on OAT and/or who actively use drugs.
- All medical staff and substance use counselors should receive basic HCV-related education.
- HCV-related literature should be available to patients on site.

Make regular HCV support groups available onsite
- Ideally, support groups should be cofacilitated by staff members (medical or nonmedical) and patients.
- Onsite HCV peer programs for patients who cofacilitate support groups should be considered.

Provide education on substance use disorders and provide community-based drug treatment resources to HCV specialists such as hepatology and infectious diseases physicians.
- Efforts must be undertaken to reduce the shame and stigma of substance use, opiate agonist treatment, and HCV, all of which are barriers to engaging HCV-infected patients in care.

Staging: Primary care and drug treatment providers not providing onsite HCV treatment must still have a basic understanding of HCV evaluation and management to help facilitate appropriate off-site care.
- Liver biopsies are not necessary to stage liver disease. Patients should be made aware of this.
- Use noninvasive staging methods such as the Aspartate Aminotransferase Platelet Ratio Index or Fibrosis-4 (readily available with basic laboratory tests including aspartate aminotransferase, alanine aminotransferase, and platelets) to determine advanced fibrosis and cirrhosis to increase the completion of disease assessment in patients on OAT and people who are currently using drugs.
- An attempt should be made to engage all patients with HCV in care, however if the Aspartate Aminotransferase Platelet Ratio Index score is greater than 2 or the Fibrosis-4 score is greater than 3.25, patients need to be educated about the possibility of cirrhosis and a more active process must be in place to get these patients into treatment.

Linkage to HCV treatment: Provide care and treatment via multidisciplinary teams, including HCV providers (practitioners with expertise in HCV treatment, which may include hepatology, gastroenterology, infectious diseases, and/or trained primary care providers), addiction specialists and addiction counselors, psychiatric services, and social support (including peer support groups if available).
- Use telemedicine to more readily facilitate these team efforts.
- Establish working relationship with HCV providers and communicate with HCV providers in real-time if issues arise (eg, side effects or insurance problems that may lead to loss of access to medications).

Linkage to HCV provider will be key for off-site treatment
- Establish a working relationship with an HCV provider who understands this patient population.
- Use case management and peers to support linkage.
- Peer accompaniment to appointments can be beneficial.

Encourage patients who are currently using drugs to start substance use treatment because HCV treatment in conjunction with addiction treatment improves the rates of treatment completion.
- Do not withhold HCV treatment from patients who defer substance use treatment.
- Patients who are currently using drugs can be successfully treated for HCV and should be considered for treatment on a case-by-case basis. Motivation and engagement should help to decide about treatment readiness, not patterns of drug use.

Onsite HCV treatment: Consider establishing onsite treatment at OTP or primary care clinics with OAT.
- Evaluate HCV infection and treatment options by following an established protocol based on the latest established HCV guidelines. Use hcvguidlines.org as a resource.
- All DAAs can be used in patients on OAT without dose alterations and there are data to support the efficacy and safety of these regimens in this specific population.
- Consider all medications taken by each patient to assess drug–drug interactions with DAAs.
- For those with cirrhosis, HCC screening every 6 months with ultrasound examination and refer to gastroenterology for upper endoscopy to screen for varices.
- Establish a community of HCV providers to discuss issues as they arise, for example, side effect management, drug–drug interactions, and so on.
- Refer to HCV specialists for treating complicated cases (eg, autoimmune hepatitis; decompensated cirrhosis; any case that provider is not comfortable with).

Train nonmedical staff at OTPs to administer HCV therapy in DOT at methadone pickup window and monitor patients for side effects.
- Substance abuse counselors should know the HCV status of each patient and be able to provide basic HCV-related case management, and know what services are available on site.
- Substance abuse counselors should be able to identify lapse or relapse to drug and/or alcohol use and provide support; help with adherence to HCV visits and medications; and be aware of emerging psychiatric conditions while patients are on HCV therapy

REFERENCES

1. Ly KN, Xing J, Klevens RM, et al. The increasing burden of mortality from viral hepatitis in the United States between 1999 and 2007. Ann Intern Med 2012; 156(4):271–8.

2. Armstrong GL, Wasley A, Simard EP, et al. The prevalence of hepatitis C virus infection in the United States, 1999 through 2002. Ann Intern Med 2006; 144(10):705–14.

3. Kanwal F, Hoang T, Kramer JR, et al. Increasing prevalence of HCC and cirrhosis in patients with chronic hepatitis C virus infection. Gastroenterology 2011;140(4):1182–8.e1.

4. Chak E, Talal AH, Sherman KE, et al. Hepatitis C virus infection in USA: an estimate of true prevalence. Liver Int 2011;31(8):1090–101.
5. Backus LI, Boothroyd DB, Phillips BR, et al. A sustained virologic response reduces risk of all-cause mortality in patients with hepatitis C. Clin Gastroenterol Hepatol 2011;9(6):509–16.e1.
6. van der Meer AJ, Veldt BJ, Feld JJ, et al. Association between sustained virological response and all-cause mortality among patients with chronic hepatitis C and advanced hepatic fibrosis. Jama 2012;308(24):2584–93.
7. Chatterjee S, Tempalski B, Pouget ER, et al. Changes in the prevalence of injection drug use among adolescents and young adults in large U.S. metropolitan areas. AIDS Behav 2011;15(7):1570–8.
8. Nelson PK, Mathers BM, Cowie B, et al. Global epidemiology of hepatitis B and hepatitis C in people who inject drugs: results of systematic reviews. Lancet 2011;378(9791):571–83.
9. Suryaprasad AG, White JZ, Xu F, et al. Emerging epidemic of hepatitis C virus infections among young nonurban persons who inject drugs in the United States, 2006-2012. Clin Infect Dis 2014;59(10):1411–9.
10. Substance Abuse and Mental Health Services Administration (SAMHSA). National Survey of substance abuse treatment services (N-SSATS): 2012. Data on substance abuse treatment facilities. Rockville (MD): Substance Abuse and Mental Health Services Administration; 2013.
11. Maxwell JC, McCance-Katz EF. Indicators of buprenorphine and methadone use and abuse: what do we know? Am J Addict 2010;19(1):73–88.
12. Kresina TF, Litwin AH, Marion I, et al. United States government oversight and regulation of medication assisted treatment for the treatment of opioid dependence. J Drug Policy Anal 2009;2(1):1941–2851.
13. Drug Enforcement Administration (DEA). Buprenorphine. Drug Enforcement Administration Office of Diversion Control. 2013.
14. Harris KA Jr, Arnsten JH, Litwin AH. Successful integration of hepatitis C evaluation and treatment services with methadone maintenance. J Addict Med 2010; 4(1):20–6.
15. Litwin AH, Soloway I, Gourevitch MN. Integrating services for injection drug users infected with hepatitis C virus with methadone maintenance treatment: challenges and opportunities. Clin Infect Dis 2005;40(Suppl 5):S339–45.
16. Martinez AD, Dimova R, Marks KM, et al. Integrated internist - addiction medicine - hepatology model for hepatitis C management for individuals on methadone maintenance. J Viral Hepat 2012;19(1):47–54.
17. Litwin AH, Agyemang L, Akiyama M, et al. The PREVAIL study: intensive models of HCV care for people who inject drugs the International Liver Congress™. Amsterdam: European Association for the Study of the Liver (EASL); 2017.
18. Dore GJ, Altice F, Litwin AH, et al. Elbasvir-Grazoprevir to treat hepatitis C virus infection in persons receiving opioid agonist therapy: A randomized trial. Annals of internal medicine 2016;165:625–34.
19. Treloar C, Newland J, Rance J, et al. Uptake and delivery of hepatitis C treatment in opiate substitution treatment: perceptions of clients and health professionals. J Viral Hepat 2010;17(12):839–44.
20. Edlin BR, Seal KH, Lorvick J, et al. Is it justifiable to withhold treatment for hepatitis C from illicit-drug users? N Engl J Med 2001;345(3):211–5.
21. Astone JM, Strauss SM, Hagan H, et al. Outpatient drug treatment program directors' hepatitis C-related beliefs and their relationship to the provision of HCV services. Am J Drug Alcohol Abuse 2004;30(4):783–97.

22. Davis GL, Rodrigue JR. Treatment of chronic hepatitis C in active drug users. N Engl J Med 2001;345(3):215–7.

23. Mehta SH, Genberg BL, Astemborski J, et al. Limited uptake of hepatitis C treatment among injection drug users. J Community Health 2008;33(3):126–33.

24. Grebely J, Genoway KA, Raffa JD, et al. Barriers associated with the treatment of hepatitis C virus infection among illicit drug users. Drug Alcohol Depend 2008;93(1–2):141–7.

25. Treloar C, Rance J, Backmund M. Understanding barriers to hepatitis C virus care and stigmatization from a social perspective. Clin Infect Dis 2013; 57(Suppl 2):S51–5.

26. Barua S, Greenwald R, Grebely J, et al. Restrictions for Medicaid reimbursement of sofosbuvir for the treatment of hepatitis C virus infection in the United States. Ann Intern Med 2015;163(3):215–23.

27. Hellard M, Doyle JS, Sacks-Davis R, et al. Eradication of hepatitis C infection: the importance of targeting people who inject drugs. Hepatology 2014;59(2): 366–9.

28. Martin NK, Vickerman P, Foster GR, et al. Can antiviral therapy for hepatitis C reduce the prevalence of HCV among injecting drug user populations? A modeling analysis of its prevention utility. J Hepatol 2011;54(6):1137–44.

29. Hagan LM, Schinazi RF. Best strategies for global HCV eradication. Liver Int 2013;33(Suppl 1):68–79.

30. American Association for the Study of Liver Diseases, Infectious Diseases Society of America. Recommendations for testing, managing, and treating hepatitis C. 2014. Available at: http://www.hcvguidelines.org/. Accessed March 21, 2018.

31. Aspinall EJ, Corson S, Doyle JS, et al. Treatment of hepatitis C virus infection among people who are actively injecting drugs: a systematic review and meta-analysis. Clin Infect Dis 2013;57(Suppl 2):S80–9.

32. Hellard M, Sacks-Davis R, Gold J. Hepatitis C treatment for injection drug users: a review of the available evidence. Clin Infect Dis 2009;49(4):561–73.

33. Merck & Co. VICTRELIS (boceprevir) highlights of US prescribing information. 2013.

34. Incorporated VP. INCIVEK (telaprevir) highlights of US prescribing information. 2013.

35. Fried MW, Shiffman ML, Reddy KR, et al. Peginterferon alfa-2a plus ribavirin for chronic hepatitis C virus infection. N Engl J Med 2002;347(13):975–82.

36. Manns MP, McHutchison JG, Gordon SC, et al. Peginterferon alfa-2b plus ribavirin compared with interferon alfa-2b plus ribavirin for initial treatment of chronic hepatitis C: a randomised trial. Lancet 2001;358(9286):958–65.

37. Alvarez-Uria G, Day JN, Nasir AJ, et al. Factors associated with treatment failure of patients with psychiatric diseases and injecting drug users in the treatment of genotype 2 or 3 hepatitis C chronic infection. Liver Int 2009;29(7):1051–5.

38. Dimova RB, Zeremski M, Jacobson IM, et al. Determinants of hepatitis C virus treatment completion and efficacy in drug users assessed by meta-analysis. Clin Infect Dis 2013;56(6):806–16.

39. Ebner N, Wanner C, Winklbaur B, et al. Retention rate and side effects in a prospective trial on hepatitis C treatment with pegylated interferon alpha-2a and ribavirin in opioid-dependent patients. Addict Biol 2009;14(2):227–37.

40. Grebely J, Raffa JD, Meagher C, et al. Directly observed therapy for the treatment of hepatitis C virus infection in current and former injection drug users. J Gastroenterol Hepatol 2007;22(9):1519–25.

41. Litwin AH, Harris KA Jr, Nahvi S, et al. Successful treatment of chronic hepatitis C with pegylated interferon in combination with ribavirin in a methadone maintenance treatment program. J Subst Abuse Treat 2009;37(1):32–40.

42. Sasadeusz JJ, Dore G, Kronborg I, et al. Clinical experience with the treatment of hepatitis C infection in patients on opioid pharmacotherapy. Addiction 2011; 106(5):977–84.

43. Schulte B, Schutt S, Brack J, et al. Successful treatment of chronic hepatitis C virus infection in severely opioid-dependent patients under heroin maintenance. Drug Alcohol Depend 2010;109(1–3):248–51.

44. Seidenberg A, Rosemann T, Senn O. Patients receiving opioid maintenance treatment in primary care: successful chronic hepatitis C care in a real world setting. BMC Infect Dis 2013;13:9.

45. Stein MR, Soloway IJ, Jefferson KS, et al. Concurrent group treatment for hepatitis C: implementation and outcomes in a methadone maintenance treatment program. J substance abuse Treat 2012;43(4):424–32.

46. Mauss S, Klinker H. Drug-drug interactions in the treatment of HCV among people who inject drugs. Clin Infect Dis 2013;57(Suppl 2):S125–8.

47. Melin P, Chousterman M, Fontanges T, et al. Effectiveness of chronic hepatitis C treatment in drug users in routine clinical practice: results of a prospective cohort study. Eur J Gastroenterol Hepatol 2010;22(9):1050–7.

48. Poordad F, Lawitz E, Gordon S, et al. Concomitant medication use (drug interactions) in patients with hepatitis C genotype 1 treated with boceprevir combination therapy [Abstract]. The American Association for the Study of Liver Diseases 62nd Annual Meeting 2011, San Francisco; Nov 6-9. 2011.

49. Litwin AH. Triple therapy in opiate addicts – first results in the United States. Amsterdam: European Association for the Study of the Liver; 2013.

50. Grebely J, Mauss S, Brown A, et al. Efficacy and safety of ledipasvir/sofosbuvir with and without ribavirin in patients with chronic HCV genotype 1 infection receiving opioid substitution therapy: analysis of phase 3 ION trials. Clin Infect Dis 2016;63(11):1405–11.

51. Grebely J, Dore GJ, Zeuzem S, et al. Efficacy and safety of sofosbuvir/velpatasvir in patients with chronic hepatitis C virus infection receiving opioid substitution therapy: analysis of phase 3 ASTRAL trials. Clin Infect Dis 2016; 63(11):1479–81.

52. Lalezari J, Sullivan JG, Varunok P, et al. Ombitasvir/paritaprevir/r and dasabuvir plus ribavirin in HCV genotype 1-infected patients on methadone or buprenorphine. J Hepatol 2015;63(2):364–9.

53. Kowdley KV, Lawitz E, Poordad F, et al. Phase 2b trial of interferon-free therapy for hepatitis C virus genotype 1. N Engl J Med 2014;370(3):222–32.

54. Dore GJ, Altice F, Litwin AH, et al. Elbasvir-grazoprevir to treat hepatitis C virus infection in persons receiving opioid agonist therapy: a randomized trial. Ann Intern Med 2016;165(9):625–34.

55. Schütz A, Moser S, Marchart K, et al. Direct observed therapy of chronic hepatitis C with interferon-free all-oral regimens at a low-threshold drug treatment facility-a new concept for treatment of patients with borderline compliance receiving opioid substitution therapy. Am J Gastroenterol 2016;111:903–5.

56. Scherz N, Brunner N, Bruggmann P. Direct-acting antivirals for hepatitis C in patient in opioid substitution treatment and heroin assisted treatment: real-life data. J Hepatol 2017;66:S726.

57. Boyle A. Partial directly observed therapy with ombitasvir/paritaprevir based regimens allows for successful treatment of patients on daily supervised methadone. J Hepatol 2017;66:S282.

58. Moser S. Directly observed therapy with sofosbuvir/ledipasvir for 8 weeks is highly effective in treatment-naïve, precirrhotic genotype 1 patients with borderline compliance receiving opioid agonist therapy. J Hepatol 2017;66:S740.

59. Norton BL, Fleming J, Steinman M, et al. High HCV cure rates for drug users treated with DAAs at an urban primary care clinic. Boston: CROI; 2016.

60. Perut V, Labalette C, Sogni P, et al. Access to care of patients with chronic hepatitis C virus infection in a university hospital: is opioid dependence a limiting condition? Drug and alcohol dependence 2009;104(1–2):78–83.

61. Bachhuber MA, Cunningham CO. Changes in testing for human immunodeficiency virus, sexually transmitted infections, and hepatitis C virus in opioid treatment programs. JAMA 2013;310(24):2671–2.

62. Litwin AH, Kunins HV, Berg KM, et al. Hepatitis C management by addiction medicine physicians: results from a national survey. J substance abuse Treat 2007;33(1):99–105.

63. Centers for Medicare and Medicaid Services (CMS). Proposed decision memo for screening for hepatitis C virus (HCV) in adults (CAG-00436N). 2014. Available at: http://www.cms.gov/medicare-coverage-database/details/nca-proposed-decision-memo.aspx?NCAId=272 2014. Accessed on March 27, 2014.

64. Norton BL, Park L, McGrath LJ, et al. Health care utilization in HIV-infected patients: assessing the burden of hepatitis C virus coinfection. AIDS Patient Care STDS 2012;26(9):541–5.

65. Talal AH, Dimova RB, Seewald R, et al. Assessment of methadone clinic staff attitudes toward hepatitis C evaluation and treatment. J substance abuse Treat 2013;44(1):115–9.

66. Surjadi M, Torruellas C, Ayala C, et al. Formal patient education improves patient knowledge of hepatitis C in vulnerable populations. Dig Dis Sci 2011;56(1):213–9.

67. Reimer J, Schmidt CS, Schulte B, et al. Psychoeducation improves hepatitis C virus treatment during opioid substitution therapy: a controlled, prospective multicenter trial. Clin Infect Dis 2013;57(Suppl 2):S97–104.

68. Robaeys G, Grebely J, Mauss S, et al. Recommendations for the management of hepatitis C virus infection among people who inject drugs. Clin Infect Dis 2013;57(Suppl 2):S129–37.

69. Batki SL, Canfield KM, Ploutz-Snyder R. Psychiatric and substance use disorders among methadone maintenance patients with chronic hepatitis C infection: effects on eligibility for hepatitis C treatment. The Am J Addict 2011;20(4):312–8.

70. Batki SL, Canfield KM, Smyth E, et al. Hepatitis C treatment eligibility and comorbid medical illness in methadone maintenance (MMT) and non-MMT patients: a case-control study. J Addict Dis 2010;29(3):359–69.

71. Litwin AH, Berg KM, Li X, et al. Rationale and design of a randomized controlled trial of directly observed hepatitis C treatment delivered in methadone clinics. BMC Infect Dis 2011;11:315.

72. Robaeys G, Nevens F, Starkel P, et al. Previous intravenous substance use and outcome of liver transplantation in patients with chronic hepatitis C infection. Transplant Proc 2009;41(2):589–94.

73. Sylvestre DL, Clements BJ. Adherence to hepatitis C treatment in recovering heroin users maintained on methadone. Eur J Gastroenterol Hepatol 2007; 19(9):741–7.

74. Litwin A, Yu K, Wong J, et al. High rates of sustained virological response in people who inject drugs treated with sofosbuvir-based regimens. 4th International Symposium on Hepatitis Care in Substance Users; 2015; Sydney.

75. Dore G, Grebely J, Altice F, et al. Adherence and drug use in HCV-infected persons who inject drugs (PWID) on Opioid Agonist Therapy (OAT) receiving Grazoprevir + Elbasvir (GZR/EBR) Fixed Dose Combination (FDC) for 12 Weeks. 4th International Symposium on Hepatitis Care in Substance Users; 2015; Sydney.

76. Ghany MG, Strader DB, Thomas DL, et al. Diagnosis, management, and treatment of hepatitis C: an update. Hepatology 2009;49(4):1335–74.

77. Grady BP, Schinkel J, Thomas XV, et al. Hepatitis C virus reinfection following treatment among people who use drugs. Clin Infect Dis 2013;57(Suppl 2): S105–10.

78. Grebely J, Hajarizadeh B, Dore GJ. Direct-acting antiviral agents for HCV infection affecting people who inject drugs. Nat Rev Gastroenterol Hepatol 2017; 14(11):641–51.

79. Martin NK, Vickerman P, Grebely J, et al. Hepatitis C virus treatment for prevention among people who inject drugs: modeling treatment scale-up in the age of direct-acting antivirals. Hepatology 2013;58(5):1598–609.

80. Bruggmann P, Litwin AH. Models of care for the management of hepatitis C virus among people who inject drugs: one size does not fit all. Clin Infect Dis 2013; 57(Suppl 2):S56–61.

81. Roose RJ, Cockerham-Colas L, Soloway I, et al. Reducing barriers to hepatitis C treatment among drug users: an integrated hepatitis C peer education and support program. J Health Care Poor Underserved 2014;25(2):652–62.

82. Arora S, Thornton K, Murata G, et al. Outcomes of treatment for hepatitis C virus infection by primary care providers. N Engl J Med 2011;364(23):2199–207.

83. Hilsden RJ, Macphail G, Grebely J, et al. Directly observed pegylated interferon plus self-administered ribavirin for the treatment of hepatitis C virus infection in people actively using drugs: a randomized controlled trial. Clin Infect Dis 2013; 57(Suppl 2):S90–6.

84. Grebely J, Genoway K, Khara M, et al. Treatment uptake and outcomes among current and former injection drug users receiving directly observed therapy within a multidisciplinary group model for the treatment of hepatitis C virus infection. Int J Drug Policy 2007;18(5):437–43.

85. Bruce RD, Eiserman J, Acosta A, et al. Developing a modified directly observed therapy intervention for hepatitis C treatment in a methadone maintenance program: implications for program replication. Am J Drug Alcohol Abuse 2012; 38(3):206–12.

86. Waizmann M, Ackermann G. High rates of sustained virological response in hepatitis C virus-infected injection drug users receiving directly observed therapy with peginterferon alpha-2a (40KD) (PEGASYS) and once-daily ribavirin. J substance abuse Treat 2010;38(4):338–45.

87. Berk SI, Litwin AH, Arnsten JH, et al. Effects of pegylated interferon alfa-2b on the pharmacokinetic and pharmacodynamic properties of methadone: a prospective, nonrandomized, crossover study in patients coinfected with hepatitis C and HIV receiving methadone maintenance treatment. Clin Ther 2007;29(1): 131–8.

88. Kraus MR, Schafer A, Schottker K, et al. Therapy of interferon-induced depression in chronic hepatitis C with citalopram: a randomised, double-blind, placebo-controlled study. Gut 2008;57(4):531–6.

89. Bruce RD, Moody DE, Altice FL, et al. A review of pharmacological interactions between HIV or hepatitis C virus medications and opioid agonist therapy: implications and management for clinical practice. Expert Rev Clin Pharmacol 2013; 6(3):249–69.

90. Ogbuagu O, Friedland G, Bruce RD. Drug interactions between buprenorphine, methadone and hepatitis C therapeutics. Expert Opin Drug Metab Toxicol 2016; 12(7):721–31.

91. Hancock MM, Prosser CC, Ransibrahmanakul K, et al. Liver transplant and hepatitis C in methadone maintenance therapy: a case report. Subst Abuse Treat Prev Policy 2007;2:5.

92. Alavian SM, Mirahmadizadeh A, Javanbakht M, et al. Effectiveness of methadone maintenance treatment in prevention of hepatitis C virus transmission among injecting drug users. Hepat Mon 2013;13(8):e12411.

93. Martin NK, Hickman M, Hutchinson SJ, et al. Combination interventions to prevent HCV transmission among people who inject drugs: modeling the impact of antiviral treatment, needle and syringe programs, and opiate substitution therapy. Clin Infect Dis 2013;57(Suppl 2):S39–45.

94. Gossop M, Marsden J, Stewart D, et al. Outcomes after methadone maintenance and methadone reduction treatments: two-year follow-up results from the National Treatment Outcome Research Study. Drug and alcohol dependence 2001;62(3):255–64.

95. Centers for Disease Control and Prevention. Hepatitis C virus infection among adolescents and young adults: Massachusetts, 2002-2009. MMWR Morb Mortal Wkly Rep 2011;60(17):537–41.

96. Mauss S, Berger F, Goelz J, et al. A prospective controlled study of interferon-based therapy of chronic hepatitis C in patients on methadone maintenance. Hepatology 2004;40(1):120–4.

97. Luo X, Trevejo J, van Heeswijk RP, et al. Effect of telaprevir on the pharmacokinetics of buprenorphine in volunteers on stable buprenorphine/naloxone maintenance therapy. Antimicrob Agents Chemother 2012;56(7):3641–7.

98. van Heeswijk R, Verboven P, Vandevoorde A, et al. Pharmacokinetic interaction between telaprevir and methadone. Antimicrob Agents Chemother 2013;57(5): 2304–9.

99. Hulskotte EG, Bruce RD, Feng HP, et al. Pharmacokinetic interaction between HCV protease inhibitor boceprevir and methadone or buprenorphine in subjects on stable maintenance therapy. Eur J Clin Pharmacol 2015;71(3):303–11.

100. Ouwerkerk-Mahadevan S, Snoeys J, Peeters M, et al. Drug-drug interactions with the NS3/4A protease inhibitor simeprevir. Clin Pharmacokinet 2016;55(2): 197–208.

101. Denning JM, CM CD, Fang L, et al. Lack of effect of the nucleotide analog polymerase inhibitor PSI-7977 on methadone pharmacokinetics and pharmacodynamics. San Francisco (CA): American Association for the study of Liver Diseases; 2011.

102. German P, Pang P, Fang L, et al. Drug-drug interaction profile of the fixed-dose combination tablet ledipasvir/sofosbuvir. Boston: American Association for the study of Liver Diseases; 2014.

103. Menon RM, Badri PS, Wang T, et al. Drug-drug interaction profile of the all-oral anti-hepatitis C virus regimen of paritaprevir/ritonavir, ombitasvir, and dasabuvir. J Hepatol 2015;63(1):20–9.

104. Garimella T, Wang R, Luo WL, et al. Assessment of drug-drug interactions between daclatasvir and methadone or buprenorphine-naloxone. Antimicrob Agents Chemother 2015;59(9):5503–10.

105. Fraser IP, Yeh W, Reitmann C, et al. Lack of PK interaction between the HCV protease inhibitor MK-5172 and methadone or buprenorphine/naloxone in subjects on opiate maintenance therapy. 8th International Workshop on Clinical Pharmacology of Hepatitis Therapy; June, 2013; Cambridge, MA.

106. Marshall W, Jumes P, Yeh W. Lack of PK interaction between the hepatitis c virus nonstructural protein 5a inhibitor MK-8742 and methadone in subjects on stable opiate maintenance therapy. HEPDART, Big Island, Hawaii, December 8-12, 2013.

107. Merck and Co. Inc, Zepatier (elbasvir and grazoprevir) tablets for oral use: US Prescribing information 2016. Available at: https://http://www.merck.com/product/usa/pi_circulars/z/zepatier/zepatier_pi.pdf. Accessed February 25, 2017.

108. Grebely J, Dore G, Aspinall R, et al. Sofosbuvir/velpatasvir for 12 weeks is well tolerated and results in high SVR12 rates in people receiving opioid substitution therapy. Barcelona (Spain): European Association for the study of the Liver; 2016.

Strategies to Reduce Hepatitis C Virus Reinfection in People Who Inject Drugs

Marianne Martinello, MBBS, FRACP, PhD*,
Gregory J. Dore, BSc, MBBS, MPH, FRACP, PhD,
Gail V. Matthews, MBChB, MRCP (UK), FRACP, PhD,
Jason Grebely, BSc, PhD

KEYWORDS

- Hepatitis C • Direct-acting antiviral • DAA • Injecting drug use • HIV • Reinfection

KEY POINTS

- Reinfection will occur after direct-acting antiviral therapy in people with ongoing risk behaviors for acquisition.
- The possibility of hepatitis C virus reinfection should be discussed before, during, and after direct-acting antiviral treatment.
- After achieving sustained virologic response, individuals reporting ongoing risk behaviors for transmission/reinfection should be followed at least annually, with liver function tests and hepatitis C virus RNA.
- Education should include discussions of hepatitis C virus transmission, reinfection risk, and harm reduction strategies.
- Retreatment for reinfection should be offered, without stigma or discrimination.

INTRODUCTION

Globally, 71 million people are estimated to be living with chronic hepatitis C virus (HCV) infection, with approximately 2 million new infections annually.[1,2] The majority of new and existing HCV infections in high-income countries occur among people who inject drugs (PWID) with HCV antibody prevalence estimated at 52% (42%–62%).[3]

One of the goals of the United Nations 2030 Agenda for Sustainable Development and the World Health Organization Viral Hepatitis Strategy is the elimination

Disclosure Statement: See last page of article.
Viral Hepatitis Clinical Research Program, Kirby Institute, Level 5, Wallace Wurth Building, High Street, UNSW Sydney, Kensington NSW 2052, Australia
* Corresponding author.
E-mail address: mmartinello@kirby.unsw.edu.au

Infect Dis Clin N Am 32 (2018) 371–393
https://doi.org/10.1016/j.idc.2018.02.003
0891-5520/18/© 2018 Elsevier Inc. All rights reserved.

id.theclinics.com

of viral hepatitis as a public health threat.[4,5] To realize this goal, strategies to enhance HCV diagnosis, treatment uptake, and prevention are required. Modeling supports HCV treatment scale-up among populations at greatest risk of transmission to reduce incidence and prevalence, including among recent PWID.[6–8] Interferon-based HCV treatment uptake among PWID was low with multiple barriers to care at the patient, provider, system, and societal levels.[9] Concerns regarding adherence, social instability, treatment-related adverse effects, psychiatric comorbidity, and the potential for reinfection have limited interferon-based treatment initiation among PWID.[9,10]

The development and availability of highly effective, well tolerated interferon-free direct-acting antiviral (DAA) therapy has revolutionized HCV therapeutics and provides the therapeutic tools required to strive for elimination.[11,12] One challenge to achieving HCV elimination through therapeutic intervention is reinfection. There is concern that HCV reinfection may compromise HCV treatment outcomes in populations with ongoing risk behaviors, with the risk of reinfection cited as a reason for not offering treatment to PWID.[13,14]

This review summarizes the literature regarding reinfection after successful HCV treatment among PWID, discusses strategies to reduce HCV infection and reinfection, and highlights the potential individual- and population-level impact of DAA treatment-scale up on HCV elimination.

Paul, a 54-year-old man, presents for review with his methadone prescriber and asks to discuss the "new treatments" for chronic HCV infection.

Paul was diagnosed with chronic genotype 1a HCV infection in 1992. He is treatment naive. There is no evidence of significant fibrosis, with recent liver stiffness measurement 5.5 kPa. Quantitative HCV RNA is 6,798,242 IU/mL with and alanine aminotransferase level of 54 U/L.

He reports first injecting heroin in 1979; currently, he injects once per week. He is on methadone 65 mg/d.

After discussion, he is commenced on sofosbuvir/ledipasvir for 12 weeks.

EFFICACY OF DIRECT-ACTING ANTIVIRAL THERAPY FOR CHRONIC HEPATITIS C VIRUS INFECTION AMONG PEOPLE WHO INJECT DRUGS

DAA therapy is safe and effective among PWID and people receiving opioid substitution therapy (OST; **Tables 1** and **2**).[15] However, the majority of phase II and III clinical trials examining DAA efficacy have excluded people with recent drug use.

A small number of clinical trials have been conducted among people who report recent drug use[16–19] (see **Table 1**). In the C-EDGE CO-STAR trial (A Phase III Randomized Clinical Trial to Study the Efficacy and Safety of the Combination Regimen of MK-5172/MK-8742 in Treatment-Naïve Subjects With Chronic HCV GT1, GT4, and GT6 Infection Who Are on Opiate Substitution Therapy), the efficacy and safety of grazoprevir/elbasvir for 12 weeks in chronic HCV genotypes 1, 4, and 6 was assessed among people receiving OST (n = 301), the majority of whom reported drug use during treatment and follow-up.[16] Most (58%) had a positive urine drug screen at treatment initiation with stable patterns of drug use noted throughout treatment. At treatment initiation (immediate treatment arm), recent use of benzodiazepines, opiates, cocaine, or amphetamines/methamphetamines was seen in 25%, 22%, 10%, and 5%, respectively. SVR at 12 weeks (SVR12) was 92%,

Table 1
Clinical trials of DAA therapy among people receiving opioid substitution therapy and people who inject drugs

Study	n	OST Use (%)	Recent Drug Use (%)	Recent IDU (%)	Genotype	Cirrhosis (%)	DAA Regimen/s	Duration (wk)	SVR (ITT) (%)
People receiving OST									
Recent drug use excluded									
Puoti et al,[85] 2014[a]	56	100	0	0	1	2	PrOD + RBV	12–24	96
Lalezari et al,[86] 2015	38	100	0	0	1	0	PrOD + RBV	12	97
Grebely et al,[87] 2016	70	100	0	0	1	10	SOF/ LDV ± RBV	8–24	94
Grebely et al,[88] 2016	51	100	0	0	1–4	25	SOF/VEL	12	96
Grebely et al,[89] 2017[a]	149	100	0	0	1	17	PrOD ± RBV	12	94
Grebely et al,[90] 2017[a]	49	100	0	0	1–4	50	SOF/VEL/ VOX	12	96
Recent drug use permitted									
Dore et al,[16] 2016	296	100	46[b]	NA	1, 4, 6	21	GZR/EBR	12	91
Moser et al,[17] 2017[a]	40	100	NA	NA	1	0	SOF/LDV	8	100
People who inject drugs									
History of injecting drug use									
Sulkowski et al,[18] 2017[a]	110	NA	25	21[c]	1	NA	SOF/ LDV ± RBV	12	90 (88/98)[e]
Recent injecting drug use									
Grebely et al,[19] 2017[a]	103	57	100[d]	100[d]	1–4	9	SOF/VEL	12	94

Abbreviations: DAA, direct-acting antiviral; EBR, elbasvir; GZR, grazoprevir; IDU, injecting drug use; ITT, intention-to-treat; LDV, ledipasvir; NA, not available; OST, opioid substitution therapy; PrOD, paritaprevir, ritonavir, ombitasvir, and dasabuvir; RBV, ribavirin; SOF, sofosbuvir; SVR, sustained virologic response; VEL, velpatasvir; VOX, voxilaprevir.
[a] Conference abstract.
[b] Any 1 positive urine drug screen result at baseline for amphetamines, barbiturates, benzodiazepines, cocaine, other opioids, phencyclidine, and propoxyphene.
[c] Current use.
[d] In the last 6 months.
[e] SVR was calculated among those initiating treatment and due for 12-week posttreatment follow-up at the time of analysis.

Table 2
Cohort studies of DAA therapy among people receiving opioid substitution therapy and people who inject drugs

Study	n	OST (%)	Recent Drug Use (%)	Recent IDU (%)	Genotype	Cirrhosis (%)	DAA Regimen/s	Duration (wk)	SVR (ITT)
People receiving OST									
Christensen et al,[91] 2016[a]	739	100	NA	NA	1–4	28	SOF/LDV ± RBV (n = 377) SOF + RBV (n = 108) SOF + DAC ± RBV (n = 98) SOF + PEG + RBV (n = 69) PrO ± D ± RBV (n = 72) SOF + SIM ± RBV (n = 15)	8–24	85% (450/528)[d]
Schütz et al,[92] 2016	15	100	NA	NA	1, 3	33	SOF/LDV (n = 11) SOF + DAC (n = 4)	8–24	100%
Scherz et al,[93] 2017[a]	50	100	NA	12	1–4	60	SOF/LDV ± RBV (n = 21) SOF + DAC ± RBV (n = 17) GZR/EBR (n = 5) PrOD (n = 4) SOF + RBV (n = 2) SOF + SIM (n = 1)	8–24	98% (39/40)[d]
Dillon et al,[94] 2017[a]	37	100	NA	NA	1, 4	26	SIM + DAA ± RBV	12–24	83%
Butner et al,[95] 2016	75	87	23	NA	1–4	17	SOF/LDV (n = 57) SOF + RBV (n = 12) SOF + DAC (n = 3) GZR/EBR (n = 2) PrO + RBV (n = 1)	8–24	85%
Boyle et al,[96] 2017[a]	31	100	NA	NA	1	16	PrOD + RBV	12	95% (20/21)[d]
People who inject drugs									
Conway et al,[97] 2016[a]	98	40	100	NA	NA	26	SOF/LDV ± RBV or SOF + RBV (n = 67) PrOD ± RBV (n = 31)	12–24	95%
Morris et al,[98] 2017	127	NA	NA	NA	1–3	NA	SOF/LDV (n = 66) SOF + DAC ± RBV (n = 53) PrOD ± RBV (n = 8)	8–24	80%

Study						Regimen		SVR
Norton et al,[20] 2017	56	52	67	NA	1–4	NA	SOF/LDV SOF + SIM SOF + PEG + RBV SOF + RBV	12–24	96%
Mason et al,[99] 2017	74	24	30[b]	11[b]	1–3	32	SOF/LDV ± RBV (n = 56) SOF + RBV (n = 16) SOF + DAC ± RBV (n = 1) GZR/EBR (n = 1)	8–24	87% (60/69)[d]
Read et al,[23] 2017	72	25	NA	75[e]	1–3	10	SOF/LDV (n = 38) SOF + DAC (n = 28) PrOD ± RBV (n = 6)	8–24	82%
Litwin et al,[100] 2017[a]	150	100	65	NA	1	27	TVR + PEG + RBV (n = 3) SOF + PEG + RBV (n = 15) SOF + RBV (n = 17) SOF + SIM (n = 11) SOF/LDV (n = 104)	8–24	94%
Boglione et al,[22] 2017	174	34	100[c]	100[c]	1–4	63	SOF + DAC ± RBV (n = 56) SOF/LDV (n = 54) PrOD ± RBV (n = 26) SOF + SIM ± RBV (n = 20) SIM + PEG + RBV (n = 9) SOF + RBV (n = 7) SOF + PEG + RBV (n = 2)	8–24	93%
Bouscaillou et al,[21] 2017[a]	244	NA	100	100	1–3	54	SOF + PEG + RBV (n = 106) SOF + RBV (n = 130) SOF/LDV ± RBV (n = 8)	12–24	88%

Abbreviations: DAA, direct-acting antiviral (unspecified); DAC, daclatasvir; EBR, elbasvir; GZR, grazoprevir; IDU, injecting drug use; ITT, intention-to-treat; LDV, ledipasvir; NA, not available; OST, opioid substitution therapy; PEG, pegylated interferon alfa; PrOD, paritaprevir, ritonavir, ombitasvir, and dasabuvir; RBV, ribavirin; SVR, sustained virologic response; SIM, simeprevir; SOF, sofosbuvir.

[a] Conference abstract.
[b] In the last 30 d.
[c] In the last year.
[d] SVR was calculated among those initiating treatment and due for 12-week posttreatment follow-up at the time of analysis.

with similar adherence and efficacy to the other C-EDGE phase III studies that excluded people with recent drug use.

The SIMPLIFY trial (A Phase II, Open-label, Single Arm, Multicentre, International Trial of Sofosbuvir (SOF) and GS-5816 for People With Chronic Hepatitis C Virus Infection and Recent Injection Drug Use) evaluated the efficacy and safety of sofosbuvir/velpatasvir for 12 weeks in chronic HCV genotypes 1 through 4 among PWID reporting recent injecting drug use (defined as use within 6 months of enrollment; n = 103).[19] Injecting drug use within 30 days of enrollment was reported by 74%. SVR12 was 94%, with no virologic failures or relapse observed. There are other ongoing clinical trials examining DAA efficacy among current PWID, including HERO (Patient-Centered Models of HCV Care for People Who Inject Drugs; NCT02824640; sofosbuvir/velpatasvir).

Observational cohort studies have evaluated DAA therapy in "real-world" populations, with high efficacy in cohorts of people who use drugs (PWUD; see **Table 2**). In a single-center US cohort of PWUD (defined as people receiving OST, people reporting recent drug use, or people with a positive urine drug screen) treated with interferon-free DAA therapy, SVR12 was 96%, compared with 95% in non-PWUD.[20] These real-world cohort studies highlight the importance of posttreatment follow-up and assessment. In 2 single-center cohorts of current PWID recruited from Georgia[21] and Italy,[22] SVR12 was 88% and 93%, respectively, with the majority of treatment failures owing to early treatment cessation (with interferon-containing regimens) or loss to follow-up. Similarly, among a cohort of PWID in Sydney (of whom 75% reported injecting drug use within 6 months of enrollment), SVR12 by intention-to-treat analysis was 82%, with all treatment failure owing to loss to follow-up (SVR 12 by per-protocol analysis, 100%).[23] Appropriate review during and after treatment will allow characterization of treatment response and further opportunities for interventions, which may reduce the risk of reinfection.

Paul completes 12 weeks of sofosbuvir/ledipasvir. He tolerates therapy very well, reporting only a mild headache at treatment initiation, which rapidly subsides. He reports excellent adherence, missing only 1 pill during the 12 weeks of therapy.

Paul achieves SVR12.

He is very pleased with the result and feels "the best [he] has in years."

He reports injecting heroin once during the treatment period, but denies any drug use after treatment.

REINFECTION AFTER TREATMENT FOR HEPATITIS C VIRUS
Are All People Who Inject Drugs at "High Risk" of Reinfection?

The risk of reinfection has been cited as a reason for not offering HCV treatment to PWID.[13] However, PWID are diverse, with varying risk profiles. Subpopulations of PWID include those who report injecting an illicit drug at least once (lifetime PWID) and those who continue to inject drugs (recent or current PWID, with definitions varying between use in the preceding 1 and 12 months).[24] Among lifetime PWID, there also exists a group of people receiving OST, some of whom may also be recent PWID. It is crucial to accurately define the individual and population of interest to determine reinfection risk after DAA therapy.

In a metaanalysis, Simmons and colleagues[25] examined the risk of HCV recurrence after interferon-based treatment-induced SVR in 3 different populations, defined by their perceived risk of reinfection—HCV monoinfected "low risk" (no recognized risk factors for reinfection), HCV monoinfected "high risk" (lifetime and/or recent injecting drug use, incarceration), and human immunodeficiency virus (HIV)/HCV coinfection. Reinfection incidence was 0.0 per 100 person-years (95% confidence interval [CI], 0.0–0.0) in those deemed "low risk," 1.9 per 100 person-years (95% CI, 1.1–2.8) in those deemed "high risk" and 3.2 per 100 person-years (95% CI, 0.0–12.3) in those with HIV/HCV coinfection. Regardless of the risk category, reinfection incidence was low. However, it was unclear what proportion of those included in the high-risk group continued to demonstrate behaviors after achieving SVR, which posed a risk for HCV reinfection.

Hepatitis C Virus Reinfection After Interferon-Based Treatment Among People Who Inject Drugs

The reported reinfection incidence after interferon-based therapy for chronic HCV has generally been low among lifetime PWID (reinfection incidence of 0–5 per 100 person-years; **Table 3**).[25,26] However, uncertainty persists, because many of the primary studies reported to date suffer from small sample size, differing methodologies, and frequent exclusion of people reporting recent injecting drug use, with considerable selection bias in those PWID deemed suitable for interferon-based treatment. As a result, few cases of reinfection have been observed, with high variability in reinfection incidence.

Unsurprisingly, the risk of HCV reinfection seems to be significantly higher in people treated for HCV infection who report ongoing risk behavior, with reinfection incidence in those reporting injecting drug use after treatment ranging between 0.0 and 33.0 per 100 person-years[26–32] (see **Table 3**). In a metaanalysis examining reinfection incidence among PWUD (recent and lifetime), the overall reinfection incidence was 2.4 per 100 person-years (95% CI, 0.9, 6.1), increasing to 6.4 per 100 person-years (95% CI, 2.5–16.7) in those who reported injecting drug use after achieving SVR.[26]

Several recent studies have demonstrated the impact of ongoing injecting drug use after treatment on HCV reinfection incidence. Among a Norwegian cohort of PWID followed for 7 years after achieving SVR, the overall reinfection incidence was 2.0 per 100 person-years (95% CI, 1.0–3.5); among PWID reporting injecting drug use after achieving SVR, reinfection incidence was 5.8 per 100 person-years (95% CI, 3.0–10.2).[30] In Scotland, reinfection incidence among lifetime PWID after SVR was 1.7 per 100 person-years (95% CI, 0.7–3.5).[29] Among PWID who had been hospitalized for an opiate or injection-related cause after achieving SVR, the reinfection incidence was higher at 5.7 per 100 person-years (95% CI, 1.8–13.3). Among a Spanish cohort of HIV/HCV coinfected individuals (86% lifetime PWID), the overall reinfection incidence was 1.2 per 100 person-years (95% CI, 0.3–3.1), increasing to 8.7 per 100 person-years (95% CI, 4.8–23.7) among those who used heroin and/or cocaine during follow-up.[33] In an Australian and New Zealand cohort of individuals treated for recent HCV infection (duration of HCV infection of <18 months), the reinfection incidence was 7.4 per 100 person-years (95% CI, 4.0–13.8), increasing to 15.5 per 100 person-years (95% CI, 7.8–31.1) in those who reported injecting drug use at end of or after treatment.[34]

Additionally, specific drug use behaviors, including frequency of injection drug use and predominant type of drug injected, impact HCV reinfection risk. Among

Table 3
HCV reinfection incidence after treatment-induced clearance among PWID

Author, Year	Study Population	Subjects (n)	Reinfection (n)	Reinfection Incidence per 100 Person-Years (95% CI) Overall	IDU After Treatment
Metaanalyses					
Simmons et al,[25] 2016	Chronic HCV "High risk"[c]	771	36	1.9 (1.1–2.8)	NA
Aspinall et al,[26] 2013	Chronic HCV PWUD	131	7	2.4 (0.9–6.1)	6.4 (2.5–16.7)
Primary studies					
Reinfection after treatment for chronic HCV infection					
Young et al,[35] 2017	Chronic HCV HIV positive (100%) Lifetime (74%) and recent (14%) PWID GBM (33%)	257	18	3.1	High frequency: 5.8 (1.8–13.4)[d] Low frequency: 2.6 (0.6–6.6)[d]
Islam et al,[44] 2017	Chronic HCV Lifetime PWID (100%)	595	30	1.1 (0.8–1.6)	NA
Elsherif et al,[101] 2017	Chronic HCV Lifetime PWID (100%)	219	13	1.1	NA
Dore et al,[36] 2016	Chronic HCV OST (100%) Recent PWUD (58%)	301	6	4.0 (1.7–8.0)	NA
Midgard et al,[30] 2016	Chronic HCV Lifetime (100%) and recent (39%) PWID	94	12	2.0 (1.0–3.5)	5.8 (3.0–10.2)

Study	Population				
Weir et al,[29] 2016	Chronic HCV Lifetime PWID (100%)	277	7	1.7 (0.7–3.5)	5.7 (1.8–13.3)
Pineda et al,[33] 2015	Chronic HCV HIV positive (100%) Lifetime PWID (86%)	84	4	1.2 (0.3–3.1)	8.7 (4.8–23.7)
Conway et al,[102] 2013[a]	Chronic HCV Recent PWID (100%)	70	4	2.9 (1.1–7.2)	—
Deshaies[103] 2013[a]	Chronic HCV Recent PWID (100%)	20	2	6.3 (1.7–20.3)	—
Edlin et al,[104] 2013[a]	Chronic HCV Recent PWID (100%)	15	1	2.2 (3.9–11.5)	—
Hilsden et al,[105] 2013[a]	Chronic HCV Recent PWUD (100%)	23	1	2.8 (0.0–14.5)	NA
Marco et al,[27] 2013[a]	Chronic HCV Incarcerated (100%) Lifetime (81%) and recent (10%) PWID HIV positive (15%)	119	9	5.3	33.0
Ruzić et al,[106] 2013[a]	Chronic HCV Former PWID (100%)	20	0	0.0 (0.0–3.7)	NA
Grady et al,[107] 2012[a]	Chronic HCV Recent PWUD (100%)	42	1	0.8 (0.0–3.7)	3.1 (0.1–17.3)
Manolakopoulos et al,[108] 2012[a]	Chronic HCV Lifetime PWID (100%) Recent PWID (57%)	61	5	4.1 (1.8–9.2)	—

(continued on next page)

Table 3
(continued)

Author, Year	Study Population	Subjects (n)	Reinfection (n)	Reinfection Incidence per 100 Person-Years (95% CI)	
				Overall	IDU After Treatment
Grebely et al,[31] 2010[a,b]	Chronic HCV Lifetime (100%) and recent (54%) PWID	35	2	3.2 (0.4–11.6)	5.3 (0.6–19.2)
Currie et al,[32] 2008[a,b]	Chronic HCV Lifetime PWID (100%)	9	1	2.6 (0.1–14.7)	28.6 (0.7–159.2)
Backmund,[28] 2004[a,b]	Chronic HCV Lifetime PWID (100%)	18	2	3.9 (0.5–14.2)	8.4 (1.0–30.4)
Dalgard et al,[109] 2002[a,b]	Chronic HCV Lifetime PWID (100%)	27	1	0.9 (0.0–4.7)	2.5 (0.0–13.9)
Reinfection after treatment for acute HCV infection					
Martinello et al,[34] 2017	Recent HCV[e] Lifetime (69%) and recent (49%) PWID HIV-positive GBM (53%)	120	10	7.4 (4.0–13.8)	15.5 (7.8–31.1)

Abbreviations: CI, confidence interval; GBM, gay and bisexual men; HCV, hepatitis C virus; HIV, human immunodeficiency virus; NA, not available; OST, opiate substitution therapy; PWID, people who inject drugs; PWUD, people who use drugs.

[a] Studies included in a metaanalysis performed by Simmons and colleagues.[25]
[b] Studies included in a metaanalysis performed by Aspinall and colleagues.[26]
[c] HCV monoinfected "high risk" defined in the metaanalysis as people with recognized risk factors for reinfection, including former or recent injecting drug use (12 studies [n = 617]; 8 studies included recent PWID or PWUD) and history of incarceration (2 studies [n = 154]).
[d] 95% credible interval (CrI).
[e] Recent HCV infection, duration of infection less than 18 months.

a Canadian HIV/HCV coinfection cohort followed after achieving SVR (lifetime PWID 74%, recent PWID 14%), the reinfection risk was highest among PWID who reported high-frequency injecting drug use after treatment (defined as "any self-reported use of injection cocaine or methamphetamine in the last 6 months"), followed by gay and bisexual men (GBM) reporting high-risk sexual behaviors (defined as "more than one sexual partner and <100% condom use in the preceding 6 months") and PWID reporting low-frequency injection drug use (defined as "self-report of any other injection drug").[35] Similarly, in the aforementioned Australian and New Zealand cohort, reinfection among PWID was associated with needle and syringe sharing and methamphetamine use after treatment.[34] A high reinfection incidence after treatment for HCV infection in individuals with ongoing risk behavior emphasizes the need for posttreatment surveillance, harm reduction strategies, and education.

Hepatitis C Virus Reinfection After Direct-Acting Antiviral Agent Treatment Among People Who Inject Drugs

The risk of reinfection after DAA therapy among PWID is being assessed. A 3-year posttreatment extension of the C-EDGE COSTAR study examining reinfection and drug use behavior is underway (NCT02105688). To date, 8 cases of reinfection have been identified, including 5 cases detected at posttreatment week 8, for a reinfection incidence of 4.0 per 100 person-years (95% CI, 1.7–8.0).[36] Of interest, 3 of these 5 early reinfection cases experienced spontaneous clearance. In the SIMPLIFY study among recent PWID, 1 case of reinfection was demonstrated before posttreatment week 12 (reinfection incidence of 2.7 per 100 person-years [95% CI, 0.1–13.8]).[19] Because clinical trials have largely excluded those at greatest risk of ongoing transmission, including people reporting recent injecting drug use, further evidence is required to robustly evaluate the long-term outcomes after DAA therapy, including reinfection incidence and drug use behavior, with sufficient follow-up time and HCV RNA testing at regular intervals.

HCV reinfection is confirmed, with repeated laboratory results showing detectable HCV RNA (1,342,311 IU/mL) with a genotype switch to 3a.

Paul reports that he started using heroin again about 4 months ago. Although he usually injects alone, he reports injecting on a couple of occasions with some old acquaintances. He used his own sterile needle and syringe, but was not sure about the other equipment. He is "embarrassed" about the result. He thinks he has "let [himself] and everyone else down."

After a period of observation for spontaneous clearance, Paul undergoes retreatment with sofosbuvir/velpatasvir, and achieves SVR12. He remains in follow-up.

Paul's results at 6 and 12 months after treatment				
	End of Treatment	12 wk After Treatment (SVR12)	24 wk After Treatment (SVR 24)	48 wk After Treatment
Alanine aminotransferase, U/L	25	12	15	321
Hepatitis C virus RNA (qualitative)	TND	TND	TND	Detected

STRATEGIES TO REDUCE HEPATITIS C VIRUS (RE)INFECTION AMONG PEOPLE WHO INJECT DRUGS

As DAA treatment scale-up expands among populations with ongoing risk behaviors for reacquisition (including recent PWID and HIV-positive GBM), acknowledgment that HCV reinfection can and will occur is essential. Although still unknown, the rate of HCV reinfection after DAA therapy may mirror the incidence of primary infection among current PWID in a given location.

Efforts directed at addressing, preventing, and managing HCV reinfection should be incorporated into individual- and population-level HCV strategies, with multicomponent interventions likely to be most effective[37] (**Box 1**). At an individual level, the treating clinician should conduct a reinfection risk assessment on initiating DAA therapy. Potential constructive management options include acknowledging the potential for reinfection, education and counseling regarding HCV transmission and drug use, optimizing harm reduction,[37–45] treating the individual and their injecting (or sexual) partner or people in their network,[46] management of medical and psychiatric comorbidity,[44] posttreatment surveillance[47] and rapid retreatment of reinfection. At a population level, appropriate health care provision with universal access to care and treatment, political will, sufficient funding, and alleviation of the stigma associated with HCV infection and drug use should assist in efforts to reduce HCV primary and reinfection incidence.

Harm Reduction Services

Access to OST and high-coverage needle and syringe programs (NSP; often defined as 100% of total injections performed using a sterile needle/syringe) will be crucial to minimize reinfection risk, with the reduction in HCV incidence greater in combination than with either intervention alone.[37–40,42–45] However, despite evidence for harm reduction strategies in reducing bloodborne virus transmission among PWID, global access to services is suboptimal. In 2009, NSP coverage was estimated at 22 sterile needles/syringes per PWID per year and OST coverage estimated at 8 OST recipients per 100 PWID.[48] Significant regional variation existed, with the highest NSP coverage in Australia and New Zealand (202 needles/syringes per PWID per year) and the highest OST coverage in Western Europe (61 OST recipients per 100 PWID).[48] In contrast, very low NSP coverage was seen in Latin America and the Caribbean

---

Box 1
What will be required to limit the impact of HCV reinfection?

Strategies to reduce HCV (re)infection among people who inject drugs
- Harm reduction[37–45]
  - Opioid substitution therapy
  - High-coverage needle and syringe program
- Integrated care[44,46,50]
  - Mental health assessment
- Education[51,52]
  - Counseling
  - Peer support
- Posttreatment surveillance[47,56–58]
  - Regular HCV RNA testing
- Retreatment of reinfection

Abbreviation: HCV, hepatitis C virus.

(0.3 needles/syringes per PWID per year), the Middle East and North Africa (0.5 needles/syringes per PWID per year), and sub-Saharan Africa (0.1 needles/syringes per PWID per year).

The implementation of broad harm reduction services has had demonstrable benefit in reducing HCV incidence among PWID. Low or declining HCV incidence has been demonstrated among PWID in Australia and the Netherlands, whereas high incidence persists among PWID in the United States and Canada.[49] In contrast with North America, government-supported harm reduction programs (NSP followed by OST) were established in Australia and the Netherlands in the 1980s and have been maintained. Similarly, a marked reduction in HCV incidence was demonstrated among PWID in Scotland between 2008 and 2012 after changes to government policy and provision of harm reduction interventions.[45] Although many countries have not achieved an adequate level of coverage to curb HCV transmission, the Scottish example highlights the potential positive impact of broad harm reduction strategies in only a short period in the context of political will, widespread availability, and high end-user uptake. The implementation of evidence-based harm reduction programs is necessary to reduce primary HCV infection and reinfection after treatment among PWID.

Integrated Care

HCV treatment should not occur in isolation. Substance use, mental health, and medical comorbidity should be addressed concurrently, with lower HCV reinfection risk seen among recent PWID receiving OST and mental health counseling services.[44] Holistic models of care external to traditional tertiary hospital clinics may more effectively facilitate the ongoing health care needs of PWID and reduce the risk of reinfection. Acknowledgment of the individual circumstances of PWID as opposed to rigid criteria will aid in the success of long-term HCV management strategies and drug user health overall.

HCV care and treatment among PWID is feasible and successful across a broad range of multidisciplinary health care settings.[50] In an effort to expand DAA uptake and access, different models of care are being assessed. In a multicenter, randomised US study, the feasibility and acceptability of a patient-led model of care is being compared with directly-observed therapy in recent PWID (HERO [Patient-Centered Models of HCV Care for People Who Inject Drugs]; NCT02824640). In Scotland, a cluster randomised trial is assessing the impact of pharmacy-led directly observed HCV DAA therapy versus conventional nurse-led HCV therapy for people receiving OST (SuperDOT-C [A Cluster Randomised Trial of Pharmacy Led HCV Therapy Versus Conventional Treatment Pathways for HCV Positive Patients Receiving Daily OST in Pharmacies in Health Boards Within NHS Scotland], NCT02706223).

Education and Counseling

Education and counseling can reduce high-risk injecting behaviors among people with HCV infection.[51,52] Although injecting risk behavior decreased after interferon-based treatment,[53,54] it is unclear what will occur in the era of DAA therapy. It is possible that the optimism developed by broad access to DAA therapy may be associated with an increase in risk behavior among PWID, as seen among GBM after the introduction of HIV combination antiretroviral therapy.[55] Education should be offered to PWID commencing DAA therapy by health care providers, peer support workers, and community drug user organizations. Consulting and involving community drug user organizations in the design and implementation of HCV reinfection prevention strategies will be essential, ensuring public health efforts meet the needs of the target population.

Additionally, education needs to be delivered to health care providers regarding contemporary best practice in the care and management of HCV infection among PWID. Many medical practitioners have previously reported being unwilling to treat PWUD, with reinfection, adherence, and medication cost listed as important concerns when determining an individual's suitability for HCV treatment.[13] Concerns regarding reinfection should not be a deterrent to HCV treatment.

Posttreatment Surveillance and Treatment of Reinfection

People at risk for HCV reinfection should have at least annual monitoring with HCV RNA and alanine aminotransferase.[56–58] The optimal testing interval for the detection of (clinically significant) reinfection is under investigation; more frequent testing may identify a greater number of reinfections[47] and provide the potential for earlier retreatment. Routine posttreatment surveillance and adherence to international guidelines should ensure that reinfection is diagnosed within the first year of reacquisition. However, recent data would suggest that monitoring for HCV reinfection after treatment occurs infrequently, with only 61% of PWID in a Scottish cohort study screened at least once in 4.5 years of follow-up after achieving SVR.[29] If testing rates remain low, reinfection incidence will be underreported and the impact of DAA treatment scale-up will be unclear.

One of the barriers to testing for reinfection may be jurisdictional limitations on DAA access, driven largely by the current high cost of treatment.[59,60] DAA retreatment should be made available to all people with reinfection, without stigma or discrimination. Key health care bodies and medical societies should consider implicit recommendations regarding retreatment of reinfection so as help facilitate reimbursement by payers.

An additional barrier to testing may be the number of competing health, family, financial, or drug use priorities. A monitoring and diagnostic algorithm that incorporates rapid point-of-care HCV RNA testing[61,62] conducted in settings appropriate to and frequently used by PWID may facilitate testing, diagnosis, and expedient retreatment of reinfection.

In the future, prevention of HCV (re)infection may include a prophylactic vaccine strategy. A double-blind, randomized, placebo-controlled clinical trial of a prophylactic HCV vaccine (AdCh3NSmut-MVANSMut HCV vaccine) among recent PWID at high risk for HCV infection is underway in the United States (NCT01436357 [A Staged Phase I/II Study, to Assess Safety, Efficacy and Immunogenicity of a New Hepatitis C Prophylactic Vaccine Based on Sequential Use of AdCh3NSmut1 and MVA-NSmut]). Ideally, an effective vaccine would provide long-term protection.

Screening and Targeted Strategies in High-Risk Populations

All PWID should be screened for HCV with anti-HCV antibody.[56–58] In the context of ongoing injection drug use, 6 to 12 monthly screening should be performed with anti-HCV antibody to assess for incident primary infection[56–58] and with HCV RNA to assess for reinfection.

Certain populations, including young PWID, incarcerated PWID, and HIV-positive GBM, may require targeted screening and interventions to prevent ongoing transmission and reinfection. The high primary HCV incidence persists among young adult[39,63–67] and incarcerated[68–71] PWID, with HCV acquisition risk greatest among young adult PWID in the first years of unsafe injection practices.[72,73] Young female PWID are at greater risk of HCV acquisition than men,[74,75] potentially related to high-risk injecting behaviors in the setting of coexisting sexual and injecting relationships.[74,76] The high incidence among young adult and incarcerated PWID highlights the importance of treating the individual within the context of their injecting (and sexual) network to gain the greatest individual and population-level benefit. In Melbourne, Australia, the TAP study (NCT02363517 [The Treatment And Prevention (TAP) Study: Treating People Who Inject Drugs (PWID) in Community-based Settings Using a Social Network Approach]) is assessing a social network-based approach ("bring a friend") to HCV treatment among PWID. Among people who are incarcerated, large trials are being conducted in prisons in Australia (STOP-C [A Pilot Study to Assess the Feasibility of Hepatitis C Virus (HCV) Treatment as Prevention With Interferon-free Direct Acting Antivirals (DAAs) in the Prison Setting]; NCT02064049) and Spain (JAILFREE-C [Program of Screening, Prevention and Elimination of Hepatitis C in Penitentiary Institutions in Cantabria]; NCT02768961).

Populations at risk for reinfection, such as recent PWID and HIV-positive GBM, are not mutually exclusive.[34,77] HIV-positive GBM who inject drugs are at significantly higher risk of HCV (re)infection than HIV-positive GBM who do not inject drugs.[34,44] However, different drug use and sexual behaviors and levels of health care engagement may necessitate different public health strategies. Increasing use of (meth) amphetamine among HIV-positive GBM who inject drugs contrasts with much of the literature surrounding opiate use in HCV monoinfected populations. Although robust evidence exists for HCV infection prevention among people who use opioids, little evidence exists for those who predominantly inject (meth)amphetamine or cocaine, with no pharmacotherapies available. Education regarding high-risk sexual behaviors consistent with currently recommended HIV prevention strategies is warranted, although evidence supporting the success of these strategies in limiting HCV transmission is lacking.[78] The evaluation of novel prevention strategies should be a priority.

Stigma, Discrimination, and the Criminalization of Drug Use

The criminalization of drug use and restrictive drug law enforcement policies hinder access to and provision of HCV prevention services, which in turn may drive increased risk behaviors (including needle and syringe sharing) and HCV transmission.[79] In jurisdictions with repressive drug policies, PWID may end up in prison, where the risk of HCV (re)infection is often high and prevention measures are absent.

Treatment as Prevention and the Impact of Reinfection

The burden of disease attributable to HCV is high among PWID. Mathematical modeling suggests that substantial reductions in HCV incidence and prevalence could be achieved by targeted DAA treatment scale-up among those at greatest risk for ongoing transmission.[80,81] Using HCV treatment uptake data from 7 sites in the United Kingdom, Martin and colleagues[81] demonstrated that treating 26 per 1000 HCV-infected PWID per annum with DAA therapy could achieve a 15% to 50% decrease in the chronic HCV prevalence within 10 years. Despite the cost of DAA therapy, treating recent PWID with early liver disease seems to be cost effective compared with delaying until cirrhosis, given the decrease in liver-related complications and additional benefit of averting secondary infections.[6,82,83]

Rapid DAA treatment scale-up among PWID will be required to gain the greatest population-level benefit (Fig. 1). Given the high efficacy, a rapid scale-up of DAA therapy (>8% per year) among PWID will markedly increase the population susceptible to HCV reinfection in the short term.[84] Although initially this strategy will lead to an increase in the number of people with HCV reinfection, as the HCV RNA prevalence decreases overall, the number with reinfection will also decrease. The incidence of HCV reinfection after DAA-based treatment needs careful evaluation. Sufficient follow-up

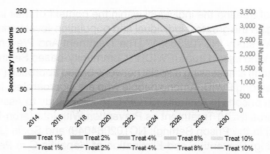

Fig. 1. Modeling the effect of HCV treatment on reinfection in people who inject drugs (PWID). Mathematical modeling was used to evaluate the effect of increased treatment on hepatitis C virus (HCV) reinfection among PWID in Australia. Each line represents the expected number of individuals with HCV reinfection (secondary infections, left axis) in each year, based on a given annual HCV treatment scenario. The colored lines represent the annual proportion of PWID treated per year. Permission to reproduce the image has been obtained from the author.[84] (*Courtesy of* Homie Razavi, PhD, Denver, CO, with permission; and *Reproduced from* Razavi H. Reducing a country's HCV-disease burden. The 4th International Symposium on Hepatitis in Substance Users (INHSU 2015). Sydney, Australia, October 7–9, 2015, with permission.)

time with regular HCV RNA testing after treatment will be required to appropriately evaluate reinfection incidence.

SUMMARY

Given the global burden of HCV-related disease among PWID, strategies to enhance HCV assessment, (re)treatment, and prevention are urgently needed. The incidence of HCV reinfection after DAA-based treatment is unknown and needs careful evaluation as access to treatment among populations at risk of ongoing transmission increases. Access to interventions known to prevent or reduce the risk of HCV (re)infection, including OST and high-coverage NSPs,[38–42] is crucial. Education regarding the potential for reinfection after treatment by health providers, peer support workers, and community drug user organizations should be routinely offered. The evaluation of novel prevention and retreatment strategies should be a priority.

Ultimately, the population-level impact of DAA therapy will require facilitating global access to HCV screening, care, and treatment. Overcoming barriers imposed by high drug pricing, drug use, and liver disease stage restrictions and stigma are central to achieving HCV elimination.[59] The risk of HCV reinfection after treatment in individuals with ongoing risk behaviors at risk for transmission emphasizes the need for posttreatment surveillance, harm reduction strategies, and education. However, reinfection must not be considered an impediment to treatment, if HCV elimination is to be achieved.

DISCLOSURE STATEMENT

The Kirby Institute is funded by the Australian Government Department of Health and Aging. The views expressed in this publication do not necessarily represent the position of the Australian Government. The content is solely the responsibility of the authors. None of the authors has commercial relationships that might pose a conflict of interest in connection with this article. J. Grebely and G.V. Matthews are supported through NHMRC Career Development Fellowships. G.J. Dore is supported through

NHMRC Practitioner Fellowships. M. Martinello has received speaker payments from Abbvie. G.J. Dore is an advisory board member and has received honoraria from Roche, Merck, Janssen, Gilead Sciences Inc, Bristol-Myers Squibb, and Abbvie; has received research grant funding from Roche, Merck, Janssen, Gilead Sciences Inc, Bristol-Myers Squibb, Vertex, Boeringher Ingelheim, and Abbvie; and travel sponsorship from Roche, Merck, Janssen, Gilead Sciences Inc, and Bristol-Myers Squibb. G.V. Matthews has received research funding, advisory board payments, and speaker payments from Gilead Sciences Inc, and research funding and speaker payments from Janssen. J. Grebely is a consultant/advisor and has received research grants from Abbvie, Bristol-Myers Squibb, Cepheid, Gilead Sciences Inc, and Merck.

REFERENCES

1. Global Hepatitis Report 2017. Geneva: World Health Organization; 2017. Licence: CC BY-NC-SA 3.0 IGO.
2. Blach S, Zeuzem S, Manns M, et al. Global prevalence and genotype distribution of hepatitis C virus infection in 2015: a modelling study. Lancet Gastroenterol Hepatol 2017;2(3):161–76.
3. Degenhardt L, Peacock A, Colledge S, et al. A global profile of people who inject drugs: Systematic reviews of characteristics, prevalence of injecting and of HIV, hepatitis B and hepatitis C. Lancet Glob Health 2017;5(12): e1192–207.
4. World Health Organization (WHO). Global health sector strategy on viral hepatitis, 2016–2021. Geneva (Switzerland). World Health Organization; 2016.
5. United Nations General Assembly. Transforming our world: the 2030 Agenda for Sustainable Development 2015. Available at: https://sustainabledevelopment. un.org/content/documents/21252030%20Agenda%20for%20Sustainable%20 Development%20web.pdf.
6. Martin NK, Vickerman P, Dore GJ, et al. Prioritization of HCV treatment in the direct-acting antiviral era: an economic evaluation. J Hepatol 2016;65(1):17–25.
7. Martin NK, Thornton A, Hickman M, et al. Can hepatitis C virus (HCV) direct-acting antiviral treatment as prevention reverse the HCV epidemic among men who have sex with men in the United Kingdom? Epidemiological and modeling insights. Clin Infect Dis 2016;62(9):1072–80.
8. Martin NK, Vickerman P, Grebely J, et al. Hepatitis C virus treatment for prevention among people who inject drugs: modeling treatment scale-up in the age of direct-acting antivirals. Hepatology 2013;58(5):1598–609.
9. Edlin BR, Kresina TF, Raymond DB, et al. Overcoming barriers to prevention, care, and treatment of hepatitis C in illicit drug users. Clin Infect Dis 2005; 40(Suppl 5):S276–85.
10. Martinello M, Hajarizadeh B, Grebely J, et al. HCV cure and reinfection among people with HIV/HCV coinfection and people who inject drugs. Curr HIV/AIDS Rep 2017;14(3):110–21.
11. Gotte M, Feld JJ. Direct-acting antiviral agents for hepatitis C: structural and mechanistic insights. Nat Rev Gastroenterol Hepatol 2016;13(6):338–51.
12. Manns MP, Buti M, Gane E, et al. Hepatitis C virus infection. Nat Rev Dis Primers 2017;3:17006.
13. Asher AK, Portillo CJ, Cooper BA, et al. Clinicians' views of hepatitis C virus treatment candidacy with direct-acting antiviral regimens for people who inject drugs. Subst Use Misuse 2016;51(9):1218–23.

14. Cunningham EB, Applegate TL, Lloyd AR, et al. Mixed HCV infection and reinfection in people who inject drugs–impact on therapy. Nat Rev Gastroenterol Hepatol 2015;12(4):218–30.
15. Grebely J, Hajarizadeh B, Dore GJ. Direct-acting antiviral agents for HCV infection affecting people who inject drugs. Nat Rev Gastroenterol Hepatol 2017; 14(11):641–51.
16. Dore GJ, Altice F, Litwin AH, et al. Elbasvir-grazoprevir to treat hepatitis C virus infection in persons receiving opioid agonist therapy: a randomized trial. Ann Intern Med 2016;165(9):625–34.
17. Moser S, Schütz A, Marchart K, et al. Directly observed therapy with sofosbuvir/ ledipasvir for 8 weeks is highly effective in treatment-naïve, precirrhotic genotype 1 patients with borderline compliance receiving opioid agonist therapy. J Hepatol 2017;66:S740.
18. Sulkowski M, Ward K, Falade-Nwulia O, et al. Randomized controlled trial of cash incentives or peer mentors to improve HCV linkage and treatment among HIV/HCV coinfected persons who inject drugs: the CHAMPS Study. J Hepatol 2017;66:S719.
19. Grebely J, Dalgard O, Conway B, et al. Efficacy and safety of sofosbuvir/velpatasvir in people with chronic hepatitis C virus infection and recent injecting drug use: the SIMPLIFY study. J Hepatol 2017;66(1):S513.
20. Norton BL, Fleming J, Bachhuber MA, et al. High HCV cure rates for people who use drugs treated with direct acting antiviral therapy at an urban primary care clinic. Int J Drug Policy 2017;47:196–201.
21. Bouscaillou J, Kikvidze T, Butsashvili M, et al. Effectiveness of DAA-based treatment of HCV in active people who inject drugs living in middle income countries (MIC): the results of a prospective cohort study in Tbilisi, Georgia. J Hepatol 2017;66:S409.
22. Boglione L, Mornese Pinna S, De Nicolo A, et al. Treatment with direct-acting antiviral agents of hepatitis C virus infection in injecting drug users: a prospective study. J Viral Hepat 2017;24(10):850–7.
23. Read P, Lothian R, Chronister K, et al. Delivering direct acting antiviral therapy for hepatitis C to highly marginalised and current drug injecting populations in a targeted primary health care setting. Int J Drug Policy 2017;47:209–15.
24. Larney S, Grebely J, Hickman M, et al. Defining populations and injecting parameters among people who inject drugs: implications for the assessment of hepatitis C treatment programs. Int J Drug Policy 2015;26(10):950–7.
25. Simmons B, Saleem J, Hill A, et al. Risk of late relapse or reinfection with hepatitis C virus after achieving a sustained virological response: a systematic review and meta-analysis. Clin Infect Dis 2016;62(6):683–94.
26. Aspinall EJ, Corson S, Doyle JS, et al. Treatment of hepatitis C virus infection among people who are actively injecting drugs: a systematic review and meta-analysis. Clin Infect Dis 2013;57(Suppl 2):S80–9.
27. Marco A, Esteban JI, Sole C, et al. Hepatitis C virus reinfection among prisoners with sustained virological response after treatment for chronic hepatitis C. J Hepatol 2013;59(1):45–51.
28. Backmund M, Meyer K, Edlin BR. Infrequent reinfection after successful treatment for hepatitis C virus infection in injection drug users. Clin Infect Dis 2004;39(10):1540–3.
29. Weir A, McLeod A, Innes H, et al. Hepatitis C reinfection following treatment induced viral clearance among people who have injected drugs. Drug Alcohol Depend 2016;165:53–60.

30. Midgard H, Bjoro B, Maeland A, et al. Hepatitis C reinfection after sustained viro-logical response. J Hepatol 2016;64(5):1020–6.
31. Grebely J, Knight E, Ngai T, et al. Reinfection with hepatitis C virus following sus-tained virological response in injection drug users. J Gastroenterol Hepatol 2010;25(7):1281–4.
32. Currie SL, Ryan JC, Tracy D, et al. A prospective study to examine persistent HCV reinfection in injection drug users who have previously cleared the virus. Drug Alcohol Depend 2008;93(1–2):148–54.
33. Pineda JA, Nunez-Torres R, Tellez F, et al. Hepatitis C virus reinfection after sus-tained virological response in HIV-infected patients with chronic hepatitis C. J Infect 2015;71(5):571–7.
34. Martinello M, Grebely J, Petoumenos K, et al. HCV reinfection incidence among individuals treated for recent infection. J Viral Hepat 2017;24(5):359–70.
35. Young J, Rossi C, Gill J, et al. Risk factors for hepatitis C virus reinfection after sustained virologic response in patients coinfected With HIV. Clin Infect Dis 2017;64(9):1154–62.
36. Dore G, Grebely J, Altice F, et al. HCV reinfection and injecting risk behavior following elbasvir/grazoprevir treatment in patients on opioid agonist therapy: Co-STAR Three Year Follow-up Study [abstract]. Hepatol-ogy 2016;64(1 Suppl):431A.
37. Hagan H, Pouget ER, Des Jarlais DC. A systematic review and meta-analysis of interventions to prevent hepatitis C virus infection in people who inject drugs. J Infect Dis 2011;204(1):74–83.
38. White B, Dore GJ, Lloyd AR, et al. Opioid substitution therapy protects against hepatitis C virus acquisition in people who inject drugs: the HITS-c study. Med J Aust 2014;201(6):326–9.
39. Tsui JI, Evans JL, Lum PJ, et al. Association of opioid agonist therapy with lower incidence of hepatitis C virus infection in young adult injection drug users. JAMA Intern Med 2014;174(12):1974–81.
40. Turner KM, Hutchinson S, Vickerman P, et al. The impact of needle and syringe provision and opiate substitution therapy on the incidence of hepatitis C virus in injecting drug users: pooling of UK evidence. Addiction 2011;106(11):1978–88.
41. Coffin PO, Rowe C, Santos GM. Novel interventions to prevent HIV and HCV among persons who inject drugs. Curr HIV/AIDS Rep 2015;12(1):145–63.
42. Nolan S, Dias Lima V, Fairbairn N, et al. The impact of methadone maintenance therapy on hepatitis C incidence among illicit drug users. Addiction 2014; 109(12):2053–9.
43. Allen EJ, Palmateer NE, Hutchinson SJ, et al. Association between harm reduc-tion intervention uptake and recent hepatitis C infection among people who inject drugs attending sites that provide sterile injecting equipment in Scotland. Int J Drug Policy 2012;23(5):346–52.
44. Islam N, Krajden M, Shoveller J, et al. Incidence, risk factors, and prevention of hepatitis C reinfection: a population-based cohort study. Lancet Gastroenterol Hepatol 2017;2(3):200–10.
45. Palmateer NE, Taylor A, Goldberg DJ, et al. Rapid decline in HCV incidence among people who inject drugs associated with national scale-up in coverage of a combination of harm reduction interventions. PLoS One 2014;9(8):e104515.
46. Hellard M, Rolls DA, Sacks-Davis R, et al. The impact of injecting networks on hepatitis C transmission and treatment in people who inject drugs. Hepatology 2014;60(6):1861–70.

47. Vickerman P, Grebely J, Dore GJ, et al. The more you look, the more you find: effects of hepatitis C virus testing interval on reinfection incidence and clearance and implications for future vaccine study design. J Infect Dis 2012; 205(9):1342–50.

48. Mathers BM, Degenhardt L, Ali H, et al. HIV prevention, treatment, and care services for people who inject drugs: a systematic review of global, regional, and national coverage. Lancet 2010;375(9719):1014–28.

49. Morris MD, Shiboski S, Bruneau J, et al. Geographic differences in temporal incidence trends of hepatitis C virus infection among people who inject drugs: the InC3 collaboration. Clin Infect Dis 2017;64(7):860–9.

50. Bruggmann P, Litwin AH. Models of care for the management of hepatitis C virus among people who inject drugs: one size does not fit all. Clin Infect Dis 2013; 57(Suppl 2):S56–61.

51. Bruneau J, Zang G, Abrahamowicz M, et al. Sustained drug use changes after hepatitis C screening and counseling among recently infected persons who inject drugs: a longitudinal study. Clin Infect Dis 2014;58(6):755–61.

52. Roux P, Le Gall JM, Debrus M, et al. Innovative community-based educational face-to-face intervention to reduce HIV, hepatitis C virus and other blood-borne infectious risks in difficult-to-reach people who inject drugs: results from the ANRS-AERLI intervention study. Addiction 2016;111(1):94–106.

53. Alavi M, Spelman T, Matthews GV, et al. Injecting risk behaviours following treatment for hepatitis C virus infection among people who inject drugs: the Australian trial in acute hepatitis C. Int J Drug Policy 2015;26(10):976–83.

54. Midgard H, Hajarizadeh B, Cunningham EB, et al. Changes in risk behaviours during and following treatment for hepatitis C virus infection among people who inject drugs: the ACTIVATE study. Int J Drug Policy 2017;47:230–8.

55. Dukers NH, Goudsmit J, de Wit JB, et al. Sexual risk behaviour relates to the virological and immunological improvements during highly active antiretroviral therapy in HIV-1 infection. AIDS 2001;15(3):369–78.

56. Grebely J, Robaeys G, Bruggmann P, et al. Recommendations for the management of hepatitis C virus infection among people who inject drugs. Int J Drug Policy 2015;26(10):1028–38.

57. AASLD-IDSA. Recommendations for testing, managing, and treating hepatitis C. 2016. Available at: http://www.hcvguidelines.org/. Accessed December 30, 2016.

58. European Association for the Study of the Liver. EASL Recommendations on Treatment of hepatitis C 2016. J Hepatol 2017;66(1):153–94.

59. Barua S, Greenwald R, Grebely J, et al. Restrictions for Medicaid reimbursement of sofosbuvir for the treatment of hepatitis C virus infection in the United States. Ann Intern Med 2015;163(3):215–23.

60. Marshall AD, Saeed S, Barrett L, et al. Restrictions for reimbursement of direct-acting antiviral treatment for hepatitis C virus infection in Canada: a descriptive study. CMAJ Open 2016;4(4):E605–e614.

61. Grebely J, Lamoury FMJ, Hajarizadeh B, et al. Evaluation of the Xpert HCV Viral Load point-of-care assay from venipuncture-collected and finger-stick capillary whole-blood samples: a cohort study. Lancet Gastroenterol Hepatol 2017;2(7): 514–20.

62. Hayes B, Briceno A, Asher A, et al. Preference, acceptability and implications of the rapid hepatitis C screening test among high-risk young people who inject drugs. BMC Public Health 2014;14:645.

63. Clatts MC, Colón-López V, Giang LM, et al. Prevalence and incidence of HCV infection among Vietnam heroin users with recent onset of injection. J Urban Health 2010;87(2):278–91.

64. Spittal PM, Pearce ME, Chavoshi N, et al. The cedar project: high incidence of HCV infections in a longitudinal study of young Aboriginal people who use drugs in two Canadian cities. BMC Public Health 2012;12:632.

65. Sacks-Davis R, Aitken CK, Higgs P, et al. High rates of hepatitis C virus reinfection and spontaneous clearance of reinfection in people who inject drugs: a prospective cohort study. PLoS One 2013;8(11):e80216.

66. Suryaprasad AG, White JZ, Xu F, et al. Emerging epidemic of hepatitis C virus infections among young nonurban persons who inject drugs in the United States, 2006–2012. Clin Infect Dis 2014;59(10):1411–9.

67. Zibbell JE, Iqbal K, Patel RC, et al. Increases in hepatitis C virus infection related to injection drug use among persons aged ≤30 years — Kentucky, Tennessee, Virginia, and West Virginia, 2006–2012. MMWR Morb Mortal Wkly Rep 2015; 64(17):453–8.

68. Snow KJ, Young JT, Preen DB, et al. Incidence and correlates of hepatitis C virus infection in a large cohort of prisoners who have injected drugs. BMC Public Health 2014;14:830.

69. Luciani F, Bretana NA, Teutsch S, et al. A prospective study of hepatitis C incidence in Australian prisoners. Addiction 2014;109(10):1695–706.

70. Larney S, Kopinski H, Beckwith CG, et al. Incidence and prevalence of hepatitis C in prisons and other closed settings: results of a systematic review and meta-analysis. Hepatology 2013;58(4):1215–24.

71. Cunningham EB, Hajarizadeh B, Bretana NA, et al. Ongoing incident hepatitis C virus infection among people with a history of injecting drug use in an Australian prison setting, 2005-2014: the HITS-p study. J Viral Hepat 2017;24(9):733–41.

72. Maher L, Jalaludin B, Chant KG, et al. Incidence and risk factors for hepatitis C seroconversion in injecting drug users in Australia. Addiction 2006;101(10): 1499–508.

73. Hagan H, Pouget ER, Des Jarlais DC, et al. Meta-regression of hepatitis C virus infection in relation to time since onset of illicit drug injection: the influence of time and place. Am J Epidemiol 2008;168(10):1099–109.

74. Tracy D, Hahn JA, Fuller Lewis C, et al. Higher risk of incident hepatitis C virus among young women who inject drugs compared with young men in association with sexual relationships: a prospective analysis from the UFO Study cohort. BMJ Open 2014;4(5):e004988.

75. Esmaeili A, Mirzazadeh A, Carter GM, et al. Higher incidence of HCV in females compared to males who inject drugs: a systematic review and meta-analysis. J Viral Hepat 2017;24(2):117–27.

76. Evans JL, Hahn JA, Page-Shafer K, et al. Gender differences in sexual and injection risk behavior among active young injection drug users in San Francisco (the UFO Study). J Urban Health 2003;80(1):137–46.

77. Matthews GV, Pham ST, Hellard M, et al. Patterns and characteristics of hepatitis C transmission clusters among HIV-positive and HIV-negative individuals in the Australian trial in acute hepatitis C. Clin Infect Dis 2011;52(6):803–11.

78. Johnson WD, Diaz RM, Flanders WD, et al. Behavioral interventions to reduce risk for sexual transmission of HIV among men who have sex with men. Cochrane Database Syst Rev 2008;(3):CD001230.

79. Grebely J, Dore GJ, Morin S, et al. Elimination of HCV as a public health concern among people who inject drugs by 2030 – What will it take to get there? J Int AIDS Soc 2017;20(1):22146.

80. Hickman M, De Angelis D, Vickerman P, et al. Hepatitis C virus treatment as prevention in people who inject drugs: testing the evidence. Curr Opin Infect Dis 2015;28(6):576–82.

81. Martin NK, Foster GR, Vilar J, et al. HCV treatment rates and sustained viral response among people who inject drugs in seven UK sites: real world results and modelling of treatment impact. J Viral Hepat 2015;22(4):399–408.

82. Zahnd C, Salazar-Vizcaya L, Dufour JF, et al. Modelling the impact of deferring HCV treatment on liver-related complications in HIV coinfected men who have sex with men. J Hepatol 2016;65(1):26–32.

83. Scott N, McBryde ES, Thompson A, et al. Treatment scale-up to achieve global HCV incidence and mortality elimination targets: a cost-effectiveness model. Gut 2017;66(8):1507–15.

84. Razavi H. Reducing a country's HCV-disease burden. The 4th International Symposium on Hepatitis in Substance Users (INHSU 2015). Sydney, Australia, October 7–9, 2015.

85. Puoti M, Cooper C, Sulkowski MS, et al. ABT-450/r/Ombitasvir plus dasabuvir with or without ribavirin in HCV genotype 1-infected patients receiving stable opioid substitution treatment: pooled analysis of efficacy and safety in phase 2 and phase 3 Trials. Hepatology 2014;60:1135a–6a.

86. Lalezari J, Sullivan JG, Varunok P, et al. Ombitasvir/paritaprevir/r and dasabuvir plus ribavirin in HCV genotype 1-infected patients on methadone or buprenorphine. J Hepatol 2015;63(2):364–9.

87. Grebely J, Mauss S, Brown A, et al. Efficacy and safety of ledipasvir/sofosbuvir with and without ribavirin in patients with chronic HCV genotype 1 infection receiving opioid substitution therapy: analysis of phase 3 ION trials. Clin Infect Dis 2016;63(11):1405–11.

88. Grebely J, Dore GJ, Zeuzem S, et al. Efficacy and safety of sofosbuvir/velpatasvir in patients with chronic hepatitis C virus infection receiving opioid substitution therapy: analysis of phase 3 ASTRAL trials. Clin Infect Dis 2016;63(11):1479–81.

89. Grebely J, Puoti M, Wedemeyer H, et al. Safety and Efficacy of ombitasvir, paritaprevir/ritonavir and dasabuvir with or without ribavirin in chronic hepatitis C patients receiving opioid substitution therapy: a pooled analysis across 12 clinical trials. J Hepatol 2017;66:S514.

90. Grebely J, Jacobson IM, Kayali Z, et al. SOF/VEL/VOX for 8 or 12 weeks is well tolerated and results in high SVR12 rates in patients receiving opioid substitution therapy. J Hepatol 2017;66:S513.

91. Christensen S, Schober A, Mauss S, et al. DAA-Treatment of HCV-infected patients on Opioid Substitution Therapy (OST): does the clinical setting matter? Data from the German Hepatitis C-Registry (DHC-R). Hepatology 2016; 64(S1):982A–3A.

92. Schutz A, Moser S, Marchart K, et al. Direct observed therapy of chronic hepatitis C with interferon-free all-oral regimens at a low-threshold drug treatment facility-a new concept for treatment of patients with borderline compliance receiving opioid substitution therapy. Am J Gastroenterol 2016;111(6):903–5.

93. Scherz N, Brunner N, Bruggmann P. Direct-acting antivirals for hepatitis C in patient in opioid substitution treatment and heroin assisted treatment: real-life data. J Hepatol 2017;66:S726.

94. Dillon J, Mauss S, Nalpas C, et al. Efficacy and safety of Simeprevir-containing hepatitis C therapy in patients on opiate substitution therapy. J Hepatol 2017;66: S520.
95. Butner JL, Gupta N, Fabian C, et al. Onsite treatment of HCV infection with direct acting antivirals within an opioid treatment program. J Subst Abuse Treat 2017; 75:49–53.
96. Boyle A, Marra F, Fox R, et al. Partial directly observed therapy with ombitasvir/paritaprevir based regimens allows for successful treatment of patients on daily supervised methadone. J Hepatol 2017;66.
97. Conway B, Raycraft T, Bhutani Y, et al. Efficacy of all-oral HCV therapy in people who inject drugs. Hepatology 2016;64(S1):990A.
98. Morris L, Smirnov A, Kvassay A, et al. Initial outcomes of integrated community-based hepatitis C treatment for people who inject drugs: findings from the Queensland Injectors' Health Network. Int J Drug Policy 2017;47:216–20.
99. Mason K, Dodd Z, Guyton M, et al. Understanding real-world adherence in the directly acting antiviral era: a prospective evaluation of adherence among people with a history of drug use at a community-based program in Toronto, Canada. Int J Drug Policy 2017;47:202–8.
100. Litwin AH, Agyemang L, Akiyama M, et al. The PREVAIL study: intensive models of HCV care for people who inject drugs. J Hepatol 2017;66:S72.
101. Elsherif O, Bannan C, Keating S, et al. Outcomes from a large 10 year hepatitis C treatment programme in people who inject drugs: no effect of recent or former injecting drug use on treatment adherence or therapeutic response. PLoS One 2017;12(6):e0178398.
102. Conway B, Wang J, Wong L, et al. HCV reinfection in high-risk illicit drug users. Paper presented at: 3rd International Symposium on Hepatitis Care in Substance Users. Vancouver, Canada, September 6, 2013.
103. Deshaies L. Treatment of hepatitis C in active intravenous drug users (IDUS): re-infection rate in TACTIC cohort. Suchtmed 2013;15(4):262–3.
104. Edlin BR, Carden MR, Getter EV, et al. Hepatitis C treatment in active injection drug users [abstract]. Hepatology 2013;58(S1):1091A–168A.
105. Hilsden RJ, Macphail G, Grebely J, et al. Directly observed pegylated interferon plus self-administered ribavirin for the treatment of hepatitis C virus infection in people actively using drugs: a randomized controlled trial. Clin Infect Dis 2013; 57(Suppl 2):S90–6.
106. Ruzić M, Fabri M, Preveden T, et al. Treatment of chronic hepatitis C in injecting drug users–a 5-year follow-up. Vojnosanit Pregl 2013;70(8):723–7.
107. Grady BP, Vanhommerig JW, Schinkel J, et al. Low incidence of reinfection with the hepatitis C virus following treatment in active drug users in Amsterdam. Eur J Gastroenterol Hepatol 2012;24(11):1302–7.
108. Manolakopoulos S, Kranidioti H, Karatapanis S, et al. Hepatitis C virus reinfection following sustained virological response in intravenous drug users [abstract]. J Hepatol 2012;56:S532.
109. Dalgard O, Bjoro K, Hellum K, et al. Treatment of chronic hepatitis C in injecting drug users: 5 years' follow-up. Eur Addict Res 2002;8(1):45–9.

Understanding and Addressing Hepatitis C Virus Reinfection Among Men Who Have Sex with Men

Thomas C.S. Martin, MD[a], Andri Rauch, MD[b],
Luisa Salazar-Vizcaya, PhD[b], Natasha K. Martin, DPhil[a,c,*]

KEYWORDS

- Hepatitis C virus • Reinfection • Prevention • Men who have sex with men

KEY POINTS

- Hepatitis C virus reinfection incidence rates among human immunodeficiency virus-infected men who have sex with men are 3 to 10 times higher than baseline incidence.
- Modeling indicates that tackling increasing incidence and high reinfection requires widespread hepatitis C virus treatment combined with behavioral interventions.
- Behavioral interventions studies addressing hepatitis C virus reinfection are required, such as the ongoing HCVree trial in Switzerland.
- Other interventions may include traditional harm reduction interventions, adapted behavioral interventions, and interventions to prevent risk related to substance use with sex.

Funding: N.K. Martin is supported by the National Institute on Drug Abuse [grant number R01 DA037773-01A1] and the University of California, San Diego Center for AIDS Research (CFAR), a National Institute of Health (NIH) funded program [grant number P30 AI036214] which is supported by the following NIH Institutes and Centers: NIAID, NCI, NIMH, NIDA, NICHD, NHLBI, NIA NIGMS, and NIDDK. The views expressed are those of the authors and not necessarily those of the National Institutes of Health.
Disclosures: T.C.S. Martin has no disclosures. N.K. Martin has received unrestricted research grants from Gilead unrelated to this work and honoraria from Merck, Gilead, and AbbVie. A. Rauch reports support to his institution for advisory boards and/or travel grants from Janssen-Cilag, MSD, Gilead Sciences, Abbvie, and Bristol-Myers Squibb, and an unrestricted research grant from Gilead Sciences. All remuneration went to his home institution and not to A. Rauch personally, and all remuneration was provided outside the submitted work.
[a] Division of Infectious Diseases and Global Public Health, Department of Medicine, University of California, San Diego, 9500 Gilman Drive La Jolla, CA 92093-0507, USA; [b] Institute for Infectious Diseases, University of Bern, Bern, Switzerland, Friedbühlstrasse 53, Personalhaus 6, 3010 Bern, Switzerland; [c] School of Social and Community Medicine, University of Bristol, Senate House, Tyndall Avenue, Bristol BS8 1TH, UK
* Corresponding author. Division of Infectious Diseases and Global Public Health, Department of Medicine, University of California, San Diego, 9500 Gilman Drive La Jolla, CA 92093-0507.
E-mail address: Natasha-martin@ucsd.edu

Infect Dis Clin N Am 32 (2018) 395–405
https://doi.org/10.1016/j.idc.2018.02.004
0891-5520/18/© 2018 Elsevier Inc. All rights reserved.

INTRODUCTION

Among people living with human immunodeficiency virus (HIV) worldwide, it has been estimated that 2.4% (interquartile range, 0.8–5.8) are coinfected with hepatitis C virus (HCV), yet this increases to 6.4% (interquartile range, 3.2–10.0) among men who have sex with men (MSM).[1] Indeed, an epidemic of HCV among HIV-infected (HIV+) men who have sex with men (MSM) has been documented in major urban centers in the United States, Europe, and Australia, with dramatic increases in HCV incidence and/or prevalence in the past decade.[2–10] This epidemic has been associated not only with injection drug use, but also with high-risk sexual practices and substance use with sex among those with no history of injection drug use.[11] Because HIV+ individuals are living longer in the era of highly active antiretoriviral therapies, the morbidity and mortality associated with viral hepatitis coinfection increases. Consequently, liver-related mortality is one of the leading non-AIDS causes of death among HIV+ individuals.[12]

The World Health Organization recently released targets for hepatitis B virus and HCV elimination, which included a 90% relative reduction in new infections and a 65% relative reduction in hepatitis-related mortality by 2030.[13] As a result, policymakers are looking for evidence-based preventions strategies to achieve these targets. Recent advanced in HCV direct-acting antiviral (DAAs) therapies have resulted in short-term (8–12 week), all-oral, highly tolerable treatments with cure rates in excess of 90% for both HCV monoinfected and HIV/HCV-coinfected individuals alike.[14] This advance has led to substantial optimism that the expansion of HCV treatment could both lead to individual cure and also to the potential prevention of onward transmission.[15] However, owing to the high cost of HCV therapy, concerns regarding reinfection continue to hamper efforts to scale-up HCV treatment for those at risk of transmission, such as MSM and people who inject drugs.

In this article, we discuss the empirical evidence surrounding HCV reinfection among MSM, modeling evidence of the importance of reinfection on achieving HCV elimination, and potential strategies to reduce reinfection.

Hepatitis C Virus Reinfection Among Men Who Have Sex with Men: Epidemiologic Evidence

Reinfection with HCV after treatment or spontaneous clearance has been demonstrated in animal models, people who inject drugs, and more recently among HIV+ MSM.[16] Indeed, several studies in the pre-DAA era have demonstrated that the reinfection incidence among HIV+ MSM in Western Europe and the United States is alarmingly high, at approximately 3 to 10 times the baseline incidence in this population.[17–20] A summary of studies of reinfection incidence rates after successful treatment is shown in **Fig. 1**.

The first of these studies, performed in Amsterdam, retrospectively identified 56 HIV+ MSM who had been successfully treated for acute HCV between 2003 and 2011.[18] There were 11 confirmed reinfections using phylogenetic analysis of the E2/HVR region of the virus, yielding a reinfection incidence of 15.2 per 100 person-years (95% confidence interval [CI], 8.0–26.5). This reinfection incidence was approximately 10 times the primary HCV infection incidence among HIV+ MSM in Amsterdam.[21] The authors also found that, for individuals who had behavioral data, those who experienced reinfection were more likely to report noninjecting recreational drug use than those who did not experience reinfection.

In London, a retrospective cohort study from 2004 to 2012 examined HCV reinfection incidence after both successful treatment and spontaneous clearance of HCV

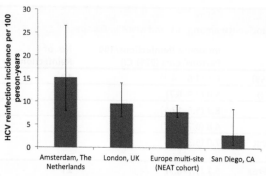

Fig. 1. Hepatitis C virus (HCV) reinfection incidence after successful treatment among human immunodeficiency virus and men who have sex with men as reported in Amsterdam, London, the NEAT cohort (European AIDS Treatment Network), and San Diego, California. (*Data from* Refs.[17–20])

infection.[19] Among 191 patients who were either treated for HCV infection or who spontaneously cleared their infection, 44 reinfections occurred, representing an incidence of 7.8 per 100 person-years (95% CI, 5.8–10.5). This reinfection rate is 6 to 7 times the observed primary incidence among HIV+ MSM in the UK (1.02–1.38 per 100py).[22] Interestingly, the authors found indications of a higher reinfection rate among those treated for HCV (9.6 per 100 person-years; 95% CI, 6.6–14.1) than among those who spontaneously cleared their infection (4.2 per 100 person-years; 95% CI, 1.7–10.0), although the difference did not reach significance. The authors hypothesized that this may be due to a degree of protective immunity developed among individuals who spontaneously clear their infection, making it less likely they become reinfected or that if any reinfection occurred it was spontaneously cleared.

In a larger multicenter study between 2002 and 2014 including 8 hospitals across Austria, France, Germany, and the UK from the NEAT cohort (European AIDS Treatment Network), nearly one-third of HIV+ MSM were reinfected with HCV within 5 years of clearing their primary infection either through successful treatment or spontaneous clearance.[17] Among 606 HIV+ MSM who cleared their primary infections, 143 were reinfected, with an overall reinfection incidence of 7.3 per 100 person-years (95% CI, 6.2–8.6).[17] The reinfection incidence per center is shown in **Table 1**. As in the London study, a trend for lower reinfection incidence after spontaneous clearance of the initial HCV infection when compared with those that were successfully treated was observed (hazard ratio, 0.62; 95% CI, 0.38–1.02; $P = .06$). Individuals who spontaneously cleared their initial infection were more likely to spontaneously clear any reinfection, supporting the possibility of protective immunity or favorable host defenses such as the IL28BCC genotype. The authors additionally found that the incidence of a second reinfection (18.8 per 100 person-years; 95% CI, 12.9–27.5) was higher compared with the incidence of first reinfection (hazard ratio, 2.5; 95% CI, 1.7–3.8), suggesting that the HCV epidemic may in part be being driven by a small group of high-risk individuals.

Outside Europe but still during the pre-DAA era, a recent retrospective study in San Diego, California, found that among 43 HIV+ MSM who had been treated successfully for their HCV infection between 2008 and 2015, 3 became reinfected, yielding a reinfection incidence of 2.9 per 100 person-years (95% CI, 0.6–8.4).[20] This compared with a local primary incidence of 1.2 per 100 person-years (95% CI, 1.0–1.4), indicating that reinfection rates may be 2- to 3-fold that of primary infection.

Table 1
HCV reinfection incidence among HIV and MSM in Europe

Center	Incidence Reinfections/100 Person-Years (95% CI)	No. of Reinfections	Person-Years of Follow-up
Dusseldorf (n = 59)	8.1 (4.6–14.3)	12	148
Hamburg (n = 73)	5.0 (2.9–8.7)	13	258
Berlin (n = 95)	8.2 (5.6–12.1)	26	316
Bonn (n = 11)	4.8 (0.7–33.7)	1	21
London – Chelwest (n = 190)	7.0 (5.3–9.1)	52	746
London – Royal Free (n = 69)	5.7 (3.7–8.7)	21	369
Paris (n = 27)	21.8 (11.3–41.8)	9	41
Vienna (n = 28)	16.8 (8.7–32.3)	9	54

Abbreviations: CI, confidence interval; HCV, hepatitis C virus; HIV, human immunodeficiency virus; MSM, men who have sex with men.

From Ingiliz P, Martin TC, Rodger A, et al. HCV reinfection incidence and spontaneous clearance rates in HIV-positive men who have sex with men in Western Europe. J Hepatol 2017;66(2):284; with permission.

The studies discussed were performed in the period that prolonged interferon-containing regimens were the standard of care. Given the shorter courses and much greater tolerability of DAA therapy, concerns have arisen that improved therapy may lead to an increase in risk-taking behavior and a higher reinfection incidence. One study to date has examined HCV reinfection in the DAA era. This was an analysis of GECCO (German Hepatitis C cohort) looking at HCV reinfection after DAA therapy between 2014 and 2016, finding that among 175 HIV+ MSM treated between February 2014 and May 2016, 7.4% (13/175) were reinfected.[23] Further work examining reinfection incidence rates in the DAA era will shed important light on this issue.

No studies have identified behavioral risks specifically associated with HCV reinfection among HIV+ MSM. However, numerous studies have explored risk behaviors associated with HCV prevalence and incidence in this population, showing that fisting,[4,9,24–26] rectal trauma with bleeding,[26] condomless receptive anal intercourse,[4,27,28] group sex,[4,26,27] injecting drug use,[9,27] sex while high on methamphetamine,[28] consumption of gamma hydroxybutyrate,[9] and recreational use of cocaine, ecstasy, gamma hydroxybutyrate, ketamine, amphetamine, or methamphetamine before or during sexual contact[25] are associated with HCV acquisition. Interventions aimed at reducing risk of HCV infection and reinfection should, therefore, target these associated risks.

Modeling the Impact of Reinfection on Achieving Hepatitis C Virus Elimination Among People Who Inject Drugs Versus Men Who Have Sex with Men Populations

A number of theoretic epidemic modeling studies have evaluated the potential impact of scaled-up HCV prevention on HCV prevalence and incidence among people who inject drugs, including the risk of reinfection. Empirical studies have shown that HCV reinfection rates among PWID are low (3% per year in the interferon-containing era).[29] Unfortunately, few studies have directly compared HCV primary incidence and reinfection rates among PWID in the same setting, but the reported rates are broadly similar to, if not lower than, the primary incidence rates. As a conservative assumption, the vast majority of epidemic models have assumed that the risk of reinfection is equal to primary infection, and have studied settings with varied incidence from 3% to 30% per year, in North America, Europe, Asia, and Australia.[30–34] In general, these studies have found that, despite the risk of reinfection, HCV incidence and prevalence can be dramatically reduced (in many settings by 90% by 2030) with scaled-up HCV treatment to rates to less than 100 per 1000 PWID annually, particularly in combination with harm reduction. As such, relatively modest levels of treatment are required to eliminate HCV despite this risk of reinfection.

Despite this encouraging evidence, a few recent epidemic modeling analyses have shown that achieving substantial reductions in HCV incidence among HIV+ MSM populations is likely to be more challenging compared with among PWID owing to the relatively high rates of existing HCV treatment combined with the increased risk of reinfection (indicating a high-risk core group) and increasing incidence over time in many settings such as Switzerland and Berlin.[22,35,36] Existing modeling studies have focused on the UK, Switzerland, Berlin, and the Netherlands, showing that achieving a greater than 80% reduction in incidence requires treating virtually all MSM upon diagnosis combined with risk reduction to prevent infection and reinfection. In the UK, a modeling study indicated that scaled-up rates of DAA therapy (from 46% to 80% treated within 1 year of diagnosis and from 7% per year to 20% per year thereafter) could decrease incidence among HIV+ MSM more than 60% by 2030, but could not meet elimination targets,[22] thus likely requiring additional behavioral interventions. Similar modeling findings in Switzerland prompted the generation of a behavioral intervention among MSM, described below.

The Swiss HCVree behavioral intervention trial and epidemic modeling

Since the mid 2000s, an outbreak of incident HCV infections among HIV+ MSM became evident in Switzerland.[10,37] This new epidemic cooccurred with an increase in self-reported condomless sex with occasional partners in this population.[10] MSM accounted for 24% and 85% of all incident HCV infections in the SHCS (Swiss HIV Cohort Study; available: www.shcs.ch) before and after 2006 respectively.[38] The health care system responded with a 10-fold increase in the HCV treatment rate.[10,35] Increasing treatment rates coincided with an increased awareness of this epidemic and the advent of better treatments, namely DAA.[39] However, such increases in the treatment rate did not result in a decreased HCV incidence among HIV+ MSM. Owing to the high costs of these drugs,[40] reimbursement in Switzerland was initially restricted to people who had reached advanced stages of liber fibrosis. This restriction inhibited the early treatment of incident infections with DAAs outside clinical trials.

Treatment reimbursement restrictions were, however, not the only barrier to tackling the intensifying epidemic. A model of HCV transmission among HIV+ MSM was developed and calibrated to Switzerland and projected the effect of treatment interventions assuming different scenarios of risk behavior. The model suggested that high rates of DAA-based treatment may fail at reducing HCV primary and reinfection incidence if sexual practices associated with transmission continue to increase among the MSM population, but could lead to a decreasing incidence if the frequency of such practices stabilizes. Moreover, the model projected that in 2030 57% of all infections would be reinfections if risk behavior increases and 23% if risk behavior stabilizes.[35]

Given these projections and the limitations imposed by regulatory reimbursement restrictions, clinicians from the SHCS engaged in a 1-year clinical trial that provided early treatment for HCV infections in MSM and prevented reinfections through risk counseling. The study includes 3 phases. First, all MSM were screened for replicating HCV infection with HCV RNA. Second, all participants infected with HCV genotypes 1 or 4 were offered treatment with grazoprevir/elbasvir with or without ribavirin. Third, HCV RNA screening will be repeated in all MSM to assess the effect of this intervention on HCV prevalence. The study started in October 2015 with the screening of 4257 MSM.[41] One hundred seventy-eight (4.8%) had a replicating HCV infection. Of those, 94% were infected with HCV genotypes 1 or 4 and were offered treatment with the study drugs. The evaluation of the treatment phase and the subsequent rescreening phase is currently ongoing. In addition to HCV treatment, enrolled patients who reported inconsistent condom use with occasional partners received four 45-minute sessions of individual sexual risk counseling at weeks 4, 6, 8, and 12. This behavioral intervention, which was specifically developed for this patient group, included detailed interviews and computer-assisted counseling similar to a previous European multicenter study targeting HIV+ MSM.[42]

Salazar-Vizcaya and coworkers subsequently used epidemic modeling to predict the potential impact of the Swiss HCVree trial (A Phase III, Multi-center, Open-label Trial to Investigate the Impact of a Treat, Counsel and Cure Strategy in Men Who Have Sex With Men With Hepatitis C Infection in the Swiss HIV Cohort Study) to assess the potential of this type of (short-term) treatment plus intensive intervention counseling. Simulations considered intensive intervention and hypothetical scenarios of treatment and risk behavior simultaneously. The model suggested that an intensive intervention would considerably decrease incidence over the intervention period, but if after intensive intervention treatment was deferred in line with reimbursement regulations, this benefit would dissipate in the long term. Interestingly, even though high treatment rates after intensive intervention led to nearly the same simulated prevalence with or without intensive intervention in the long-term, intensive intervention was predicted to save treatment costs.[43] As a consequence of the model projections, the HCVree trial was extended until the end of 2017. New incident infections as well as reinfections will be treated during this period.

Additionally, reimbursement regulations for DAA-based HCV therapy changed in May 2017, and DAA therapy is now reimbursed irrespective of fibrosis stage in all HIV+ patients. We, therefore, expect trends in risk behavior to shape the future course of HCV transmission among HIV+ MSM in Switzerland, making behavioral interventions such as the Swiss HCVree trial even more critical.

Other Interventions to Prevent Infection and Reinfection Among Men Who Have Sex with Men

In addition to behavioral interventions addressing inconsistent condom use among MSM at risk for HCV infection and reinfection (such as the Swiss HCVree trial), effective behavioral interventions targeting other HCV-related risks among MSM are urgently required.

Traditional harm reduction interventions targeting men who have sex with men who inject drugs
There is increasing evidence that traditional harm reduction interventions such as opiate substitution therapy and high coverage needle and syringe programs are effective at reducing HCV transmission among people who inject drugs. A recent Cochrane review and metaanalysis found that opiate substitution therapy reduces the risk of acquiring HCV by 50% (relative risk [RR], 0.50; 95% CI, 0.40–0.63).[44] In addition, high-coverage needle and syringe programs were found to decrease HCV acquisition by 23% (RR, 0.77; 95% CI, 0.38–1.54),[44] with a greater impact seen in Europe (RR, 0.44; 95% CI, 0.24–0.80).[44] When combining high coverage of both needle and syringe programs and opiate substitution therapy interventions, the risk of acquiring

HCV was reduced by an estimated 71% (RR, 0.29; 95% CI, 0.13–0.65).[44] Despite this evidence, the impact of harm reduction among MSM who inject drugs has not been studied specifically. Additionally, MSM who inject drugs may not self-identify as people who inject drugs, and therefore may not access traditional harm reduction services.

Adapted human immunodeficiency virus prevention interventions among men who have sex with men It is unclear whether interventions to prevent HIV transmission among MSM would be effective to prevent HCV infection among MSM. However, given the potential shared transmission routes, it is possible these interventions could be used or adapted. There is an extensive body of literature on behavioral interventions to reduce unprotected anal intercourse and HIV transmission among MSM.[45] For example, a Cochrane review and metaanalysis of 40 behavioral interventions found a reduction of occasions of or partners for unprotected anal sex by 27% (95% CI, 15%-37%) compared with no or minimal intervention.[45] One intervention, Project ECHO, targets substance using MSM and uses personalized cognitive counseling to help participants to identify and avoid risky sexual and drug-using behaviors.[46] Among HIV-negative MSM who reported sex after substance use in the past 6 months, Project ECHO reduced the number of condomless anal intercourse events with nonprimary partners by 46% (RR, 0.56; 95% CI, 0.34 - 0.92) compared with the control group.[46] Studies exploring whether interventions similar to or adapted from Project ECHO are effective for HCV prevention among MSM are warranted.

ChemSex intervention There is an emerging body of literature examining the development of educational and counseling interventions targeted at MSM who use crystal methamphetamine with sex ("ChemSex"),[47–49] which may reduce the risk of acquiring HCV among this population. ChemSex is associated with HCV infection, as well as high-risk behaviors such as multiple sexual partners, transactional sex, group sex, fisting, sharing sex toys, injecting drug use, higher alcohol consumption, and the use of 'bareback' sexual networking applications.[50]

In 1 HIV/genitourinary medicine clinic in London, after completion of HCV treatment, clinicians provide MSM with harm reduction messages, education on HCV transmission risks related to ChemSex, ChemSex packs including safe injecting equipment and educational information, and a referral to on-site, ChemSex behavior change support.[49] It has been reported that ChemSex motivations are often associated with internalized homophobia and shame surrounding homosexual sex, gay cultural/societal norms, sexual performance anxieties, and body image concerns. Successful behavioral interventions for MSM at risk of acquiring or transmitting HCV in ChemSex environments would need to address these sensitive issues.

SUMMARY

HCV reinfection rates among MSM are high (3–15 per 100 person-years), and are 3- to 10-fold higher than the rates of primary incidence, indicating a high-risk core group of MSM at risk for HCV infection and reinfection. Factors associated with HCV infection among MSM point toward a number of varied sexual and drug-related risks, which could be targeted for interventions to prevent infection and reinfection. Modeling indicates that tackling the increasing incidence and high reinfection rates requires high levels of HCV treatment combined with behavioral interventions. Enhanced testing strategies and prompt retreating of reinfection may be required to promptly diagnose reinfections and prevent further onward transmissions. Other investigators have suggested strategies such as home-based dried blot spot collection at fixed time points or after a risk event. Behavioral interventions studies addressing HCV reinfection are required, such as the HCVree trial in Switzerland. Other relevant interventions may include traditional harm reduction interventions targeting MSM who inject drugs, adapted behavioral interventions targeting HIV risks among substance-using populations, and interventions to prevent harms related to ChemSex and other risk associated with drug use with or before sexual episodes. It is likely that a suite of interventions targeting different subpopulations and risks among MSM will be required, instead of 1 blanket intervention.

REFERENCES

1. Platt L, Easterbrook P, Gower E, et al. Prevalence and burden of HCV co-infection in people living with HIV: a global systematic review and meta-analysis. Lancet Infect Dis 2016;16(7):797–808.

2. Yaphe S, Bozinoff N, Kyle R, et al. Incidence of acute hepatitis C virus infection among men who have sex with men with and without HIV infection: a systematic review. Sex Transm Infect 2012;88(7):558–64.

3. Bradshaw D, Matthews G, Danta M. Sexually transmitted hepatitis C infection: the new epidemic in MSM? Curr Opin Infect Dis 2013;26(1):66–72.

4. Danta M, Brown D, Bhagani S, et al. Recent epidemic of acute hepatitis C virus in HIV-positive men who have sex with men linked to high-risk sexual behaviours. AIDS 2007;21(8):983–91.

5. van de Laar TJ, Matthews GV, Prins M, et al. Acute hepatitis C in HIV-infected men who have sex with men: an emerging sexually transmitted infection. AIDS 2010;24(12):1799–812.

6. Hagan H, Jordan AE, Neurer J, et al. Incidence of sexually transmitted hepatitis C virus infection in HIV-positive men who have sex with men. AIDS 2015;29(17): 2335–45.

7. Jordan AE, Perlman DC, Neurer J, et al. Prevalence of hepatitis C virus infection among HIV+ men who have sex with men: a systematic review and meta-analysis. Int J STD AIDS 2017;28(2):145–59.

8. van der Helm JJ, Prins M, del Amo J, et al. The hepatitis C epidemic among HIV-positive MSM: incidence estimates from 1990 to 2007. AIDS 2011;25(8):1083–91.

9. Urbanus AT, van de Laar TJ, Stolte IG, et al. Hepatitis C virus infections among HIV-infected men who have sex with men: an expanding epidemic. AIDS 2009; 23(12):F1–7.

10. Wandeler G, Gsponer T, Bregenzer A, et al. Hepatitis C virus infections in the Swiss HIV Cohort Study: a rapidly evolving epidemic. Clin Infect Dis 2012; 55(10):1408–16.

11. Centers for Disease Control and Prevention (CDC). Sexual transmission of hepatitis C virus among HIV-infected men who have sex with men–New York City, 2005-2010. MMWR Morb Mortal Wkly Rep 2011;60(28):945–50.

12. Smith CJ, Ryom L, Weber R, et al. Trends in underlying causes of death in people with HIV from 1999 to 2011 (D: A:D): a multicohort collaboration. Lancet 2014; 384(9939):241–8.

13. WHO. Global health sector strategy on viral hepatitis, 2016-2021. Geneva (Switzerland): World Health Organization; 2016.

14. Wyles DL, Sulkowski MS, Dieterich D. Management of hepatitis C/HIV coinfection in the era of highly effective hepatitis C virus direct-acting antiviral therapy. Clin Infect Dis 2016;63(suppl_1):S3–11.

15. Martin NK, Vickerman P, Grebely J, et al. Hepatitis C virus treatment for prevention among people who inject drugs: modeling treatment scale-up in the age of direct-acting antivirals. Hepatology 2013;58(5):1598–609.
16. Grebely J, Prins M, Hellard M, et al. Hepatitis C virus clearance, reinfection, and persistence, with insights from studies of injecting drug users: towards a vaccine. Lancet Infect Dis 2012;12(5):408–14.
17. Ingiliz P, Martin TC, Rodger A, et al. HCV reinfection incidence and spontaneous clearance rates in HIV-positive men who have sex with men in Western Europe. J Hepatol 2017;66(2):282–7.
18. Lambers FA, Prins M, Thomas X, et al. Alarming incidence of hepatitis C virus reinfection after treatment of sexually acquired acute hepatitis C virus infection in HIV-infected MSM. AIDS 2011;25(17):F21–7.
19. Martin TC, Martin NK, Hickman M, et al. Hepatitis C virus reinfection incidence and treatment outcome among HIV-positive MSM. AIDS 2013;27(16):2551–7.
20. Chaillon A, Anderson C, Martin T, et al. Incidence of hepatitis C among HIV-infected men who have sex with men, 2000-2015. Seattle (WA): Conference on Retroviruses and Opportunistic Infections (CROI); 2017.
21. Vanhommerig J, Stolte IG, Lambers FA, et al. Hepatitis C virus incidence in the Amsterdam cohort study among men who have sex with men: 1984-2011. Conference on Retroviruses and Opportunistic Infections held at Boston (MA), March 3–6, 2014.
22. Martin NK, Thornton A, Hickman M, et al. Can Hepatitis C Virus (HCV) direct-acting antiviral treatment as prevention reverse the HCV epidemic among men who have sex with men in the United Kingdom? Epidemiological and modeling insights. Clin Infect Dis 2016;62(9):1072–80.
23. Ingiliz P, Christensen S, Berger F, et al. HCV reinfection after successful DAA treatment: a GECCO analysis. Seattle (WA): Conference on Retroviruses and Opportunistic Infections (CROI) 2015; 2017 [Abstract: 567].
24. Turner JM, Rider AT, Imrie J, et al. Behavioural predictors of subsequent hepatitis C diagnosis in a UK clinic sample of HIV positive men who have sex with men. Sex Transm infections 2006;82(4):298–300.
25. Matser A, Vanhommerig J, Schim van der Loeff MF, et al. HIV-infected men who have sex with men who identify themselves as belonging to subcultures are at increased risk for hepatitis C infection. PLoS One 2013;8(3):e57740.
26. Schmidt AJ, Rockstroh JK, Vogel M, et al. Trouble with bleeding: risk factors for acute hepatitis C among HIV-positive gay men from Germany—a case-control study. PLoS One 2011;6(3):e17781.
27. Witt M, Seaberg EC, Darilay A, et al. Incident hepatitis C virus infection in men who have sex with men: a prospective cohort analysis, 1984-2011. Clin Infect Dis 2013;57(1):77–84.
28. Fierer D, Factor S, Uriel A, et al. Sexual transmission of hepatitis C virus among HIV-infected men who have sex with men - New York City 2005-2010. Morb Mortal Wkly Rep 2011;60(28):945–50.
29. Simmons B, Saleem J, Hill A, et al. Risk of late relapse or reinfection with hepatitis C virus after achieving a sustained virological response: a systematic review and meta-analysis. Clin Infect Dis 2016;62(6):683–94.
30. Scott N, McBryde ES, Thompson A, et al. Treatment scale-up to achieve global HCV incidence and mortality elimination targets: a cost-effectiveness model. Gut 2017;66(8):1507–15.
31. Martin N, Hickman M, Hutchinson S, et al. Combination interventions to prevent HCV transmission among people who inject drugs: modelling the impact of

antiviral treatment, needle and syringe programmes, and opiate substitution therapy. Clin Infect Dis 2013;57(suppl 2):S39–45.

32. Gountas I, Sypsa V, Anagnostou O, et al. Treatment and primary prevention in people who inject drugs for chronic hepatitis C infection: is elimination possible in a high prevalence setting? Addiction 2017;112(7):1290–9.

33. Cousien A, Tran VC, Deuffic-Burban S, et al. Hepatitis C treatment as prevention of viral transmission and liver-related morbidity in persons who inject drugs. Hepatology 2016;63(4):1090–101.

34. Lima VD, Rozada I, Grebely J, et al. Are interferon-free direct-acting antivirals for the treatment of HCV enough to control the epidemic among people who inject drugs? PLoS One 2015;10(12):e0143836.

35. Salazar-Vizcaya L, Kouyos RD, Zahnd C, et al. Hepatitis C virus transmission among human immunodeficiency virus-infected men who have sex with men: modeling the effect of behavioral and treatment interventions. Hepatology 2016;64(6):1856–69.

36. Hullegie S, Nichols B, Rijnders B, et al. Is HCV elimination Possible? A modeling study of HIV-positive MSM. Boston: Conference on Retroviruses and Opportunistic Infections (CROI) 2016; 2016 [Abstract: #536].

37. Rauch A, Martin M, Weber R, et al. Unsafe sex and increased incidence of Hepatitis C Virus infection among HIV-infected men who have sex with men: the Swiss HIV cohort study. Clin Infect Dis 2005;41(3):395–402.

38. Wandeler G, Schlauri M, Jaquier M-E, et al. Incident Hepatitis C Virus infections in the Swiss HIV Cohort Study: changes in treatment uptake and outcomes between 1991 and 2013. Open Forum Infect Dis 2015;2(1):ofv026.

39. Béguelin C, Suter A, Bernasconi E, et al. Trends in HCV treatment uptake, efficacy and impact on liver fibrosis in the Swiss HIV Cohort Study. Liver Int 2018; 38(3):424–31.

40. Iyengar S, Tay-Teo K, Vogler S, et al. Prices, costs, and affordability of new medicines for Hepatitis C in 30 countries: an economic analysis. PLoS Med 2016; 13(5):e1002032.

41. Braun DL, Kouyos RD, Hampel BH, et al. Systematic HCV-RNA screen in HIV+ MSM reveals high numbers of potential transmitters. Boston: Conference on Retroviruses and Opportunistic Infections (CROI); 2017.

42. Nöstlinger C, Platteau T, Bogner J, et al. Implementation and operational research: computer-assisted intervention for safer sex in HIV-positive men having sex with men: findings of a European randomized multi-center trial. J Acquir Immune Defic Syndr 2016;71(3):e63–72.

43. Salazar-Vizcaya L, Kouyos RD, Fehr J, et al. On the potential of a short-term intensive intervention to interrupt HCV transmission in HIV-positive men who have sex with men: a mathematical modelling study. J Viral Hepat 2018;25(1):10–8.

44. Platt L, Reed J, Minozzi S, et al. Effectiveness of needle/syringe programmes and opiate substitution therapy in preventing HCV transmission among people who inject drugs. Cochrane Database Syst Rev 2016;2016(1) [pii:CD012021].

45. Johnson W, Diaz R, Flanders W, et al. Behavioral interventions to reduce risk for sexual transmission of HIV among men who have sex with men. Cochrane Database Syst Rev 2008;(3):CD001230.

46. Coffin PO, Santos G-M, Colfax G, et al. Adapted personalized cognitive counseling for episodic substance-using men who have sex with men: a randomized controlled trial. AIDS Behav 2014;18(7):1390–400.

47. Pakianathan MR, Lee MJ, Kelly B, et al. How to assess gay, bisexual and other men who have sex with men for chemsex. Sex Transm Infections 2016;92(8): 568–70.
48. Stuart D, Weymann J. ChemSex and care-planning: one year in practice. HIV Nurs 2015;15:24–8.
49. Stuart D. Sexualised drug use by MSM (ChemSex): a toolkit for GUM/HIV staff. HIV Nurs 2014;14(2):15.
50. Hegazi A, Lee M, Whittaker W, et al. Chemsex and the city: sexualised substance use in gay bisexual and other men who have sex with men attending sexual health clinics. Int J STD AIDS 2017;28(4):362–6.

Hepatitis C Virus Elimination in the Human Immunodeficiency Virus–Coinfected Population

Leveraging the Existing Human Immunodeficiency Virus Infrastructure

Meredith E. Clement, MD[a], Lauren F. Collins, MD[b],
Julius M. Wilder, MD, PhD[c,d], Michael Mugavero, MD, MHS[e],
Taryn Barker, MSc[f], Susanna Naggie, MD, MHS[a,d],*

KEYWORDS

- Hepatitis C infection • Elimination • Human immunodeficiency virus • Coinfection
- Care cascade • Care continuum

KEY POINTS

- Consequences of hepatitis C virus (HCV) infection are more severe in the setting of human immunodeficiency virus (HIV) coinfection, and those with HIV-HCV coinfection are a population to be prioritized for care.
- Leveraging the existing HIV infrastructure is a practical solution for expediting treatment services to coinfected patients.
- Colocalization of HCV care within HIV centers will allow centralized resources to be effectively used, optimizing the chance of an HCV cure for coinfected patients.

INTRODUCTION

More than 2 million people worldwide are coinfected with human immunodeficiency virus (HIV) and hepatitis C virus (HCV).[1] In the setting of HIV coinfection, the

---

Disclosure Statement: The authors have nothing to disclose.
[a] Division of Infectious Diseases, Duke University Medical Center, 315 Trent Drive, Hanes House, Room 181, DUMC Box 102359, Durham, NC 27710, USA; [b] Department of Medicine, Emory School of Medicine, 49 Jesse Hill Drive Southeast, Atlanta, GA 30303, USA; [c] Duke Division of Gastroenterology, Box 90120, Durham, NC 27708-0120, USA; [d] Duke Clinical Research Institute, 2400 Pratt Street, Durham, NC 27705, USA; [e] Division of Infectious Diseases, University of Alabama Birmingham, Community Care Building, 908 20th Street South, Birmingham, AL 35294, USA; [f] Clinton Health Access Initiative, 383 Dorchester Avenue, Boston, MA 02127, USA
* Corresponding author. Duke Clinical Research Institute, 2400 Pratt Street, Durham, NC 27705.
E-mail address: susanna.naggie@duke.edu

Infect Dis Clin N Am 32 (2018) 407–423
https://doi.org/10.1016/j.idc.2018.02.005
0891-5520/18/© 2018 Elsevier Inc. All rights reserved.

consequences of HCV infection are more severe, including accelerated progression to cirrhosis, liver failure, and liver-associated death.[2–4] Therefore, reaching the coinfected population with curative HCV treatment is an urgent priority.[5]

Since the inception of interferon (IFN)-based therapies, the treatment of HCV infection has been subject to many barriers.[6] Patients' medical and psychiatric comorbidities were contraindications to therapy; providers faced obstacles in determining treatment candidacy (eg, the need to obtain a liver biopsy); side effects from medications were often intolerable, and the adverse effects required close clinical and laboratory monitoring. For patients with HIV-coinfection, the limitations were even greater: disproportionately less access to care,[7,8] lower response rates to treatment,[9,10] and greater risk of adverse events, including cytopenias.[11–13]

The advent of direct-acting antiviral (DAA) therapy has been one of the greatest medical advancements of the twenty-first century. In the DAA era, treatment of HCV is achieved with excellent safety, tolerability, and efficacy. Furthermore, HIV-coinfected patients achieve cure rates comparable with monoinfected patients.[14–16] With the success of DAA regimens in HIV-HCV coinfected patients, current guidelines from the American Association for the Study of Liver Diseases/Infectious Diseases Society of America recommend that all coinfected patients be prioritized for therapy and be treated the same as patients without HIV, with special consideration given only to potential drug interactions with antiretroviral therapy.[17]

However, obstacles persist in the DAA era; medical barriers have in many cases been replaced by socioeconomic barriers.[18] In the United States, insurance status, poor clinic attendance, ongoing alcohol or substance use, or other social circumstances may impede efforts to treat. As in the IFN era, provider bias continues to impact treatment opportunities.[19] In countries other than the United States, particularly in low- and middle-income countries (LMICs), HCV diagnosis and treatment are limited by a lack of resources; however, through dedicated efforts in some LMICs, there are already early signs of success.

The objective of this review is to consider how the existing HIV infrastructure may be leveraged to inform and improve HCV treatment efforts in the coinfected population. Current gaps in HCV care relevant to the care continuum are reviewed. Successes in HIV treatment will then be applied to the HCV treatment model for coinfected patients. Finally, the authors give examples of HCV treatment strategies for coinfected patients in both domestic and international settings.

HEPATITIS C VIRUS CARE CASCADE AND IDENTIFIED GAPS

The care cascade, or continuum, is a framework for exploring the proportion of patients proceeding to successive stages of care engagement culminating in biological disease control, in the setting of HIV infection, or cure, in the setting of HCV infection. The cascade, first defined in patients with HIV,[20] has been applied to HCV infection, outlining the sequential clinical stages from screening to diagnosis to treatment to cure. The World Health Organization (WHO) profiled the global care cascade for HCV in 2015, demonstrating that stark gaps in care remain.[5] For example, only an estimated 20% of the 71 million persons living with HCV are aware of their diagnosis. As of 2015, approximately 5.4 million HCV-infected persons had been placed on treatment. Of those initiating treatment specifically in 2015 (1.1 million), about half received DAA therapy and only approximately 843,000 achieved a sustained virologic response (SVR).[5]

Other groups have outlined the HCV care cascade, demonstrating low treatment initiation and SVR achievement, especially in the IFN era. In Canadian and US cohorts, treatment rates have been 12% to 17%, with only around 7% achieving SVR.[21,22] Findings have been similar in HIV-HCV coinfected populations.[23,24] For example, in a US clinical cohort of coinfected patients evaluated from 2008 to 2012, 54% of those diagnosed were referred to care, 16% initiated treatment, and 7% were ultimately cured.[23]

Treatment uptake rates have improved in the IFN-free DAA era but are still low[19] and will need to significantly improve if we are to reach a threshold that will decrease transmission and ultimately lead to elimination. Similar to HIV infection,[25] treatment as prevention (TasP) or, as applied to HCV, cure as prevention (CasP), is possible; however, it will not occur without expanded coverage.[26,27] Additionally, given low treatment uptake rates globally, the impact of IFN-free regimens on population-level SVR will be negligible if access to treatment is not expanded.[28] As the authors discuss, strategies to improve the HIV care cascade have been deployed in many clinical settings. How these strategies can be applied to HCV infection, particularly in the context of HIV coinfection and specifically to maximize HCV cure, is largely unexplored.

CONSIDERING THE HUMAN IMMUNODEFICIENCY VIRUS CARE CASCADE AS PART OF AN HEPATITIS C VIRUS TREATMENT PARADIGM

The HIV care cascade similarly encompasses the stages of HIV care at a population level, providing a snap shot of epidemiologic estimates for successive steps toward virologic control. This widely known framework includes diagnosis, linkage to care, retention in care, adherence to antiretroviral therapy (ART), and viral suppression.[29] Although the proportion of persons living with HIV (PLWH) decreases at each successive step of the cascade, much can be learned from efforts to improve care along the continuum. Of note, dramatic differences have been observed for the HIV and HCV treatment cascades, with serostatus awareness via testing and diagnosis being substantially higher in HIV relative to HCV infection. Following this initial step on the cascade, comparable challenges have been observed for care engagement, treatment adherence, and ultimately disease control. Here the authors apply these lessons to the HCV treatment model in coinfected persons (**Fig. 1**).

Screening and Diagnosis

Higher rates of diagnosis can only be accomplished with adequate screening. In the United States, more widespread, routine HIV screening has occurred in recent years, as a result of the 2006 guidelines from the Centers for Disease Control and Prevention recommending that everyone aged 13 to 64 years undergo testing at least once in their lifetime.[30,31] Following suit, increased uptake of HCV screening among HIV-infected persons would help to identify those with coinfection.

The WHO recommends that all PLWH worldwide be screened for HCV infection.[5] In the United States, routine screening with HCV antibody is suggested for all PLWH, with more frequent screening recommended for any PLWH engaging in high-risk behaviors (eg, those using intravenous drugs or men who have sex with men [MSM]).[32] However, even complete compliance with these recommendations will be of limited value if only those who are already diagnosed with HIV and engaged in care are tested. Screening will need to be expanded more broadly to vulnerable populations not in care. Worldwide, 14 million people with HIV infection are unaware of their status.[33] Dual-routine HIV/HCV testing can lead to increased screening for both HIV and HCV, offering one potential solution.[34] One study from Pennsylvania demonstrated that integration of dual-routine HIV/HCV testing resulted in a 24% increase in the number of HCV tests performed and a 125% increase in the number of HIV tests performed

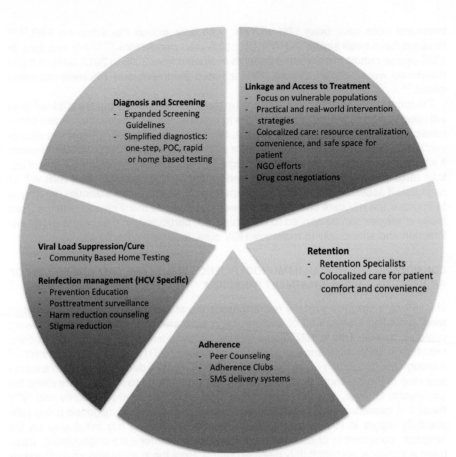

Diagnosis and Screening
- Expanded Screening Guidelines
- Simplified diagnostics: one-step, POC, rapid or home based testing

Linkage and Access to Treatment
- Focus on vulnerable populations
- Practical and real-world intervention strategies
- Colocalized care: resource centralization, convenience, and safe space for patient
- NGO efforts
- Drug cost negotiations

Viral Load Suppression/Cure
- Community Based Home Testing

Reinfection management (HCV Specific)
- Prevention Education
- Posttreatment surveillance
- Harm reduction counseling
- Stigma reduction

Retention
- Retention Specialists
- Colocalized care for patient comfort and convenience

Adherence
- Peer Counseling
- Adherence Clubs
- SMS delivery systems

Fig. 1. Leveraging HIV care strategies to augment the HCV care cascade in coinfected patients. NGO, nongovernmental organization; POC, point of care; SMS, short message service.

in primary care settings.[34] The investigators also showed subsequent increases in newly identified cases and linkage to care; similar results have been found in France.[34,35] Further studies are also evaluating the extent to which a bundled rapid HIV/HCV testing approach increases the potential for diagnosis of HIV and HCV in substance use disorder (SUD) treatment programs.[36] Such screening methods may offer a scalable and cost-effective approach to testing, particularly when targeted at high-risk populations, such as those with SUD.

Another way to facilitate screening uptake is more efficient testing. For HIV, rapid tests are now in use and results are readily available. The standard HCV test used by many clinical laboratories is an immunoassay, although rapid immunoassay tests with comparable performance are also available.[37] Self-collected tests are also available; similarly, these tests have accuracy comparable with laboratory-based antibody testing.[38]

Perhaps more importantly, tests that can eliminate the need for nucleic acid testing (NAT) confirmation may be of great value. Unlike HIV infection, positive serology for HCV does not necessarily imply chronic infection, as 15% to 50% with primary HCV infection will spontaneously clear the virus.[39] NAT testing is then required to confirm active viremia as part of a 2-step diagnostic process, although the test can be prohibitively expensive, especially in LMICs. A significant proportion of patients with positive anti-HCV do not receive NAT and are lost to follow-up.[40] Diagnostic rates of HCV in LMICs are especially poor, with fewer than 1% aware of their infection by some estimates.[41] Testing for HCV core antigen (HCVcAg) is an alternative solution to NAT, as it has high sensitivity and specificity, good correlation with HCV RNA levels, and is likely to be less expensive than NAT.[42] HCVcAg testing is especially appealing, as it could streamline the HCV care cascade by eliminating the need for 2-step diagnostic testing and reducing lost-to-follow-up rates. However, developing point-of-care (POC) HCVcAg testing may prove more difficult than developing POC NAT given the careful sample processing that is necessary and further steps that will be required (eg, signal amplification) before sufficient sensitivity can be achieved.[42] One consideration in countries with exceptionally high HCV prevalence is bypassing serologic testing altogether and screening directly with NAT. More widespread availability of efficient and cost-effective testing strategies could improve screening and, thus, diagnosis rates for HCV in HIV-infected persons worldwide. Cost-effectiveness studies should be performed to help inform different testing strategies.

Linkage to Care and Access to Therapy

In the HIV cascade, optimal linkage to care is defined as initiation of medical treatment with an HIV provider within 1 month of diagnosis documentation. Various initiatives have been designed to help link newly diagnosed HIV-infected patients to care, which may also be applicable to patients with HCV infection. One example is the Seek, Test, Treat, and Retain Data Collection and Harmonization (STTR) initiative that focused on vulnerable criminal justice populations and those with SUD in the United States. The STTR initiative enabled a standardized data collection approach and coordinated research that in turn facilitated the identification of at-risk populations and linkage to care.[43] The multisite Access to Care (A2C) initiative similarly is a multisite intervention implemented as a national evaluation strategy. A2C was designed to identify linkage to care interventions that could most readily and effectively be carried out in local and real-world settings.[44] Because many patients infected with HCV share similar burdens of psychosocial and medical challenges as those with HIV (eg, SUD, mental health disorders, institutionalization), practical strategies such as these that focus on at-risk populations may also be of particular value in linkage to HCV care.

For those with HIV who are newly diagnosed with HCV coinfection, linkage to care may be less of an issue if patients are already engaged in HIV care. However, a substantial proportion of PLWH have not been linked to care.[29] Additionally, HIV coinfection has been associated with missed appointments among HCV-infected persons; appointment-keeping behavior is an important requisite for HCV linkage and treatment initiation.[45] Furthermore, a high proportion of coinfected patients have risk factors for poor engagement, including substance use and psychiatric diseases.

Because of these additional challenges, colocalization of care (ie, treatment of HIV and HCV in one clinic) is an important approach to engaging HIV-HCV coinfected patients; this is most practicably achieved in HIV clinics, given longer-standing infrastructure and existing resources including personnel.[46] Colocalization or multidisciplinary care approaches to HCV therapy in the setting of HIV clinics provide many important benefits. First, the HIV clinic offers familiarity to patients who may be hesitant to seek out additional providers. Medical mistrust can be an important barrier to linkage to care for those with HIV-HCV coinfection,[46] and the HIV clinic is a safe space already known to patients. Second, logistical obstacles to linkage to care, such as lack of transportation, a significant hurdle for this population,[47,48] are reduced or overcome by treating HCV within the HIV clinic. Finally, HIV clinics offer the unique advantage of having readily available resources to address SUD and mental health comorbidities often faced by patients with HIV-HCV coinfection. The availability of social workers and substance abuse counselors is a critical component of HIV clinics and may help alleviate provider hesitancy in prescribing HCV regimens to those with SUD and mental health disorders. Therefore, integrating HCV care into HIV practices could lead to streamlined medical care and expanded access to treatment of coinfected populations.

Worldwide, access to ART has improved in recent decades through government initiatives as well as efforts from nongovernmental organizations (NGOs). Specifically, agencies and foundations, such as The Global Fund to Fight AIDS, Tuberculosis, and Malaria, The Clinton Health Access Initiative (CHAI), the United States President's Emergency Plan for AIDS Relief, and Unitaid, have worked toward improved access to ART, through engagement in market shaping, pooling demand, and large-scale purchase of diagnostic tests and antiretroviral drugs.[49]

Access to affordable ART in some countries has been further facilitated through the use of trade-related aspects of intellectual property rights to generically produce patented medications.[50]

For HCV, access to DAA therapy remains a significant barrier to elimination of the infection on a global scale, even when considering the substantially discounted prices being offered in most LMICs, with market prices as low as $105 in some LMICs.[51] Despite the fact that LMICs account for most HCV infections, most of the current spending on DAA therapy, upwards of $25 billion, has been from high-income countries in North America and Europe.[52,53] Concerted efforts are needed to expand access to DAA therapy in LMICs, including strategies to reduce drug costs and plans for streamlined treatment scale-up efforts.

Retention

Retention, or continuity of care, is particularly important in PLWH, as effective infection management requires lifelong treatment. Active retention efforts for patients with HIV are especially relevant for HCV-coinfected patients with severe liver fibrosis because of the long-term need for liver disease monitoring and, in many cases, hepatocellular carcinoma screening. Retention is viewed as an important quality metric within the HIV community given its independent association with ART initiation, virologic success, and decreased mortality.[54–56] For HCV, retention during initial treatment is also critical to ensure adherence to the DAA regimen. Retention efforts during HCV treatment, thus, may need to be rather intense, although for a shorter duration, relative to HIV; treating coinfected patients within the HIV clinic offers the opportunity for patients already engaged in HIV care to be more easily retained in HCV care, as the need to establish HCV care with a new clinic or provider is eliminated. In addition, many HIV clinics offer a retention specialist who helps to locate and reschedule patients who have been lost to care.[57] As discussed earlier, colocalization of HIV-HCV care within the HIV clinic would make resources, such as retention services, available for addressing HCV needs as well.

Adherence

Adherence is defined by the WHO as "the extent to which a person's behavior—taking medication, following a diet, and/or executing lifestyle changes—corresponds with agreed recommendations from a health care provider."[58] Medication adherence, specifically, refers to the way patients take a prescribed medication, including the correct medication, dose, time, duration, as well as obtaining timely refills.[59] Medication adherence is particularly important in HIV, whereby poor adherence is associated with negative outcomes, including virologic failure and resistance.[60] Several interventions aimed at improving ART adherence have shown promise,[61] with those involving peer counseling and a mobile phone short message service delivery the most widely studied and implemented to date.[62,63]

Similar to HIV, higher levels of adherence to HCV therapy translate to better outcomes.[64] For patients with HCV, adherence has been shown to be associated with several factors, including side effects, stigma, a complicated dosing schedule, and limitations of the public health care system.[65] In the DAA era, adherence is high overall but diminishes with longer treatment courses.[66] In coinfected populations, adherence to DAA regimens has been found to be high and comparable with mono-infected HCV-infected persons.[67] Specifically for patients with HIV and HCV, it is critical to review ARV adherence patterns to ensure that deviations from daily adherence, which may be sufficient to maintain HIV suppression, do not occur for HCV therapies. There remain limited data in the DAA era to determine an adherence threshold needed to maintain the SVR achieved in clinical trials and large real-world cohorts.

Viral Suppression

Viral suppression, the fifth and final step of the HIV care cascade, is the primary goal of HIV treatment. Among PLWH in the United States, 90% of those who are diagnosed, retained in care, and adhering to ART (ie, those who have completed the steps of the care continuum) are virally suppressed.[68] Worldwide, rates of viral suppression may be lower,[69,70] although often reporting is absent or viral load thresholds used to measure viral suppression are variable. In LMICs, however, interventions, such as community-based home HIV testing and counseling, have been shown to be effective in increasing viral suppression rates in HIV-infected persons.[71]

Viral suppression is an important biological marker of adherence to ART and possibly to other medical therapies. Among HIV-HCV coinfected patients, those with viral suppression are more likely to receive DAA therapy,[72] presumably because providers view adherence to ART as suggestive of a higher likelihood of adherence to DAA therapy. In HCV, achievement of viral suppression with current DAA regimens is essentially universal if patients are adherent to their regimen. Thus, similar to HIV RNA monitoring for adherence assessment, HCV RNA can also serve as a surrogate marker for adherence. Once patients have achieved HCV suppression, reassessment of HCV RNA during treatment is unnecessary unless there are concerns for changes in adherence.

LEVERAGING THE EXISTING HUMAN IMMUNODEFICIENCY VIRUS INFRASTRUCTURE

In part because of the shared steps of the care continuum and shared principles of antiviral therapies, building on the existing HIV infrastructure is a potential strategy for HCV elimination in patients with HIV and HCV coinfection. In the United States, colocalization of HIV and HCV care within the HIV clinic is an ideal approach that involves a multidisciplinary care team providing integrated services and allowing for true patient-centered care. Many colocated clinics have achieved success in treating HCV in coinfected patients.[73–76] These clinics are generally staffed by providers who are experts in HIV and HCV care (either HIV providers alone or HIV providers working together with gastroenterologists or hepatologists who treat HCV), nurses with special coinfection training, and clinic coordinators. Providers and pharmacists ensure compatibility of HIV and HCV regimens and make any necessary changes safely with appropriate monitoring. Mental health providers or collaborating mental health agencies also provide psychiatric care, counseling, case management, and addiction treatment. In addition to medical and psychosocial care, adherence counseling and patient education, including knowledge and management of side effects, are often provided by pharmacy support staff. Pharmacists and pharmacy technical assistants also help navigate financial and patient assistance programs. Staff are accustomed to such responsibilities in their HIV clinic roles and easily apply efforts to HCV management. Further advantages of colocalization include patients' familiarity with the clinic surroundings, convenience for patients and providers, and centralization of multidisciplinary services. Provider bias, which impacts the receipt of care for coinfected individuals,[72] especially for those with SUD or psychiatric disease, is likely minimized in this setting, as all staff are dedicated to the treatment of HCV infection.

In LMICs, where resources are limited, integrating HCV care into existing HIV infrastructure also has many advantages. HCV diagnosis may be facilitated by using systems already in place in HIV clinics, such as sample transport systems and viral load platforms. Access to treatment may also be expanded and expedited through the use of HIV medication supply chains. Health care workers trained in HIV testing and treatment are already knowledgeable in disease management and adherence counseling and can apply these same skillsets to help patients with HCV adhere to treatment regimens as prescribed. Finally, streamlining HCV treatment protocols in combination with HIV task-shifting models can be replicated to transfer the responsibility of HCV management and monitoring from specialists to generalist doctors, nurses, and laboratory technicians. The WHO's recommendations promote a simplified approach to HCV testing and treatment. In LMICs with developed HIV testing and treatment programs, incorporation of streamlined HCV diagnosis and management into an HIV program is a practical approach that may also serve to be cost-effective.

Such programs would begin with an assessment by ministries of health and finance and their funding partners on health priorities for that specific country.[77] Furthermore, any LMIC program focused on treating HCV must begin with a focused assessment of the prevalence of HCV and its associated risk factors within that country.[78–81] Also, similar to what was seen with HIV, consideration of societal stigmatization of HCV and potential barriers should be assessed.

REAL-WORLD HEPATITIS C VIRUS TREATMENT STRATEGIES: DOMESTIC AND INTERNATIONAL

The experiences of those already using HIV infrastructure to facilitate HCV treatment in coinfected persons provide excellent examples of success as well as challenges and lessons learned.

The authors' experience at Duke highlights some of the successes and challenges of treating coinfected patients with DAA regimens within the HIV clinic setting.[72] Treatment rates among coinfected patients increased from 1.4% in the IFN/DAA era to 18% in the IFN-free DAA, with more than 95% of those in the latter group achieving SVR. However, a large proportion remained untreated, with Caucasian race, a CD4 count of 200 or greater cells per cubic millimeter, HIV viral suppression, and the presence of cirrhosis identified as predictors of access to DAA therapy. Almost a third (31%) had not yet been evaluated for HCV treatment because of a variety of reasons, including SUD, psychiatric disease, or failure to engage in HIV care.

Falade-Nwulia and colleagues[74] described the Johns Hopkins HIV and HCV integrated clinical practice model in which comprehensive HCV care is provided within the existing HIV care infrastructure. HIV clinical care teams include a clinician, nurse, and social worker who continue to participate in care as patients are evaluated for

HCV treatment. HCV providers determine HCV disease stage and DAA therapy needs, and then pharmacy staff assess for potential drug interactions; if ART regimen changes are needed, HIV treatment is coordinated with the individual's HIV care team. For many patients, their long-standing HIV nurse conducts the DAA initiation visit. Trained pharmacists and technicians manage all DAA prescriptions, assist with prior authorization, and track all patients during the course of treatment to ensure delivery of refills. In the study by Falade-Nwulia and colleagues,[74] HCV treatment through this integrated model was highly effective among HIV-infected patients, 96.5% of whom achieved SVR; virologic success, the ultimate step in the treatment cascade, was not affected by race, SUD, or psychiatric comorbidity.

In LMICs, some early adopter countries are achieving rapid scale-up of testing and treatment through commitment from political leadership and streamlined use of diagnostic testing and medications.[5] NGOs are also critical to the success of new HCV treatment programs and have played an important role in advocating for simplified diagnostic and treatment algorithms for resource-limited contexts. The HCV Care Model in Rwanda serves as another example of DAA treatment rollout within an existing HIV infrastructure, and the experience can be contrasted to experiences in the United States. Under Rwanda Biomedical Center leadership with CHAI support, there have been many successes, including HCV screening of 67% of the HIV population enrolled in care in Rwanda in 6 months.[82] This universal screening happened relatively quickly and with the help of existing HIV staff and diagnostic and sample transport networks. Results of these screening efforts, that is, high levels of HCV coinfection of approximately 4.6%, led to increased government lobbying for donor resources for HCV care. With relatively high rates of retention in the HIV program in many LMICs after decades of donor investment, linkage to care has also happened more readily, as coinfected patients are generally reachable for expeditious DAA treatment initiation, although this has been constrained by limited availability of NAT. Finally, several places, such as Punjab State in India, Indonesia, and Myanmar, have been able to use existing HIV electronic medical record systems to inexpensively implement HCV monitoring and evaluation systems.

However, implementation in LMICs has not occurred without challenges. In several countries, CHAI faced government concerns about creating equity and stigma issues by initiating an HCV treatment program within the HIV program first. Resistance came from worry that associating HCV services with an HIV program would create stigma where previously there was very little or no stigma related to HCV. Additionally, there was concern about the public perception of providing HCV services only to those with HIV, along with fears that patients would become infected with HIV in order to receive HCV treatment. As a result, CHAI's support expanded to help governments determine how to simultaneously build service delivery models for both mono-infected patients with advanced fibrosis as well as those with HIV coinfection. Additionally, given the other significant health problems faced by LMICs, such as the burden of HIV itself, garnering support for HCV infrastructure from government officials was often challenging. Because personnel assigned to providing HCV services were often primarily dedicated to HIV care, their largest responsibility was toward the HIV program, often distracting them from the needs of developing the HCV program or limiting the opportunities for leveraging HIV infrastructure. Despite these challenges, CHAI has established promising relationships with government leadership in many LMIC governments; these collaborations continue to make progress toward HCV elimination. The authors await the end results from these partnerships to understand how such efforts will translate to broad achievement of SVR.

Unique Challenges in Hepatitis C Virus: Reinfection

Because HIV is a lifelong disease, reinfection is not an issue. However, patients can become reinfected with HCV after previous clearance, whether by spontaneous natural clearance or therapy-induced SVR. The risk of reinfection in patients with prior or ongoing high-risk behaviors, related to drug use and sexual practice, has in some instances been cited as a reason to deny curative HCV therapies to already marginalized populations.[19,83,84] However, for HCV elimination to be achieved, it is necessary that DAA therapy be especially targeted at such individuals at highest risk of ongoing transmission, despite the risk of reinfection after therapeutic cure in these subgroups. Those at high risk include persons who use drugs and HIV-positive MSM, and these groups are not mutually exclusive.[85] Although these groups were historically excluded from HCV therapeutic clinical trials, they have more recently been included in studies of DAA regimens, with excellent adherence and treatment outcomes.[14–16,86,87]

Estimates of risk of reinfection after HCV therapy-induced cure are highly subject to how populations at risk are defined (former vs active SUD) as well as the duration of HCV infection (acute/recent vs chronic). A meta-analysis by Simmons and colleagues[88] showed that summary 5-year recurrence risks after IFN-based treatment of HCV mono-infected low risk, HCV mono-infected high risk, and HIV-HCV coinfected patients were 0.95%, 10.67%, and 15.02%, respectively. The high recurrence rates for those high-risk HCV mono-infected and HIV/HCV coinfected patients were primarily driven by reinfection and not virologic relapse. For persons who use drugs, reinfection incidence is low overall, though nearly triples in those who report injection drug use after SVR.[89] Similarly, reinfection risk in HIV-positive MSM is greatest in those with ongoing risky behavior after treatment, including high-risk sexual behaviors and recreational drug use.[90–92] Lastly, individuals with acute HCV infection that is spontaneously cleared seem to be at higher risk of reinfection compared with those with chronic HCV who achieved therapy-induced SVR, again demonstrating the role of contemporary risk behaviors in ongoing transmission.[88,93,94]

The TasP strategy underscoring the widespread use of ART to minimize HIV transmission is now being considered for conquering HCV transmission. Epidemiologic modeling studies suggest that significant reductions in HCV incidence and prevalence could be attained with targeted DAA treatment scale-up among persons at highest risk of ongoing transmission.[95,96] Broadly treating persons who use drugs and HIV-positive MSM is cost-effective, given the multitude of downstream effects, including reducing our societal HCV viral load and reducing liver-related complications both in those newly and chronically infected.[97–99] The potential success of implementing a TasP or, more accurately, a CasP strategy for HCV elimination depends heavily on addressing continued high-risk behaviors during and after treatment with DAA. Therapy must be coupled with education on tactics to prevent reinfection, resources for harm minimization, and abolition of societal stigma against persons in these marginalized groups. For persons who use drugs, this entails access to opioid substitution therapy, needle and syringe exchange programs, and supervised injection sites, as such interventions clearly reduce the risk of HCV infection.[96,100,101] As incident HCV transmission among HIV-positive MSM steeply increases,[90] the efficacy of sexual behavioral interventions on transmission interruption needs further investigation, as evidence is lacking. Furthermore, active screening for reinfection in persons who remain at high risk of reexposure is critical to identify acute infection and treat early to minimize the risk of transmission.[88,102–104]

The HIV-HCV coinfected population plays a unique role in achieving HCV elimination globally. Patients with HIV-HCV not only have an accelerated natural history of liver disease, compared with HCV-monoinfected counterparts,[2] they also contribute significantly to ongoing HCV transmission[85,90] and are at high risk of reinfection.[88] The potential public health and economic gains by directly targeting this group for DAA therapy, which would reduce expensive and fatal liver-related complications and ongoing HCV transmission, are substantial. Screening and retention in care protocols for patients with HIV-HCV should be used to improve access to DAA, posttreatment surveillance, and counseling and resources on harm reduction strategies. Implementation of such protocols could be integrated into existing HIV clinic infrastructure, a safe space known to patients with experienced personnel and resources in place to address this medically and psychosocially complex patient population in need of specialized care.

SUMMARY

The WHO is calling for elimination of HCV by 2030, a task that seems daunting in light of the small proportions of HCV-infected persons achieving success, even in the early steps of the care cascade.[5] Those with HIV coinfection have been identified as a priority population, and implementing comprehensive and sustainable strategies to ensure they are diagnosed and treated is imperative. One practical strategy is to take advantage of existing HIV infrastructure and use resources already available. Currently, there are an estimated 15 million people on HIV treatment regularly visiting health centers.[105] Colocalization of HCV care within these HIV centers is an ideal approach that obviates duplication of resources, whether in the United States or abroad. In many ways, HIV-HCV coinfected patients may have access to resources, basic diagnostic and treatment resources, as well as clinical resources, including comorbidity management and treatment navigation, that HCV-mono-infected patients do not have. These resources can and should be leveraged to ensure coinfected patients have the best possible chance at cure.

REFERENCES

1. Platt L, Easterbrook P, Gower E, et al. Prevalence and burden of HCV co-infection in people living with HIV: a global systematic review and meta-analysis. Lancet Infect Dis 2016;16(7):797–808.

2. Benhamou Y, Bochet M, Di Martino V, et al. Liver fibrosis progression in human immunodeficiency virus and hepatitis C virus coinfected patients. The Multivirc Group. Hepatology 1999;30(4):1054–8.

3. Kirk GD, Mehta SH, Astemborski J, et al. HIV, age, and the severity of hepatitis C virus-related liver disease: a cohort study. Ann Intern Med 2013;158(9):658–66.

4. Lesens O, Deschênes M, Steben M, et al. Hepatitis C virus is related to progressive liver disease in human immunodeficiency virus-positive hemophiliacs and should be treated as an opportunistic infection. J Infect Dis 1999;179(5):1254–8.

5. WHO_global hepatitis report_aw.indd - 9789241565455-eng.pdf. Available at: http://apps.who.int/iris/bitstream/10665/255016/1/9789241565455-eng.pdf?ua=1. Accessed July 24, 2017.

6. North CS, Hong BA, Adewuyi SA, et al. Hepatitis C treatment and SVR: the gap between clinical trials and real-world treatment aspirations. Gen Hosp Psychiatry 2013;35(2):122–8.

7. Fleming CA, Craven DE, Thornton D, et al. Hepatitis C virus and human immunodeficiency virus coinfection in an urban population: low eligibility for interferon treatment. Clin Infect Dis 2003;36(1):97–100.

8. Restrepo A, Johnson TC, Widjaja D, et al. The rate of treatment of chronic hepatitis C in patients co-infected with HIV in an urban medical centre. J Viral Hepat 2005;12(1):86–90.

9. Torriani FJ, Rodriguez-Torres M, Rockstroh JK, et al. Peginterferon Alfa-2a plus ribavirin for chronic hepatitis C virus infection in HIV-infected patients. N Engl J Med 2004;351(5):438–50.

10. Carrat F, Bani-Sadr F, Pol S, et al. Pegylated interferon alfa-2b vs standard interferon alfa-2b, plus ribavirin, for chronic hepatitis C in HIV-infected patients: a randomized controlled trial. JAMA 2004;292(23):2839–48.

11. Mauss S. Treatment of viral hepatitis in HIV-coinfected patients-adverse events and their management. J Hepatol 2006;44(1 Suppl):S114–8.

12. Medeiros BC, Seligman PA, Everson GT, et al. Possible autoimmune thrombocytopenia associated with pegylated interferon-alpha2a plus ribavarin treatment for hepatitis C. J Clin Gastroenterol 2004;38(1):84–6.

13. Moreno L, Quereda C, Moreno A, et al. Pegylated interferon alpha2b plus ribavirin for the treatment of chronic hepatitis C in HIV-infected patients. AIDS 2004; 18(1):67–73.

14. Naggie S, Cooper C, Saag M, et al. Ledipasvir and sofosbuvir for HCV in patients coinfected with HIV-1. N Engl J Med 2015;373(8):705–13.

15. Sulkowski MS, Eron JJ, Wyles D, et al. Ombitasvir, paritaprevir co-dosed with ritonavir, dasabuvir, and ribavirin for hepatitis C in patients co-infected with HIV-1: a randomized trial. JAMA 2015;313(12):1223–31.

16. Wyles DL, Ruane PJ, Sulkowski MS, et al. Daclatasvir plus sofosbuvir for HCV in patients coinfected with HIV-1. N Engl J Med 2015;373(8):714–25.

17. AASLD/IDSA HCV Guidance Panel. Hepatitis C guidance: AASLD-IDSA recommendations for testing, managing, and treating adults infected with hepatitis C virus. Hepatology 2015;62(3):932–54.

18. Cope R, Glowa T, Faulds S, et al. Treating hepatitis C in a Ryan White-funded HIV clinic: has the treatment uptake improved in the interferon-free directly active antiviral era? AIDS Patient Care STDs 2016;30(2):51–5.

19. Collins LF, Chan A, Zheng J, et al. Direct-acting antivirals improve access to care and cure for patients with HIV and chronic HCV Infection. Open Forum Infect Dis 2018;5(1):ofx264.

20. Greenberg AE, Hader SL, Masur H, et al. Fighting HIV/AIDS in Washington, D.C. Health Aff Proj Hope 2009;28(6):1677–87.

21. Janjua NZ, Kuo M, Yu A, et al. The population level cascade of care for hepatitis C in British Columbia, Canada: the BC hepatitis testers cohort (BC-HTC). EBioMedicine 2016;12:189–95.

22. Maier MM, Ross DB, Chartier M, et al. Cascade of care for hepatitis C virus infection within the US Veterans Health Administration. Am J Public Health 2016;106(2):353–8.

23. Cachay ER, Hill L, Wyles D, et al. The hepatitis C cascade of care among HIV infected patients: a call to address ongoing barriers to care. PLoS One 2014; 9(7):e102883.

24. Tsui JI, Ko SC, Krupitsky E, et al. Insights on the Russian HCV care cascade: minimal HCV treatment for HIV/HCV co-infected PWID in St. Petersburg. Hepatol Med Policy 2016;1 [pii:13].

25. Cohen MS, Chen YQ, McCauley M, et al. Prevention of HIV-1 infection with early antiretroviral therapy. N Engl J Med 2011;365(6):493–505.

26. Durier N, Nguyen C, White LJ. Treatment of hepatitis C as prevention: a modeling case study in Vietnam. PLoS One 2012;7(4):e34548.

27. Martin NK, Vickerman P, Foster GR, et al. Can antiviral therapy for hepatitis C reduce the prevalence of HCV among injecting drug user populations? A modeling analysis of its prevention utility. J Hepatol 2011;54(6):1137–44.

28. Hajarizadeh B, Grebely J, Dore GJ. Epidemiology and natural history of HCV infection. Nat Rev Gastroenterol Hepatol 2013;10(9):553–62.

29. Kay ES, Batey DS, Mugavero MJ. The HIV treatment cascade and care continuum: updates, goals, and recommendations for the future. AIDS Res Ther 2016; 13:35.

30. Branson BM, Handsfield HH, Lampe MA, et al. Revised recommendations for HIV testing of adults, adolescents, and pregnant women in health-care settings. MMWR Recomm Rep Morb Mortal Wkly Rep Recomm Rep 2006;55(RR-14): 1–17 [quiz: CE1-4].

31. Woodring JV, Kruszon-Moran D, Oster AM, et al. Did CDC's 2006 revised HIV testing recommendations make a difference? Evaluation of HIV testing in the US household population, 2003-2010. J Acquir Immune Defic Syndr 2014; 67(3):331–40.

32. HCV/HIV adult and adolescent ARV guidelines. AIDSinfo. Available at: https:// aidsinfo.nih.gov/. Accessed July 27, 2017.

33. Global HIV/AIDS overview | HIV.gov. Available at: https://www.hiv.gov/federal-response/pepfar-global-aids/global-hiv-aids-overview. Accessed July 31, 2017.

34. Coyle C, Kwakwa H. Dual-routine HCV/HIV testing: seroprevalence and linkage to care in four community health centers in Philadelphia, Pennsylvania. Public Health Rep Wash DC 1974 2016;131(Suppl 1):41–52.

35. Bottero J, Boyd A, Gozlan J, et al. Simultaneous human immunodeficiency virus-hepatitis B-hepatitis C point-of-care tests improve outcomes in linkage-to-care: results of a randomized control trial in persons without healthcare coverage. Open Forum Infect Dis 2015;2(4):ofv162.

36. Frimpong JA, D'Aunno T, Perlman DC, et al. On-site bundled rapid HIV/HCV testing in substance use disorder treatment programs: study protocol for a hybrid design randomized controlled trial. Trials 2016;17(1):117.

37. Stockman LJ, Guilfoye SM, Benoit AL, et al. Centers for Disease Control and Prevention (CDC). Rapid hepatitis C testing among persons at increased risk for infection–Wisconsin, 2012-2013. MMWR Morb Mortal Wkly Rep 2014; 63(14):309–11.

38. Health C for D and R. Home use tests - Hepatitis C. Available at: https://www.fda.gov/MedicalDevices/ProductsandMedicalProcedures/InVitroDiagnostics/HomeUseTests/ucm125785.htm. Accessed September 10, 2017.

39. Kamal SM. Acute hepatitis C: a systematic review. Am J Gastroenterol 2008; 103(5):1283–97 [quiz: 1298].

40. Rongey CA, Kanwal F, Hoang T, et al. Viral RNA testing in hepatitis C antibody-positive veterans. Am J Prev Med 2009;36(3):235–8.

41. Global Burden of Disease Study 2013 Collaborators. Global, regional, and national incidence, prevalence, and years lived with disability for 301 acute and chronic diseases and injuries in 188 countries, 1990-2013: a systematic analysis for the Global Burden of Disease Study 2013. Lancet 2015;386(9995):743–800.

42. Freiman JM, Tran TM, Schumacher SG, et al. Hepatitis C core antigen testing for diagnosis of hepatitis C virus infection: a systematic review and meta-analysis. Ann Intern Med 2016;165(5):345–55.

43. Chandler RK, Kahana SY, Fletcher B, et al. Data collection and harmonization in HIV research: the Seek, Test, Treat, and Retain initiative at the National Institute on Drug Abuse. Am J Public Health 2015;105(12):2416–22.

44. Kim JJ, Maulsby C, Kinsky S, et al. The development and implementation of the national evaluation strategy of Access to Care, a multi-site linkage to care initiative in the United States. AIDS Educ Prev 2014;26(5):429–44.

45. Pundhir P, North CS, Fatunde O, et al. Health beliefs and co-morbidities associated with appointment-keeping behavior among HCV and HIV/HCV patients. J Community Health 2016;41(1):30–7.

46. Taylor LE. Delivering care to injection drug users coinfected with HIV and hepatitis C virus. Clin Infect Dis 2005;40(Suppl 5):S355–61.

47. Pavlova-McCalla E, Trepka MJ, Ramirez G, et al. Socioeconomic status and survival of people with human immunodeficiency virus infection before and after the introduction of highly active antiretroviral therapy: a systematic literature review. J AIDS Clin Res 2012;3(6) [pii:1000163].

48. Reif S, Golin CE, Smith SR. Barriers to accessing HIV/AIDS care in North Carolina: rural and urban differences. AIDS Care 2005;17(5):558–65.

49. 2017 Pipeline report final.pdf. Available at: http://www.pipelinereport.org/sites/default/files/2017%20Pipeline%20Report%20Final.pdf. Accessed August 10, 2017.

50. Graham CS, Swan T. A path to eradication of hepatitis C in low- and middle-income countries. Antivir Res 2015;119:89–96.

51. Negotiating affordable access to diagnostics and medicines in Punjab for HCV. WHO Southeast Asia Regional Action Plan Meeting held at New Delhi (India), April 10–12, 2017.

52. Solomon SS, Mehta SH, Srikrishnan AK, et al. Burden of hepatitis C virus disease and access to hepatitis C virus services in people who inject drugs in India: a cross-sectional study. Lancet Infect Dis 2015;15(1):36–45.

53. 2015 10-K Filings for Gilead, BMS, AbbVie, J&J, Merck and Vertex. Available at: https://www.sec.gov./. Accessed September 10, 2017.

54. Ulett KB, Willig JH, Lin H-Y, et al. The therapeutic implications of timely linkage and early retention in HIV care. AIDS Patient Care STDs 2009;23(1):41–9.

55. Mugavero MJ, Lin H-Y, Willig JH, et al. Missed visits and mortality among patients establishing initial outpatient HIV treatment. Clin Infect Dis 2009;48(2):248–56.

56. Giordano TP, Hartman C, Gifford AL, et al. Predictors of retention in HIV care among a national cohort of US veterans. HIV Clin Trials 2009;10(5):299–305.

57. Sitapati AM, Limneos J, Bonet-Vázquez M, et al. Retention: building a patient-centered medical home in HIV primary care through PUFF (Patients Unable to Follow-up Found). J Health Care Poor Underserved 2012;23(3):81–95.

58. Who | adherence to long-term therapies: evidence for action. WHO. Available at: http://www.who.int/chp/knowledge/publications/adherence_report/en/. Accessed July 25, 2017.

59. Richmond JA, Sheppard-Law S, Mason S, et al. The Australasian Hepatology Association consensus guidelines for the provision of adherence support to patients with hepatitis C on direct acting antivirals. Patient Prefer Adherence 2016; 10:2479–89.

60. Paterson DL, Swindells S, Mohr J, et al. Adherence to protease inhibitor therapy and outcomes in patients with HIV infection. Ann Intern Med 2000;133(1):21–30.

61. Haberer JE, Sabin L, Amico KR, et al. Improving antiretroviral therapy adherence in resource-limited settings at scale: a discussion of interventions and recommendations. J Int AIDS Soc 2017;20(1):21371.

62. Pop-Eleches C, Thirumurthy H, Habyarimana JP, et al. Mobile phone technologies improve adherence to antiretroviral treatment in a resource-limited setting: a randomized controlled trial of text message reminders. AIDS Lond Engl 2011; 25(6):825–34.

63. Lester RT, Ritvo P, Mills EJ, et al. Effects of a mobile phone short message service on antiretroviral treatment adherence in Kenya (WelTel Kenya1): a randomised trial. Lancet Lond Engl 2010;376(9755):1838–45.

64. Lo Re V, Teal V, Localio AR, et al. Relationship between adherence to hepatitis C virus therapy and virologic outcomes: a cohort study. Ann Intern Med 2011; 155(6):353–60.

65. Sublette VA, Smith SK, George J, et al. The hepatitis C treatment experience: patients' perceptions of the facilitators of and barriers to uptake, adherence and completion. Psychol Health 2015;30(8):987–1004.

66. Petersen T, Townsend K, Gordon LA, et al. High adherence to all-oral directly acting antiviral HCV therapy among an inner-city patient population in a phase 2a study. Hepatol Int 2015;10(2):310–9.

67. Townsend K, Petersen T, Gordon LA, et al. Effect of HIV co-infection on adherence to a 12-week regimen of hepatitis C virus therapy with ledipasvir and sofosbuvir. AIDS Lond Engl 2016;30(2):261–6.

68. Bradley H, Hall HI, Wolitski RJ, et al. Vital signs: HIV diagnosis, care, and treatment among persons living with HIV–United States, 2011. MMWR Morb Mortal Wkly Rep 2014;63(47):1113–7.

69. Nsanzimana S, Kanters S, Remera E, et al. HIV care continuum in Rwanda: a cross-sectional analysis of the national programme. Lancet HIV 2015;2(5): e208–15.

70. Maman D, Zeh C, Mukui I, et al. Cascade of HIV care and population viral suppression in a high-burden region of Kenya. AIDS Lond Engl 2015;29(12): 1557–65.

71. Barnabas RV, van Rooyen H, Tumwesigye E, et al. Initiation of antiretroviral therapy and viral suppression after home HIV testing and counselling in KwaZulu-Natal, South Africa, and Mbarara district, Uganda: a prospective, observational intervention study. Lancet HIV 2014;1(2):e68–76.

72. Collins L, Chan A, Zheng J, et al. Direct-acting antivirals improve access to care and cure for patients with HIV-HCV. Seattle (WA): CROI; 2017.

73. Clanon KA, Johannes Mueller J, Harank M. Integrating treatment for hepatitis C virus infection into an HIV clinic. Clin Infect Dis 2005;40(Suppl 5):S362–6.

74. Falade-Nwulia O, Sutcliffe C, Moon J, et al. High hepatitis C cure rates among black and non-black HIV-infected adults in an urban center. Hepatology 2017; 66(5):1402–12.

75. Kresina TF, Bruce RD, Cargill VA, et al. Integrating care for hepatitis C virus (HCV) and primary care for HIV for injection drug users coinfected with HIV and HCV. Clin Infect Dis 2005;41(Suppl 1):S83–8.

76. Kieran J, Dillon A, Farrell G, et al. High uptake of hepatitis C virus treatment in HIV/hepatitis C virus co-infected patients attending an integrated HIV/hepatitis C virus clinic. Int J STD AIDS 2011;22(10):571–6.

77. Jayasekera CR, Barry M, Roberts LR, et al. Treating hepatitis C in lower-income countries. N Engl J Med 2014;370(20):1869–71.

78. Candotti D, Sarkodie F, Allain JP. Residual risk of transfusion in Ghana. Br J Haematol 2001;113(1):37–9.

79. Marx MA, Murugavel KG, Sivaram S, et al. The association of health-care use and hepatitis C virus infection in a random sample of urban slum community residents in southern India. Am J Trop Med Hyg 2003;68(2):258–62.

80. Nelson PK, Mathers BM, Cowie B, et al. Global epidemiology of hepatitis B and hepatitis C in people who inject drugs: results of systematic reviews. Lancet Lond Engl 2011;378(9791):571–83.

81. Jafari S, Copes R, Baharlou S, et al. Tattooing and the risk of transmission of hepatitis C: a systematic review and meta-analysis. Int J Infect Dis IJID 2010; 14(11):e928–40.

82. Umutesi J, Simmons B, Makuza JD, et al. Prevalence of hepatitis B and C infection in persons living with HIV enrolled in care in Rwanda. BMC Infect Dis 2017; 17(1):315.

83. Asher AK, Portillo CJ, Cooper BA, et al. Clinicians' views of hepatitis C virus treatment candidacy with direct-acting antiviral regimens for people who inject drugs. Subst Use Misuse 2016;51(9):1218–23.

84. Wansom T, Falade-Nwulia O, Sutcliffe CG, et al. Barriers to hepatitis C virus (HCV) treatment initiation in patients with human immunodeficiency virus/HCV coinfection: lessons from the interferon era. Open Forum Infect Dis 2017;4(1): ofx024.

85. Martinello M, Hajarizadeh B, Grebely J, et al. HCV cure and reinfection among people with HIV/HCV coinfection and people who inject drugs. Curr Hiv Aids Rep 2017;14(3):110–21.

86. Norton BL, Fleming J, Bachhuber MA, et al. High HCV cure rates for people who use drugs treated with direct acting antiviral therapy at an urban primary care clinic. Int J Drug Policy 2017;47:196–201.

87. Grebely J, Mauss S, Brown A, et al. Efficacy and safety of ledipasvir/sofosbuvir with and without ribavirin in patients with chronic HCV genotype 1 infection receiving opioid substitution therapy: analysis of phase 3 ION trials. Clin Infect Dis 2016;63(11):1405–11.

88. Simmons B, Saleem J, Hill A, et al. Risk of late relapse or reinfection with hepatitis C virus after achieving a sustained virological response: a systematic review and meta-analysis. Clin Infect Dis 2016;62(6):683–94.

89. Aspinall EJ, Corson S, Doyle JS, et al. Treatment of hepatitis C virus infection among people who are actively injecting drugs: a systematic review and meta-analysis. Clin Infect Dis 2013;57(Suppl 2):S80–9.

90. Hagan H, Jordan AE, Neurer J, et al. Incidence of sexually transmitted hepatitis C virus infection in HIV-positive men who have sex with men. AIDS Lond Engl 2015;29(17):2335–45.

91. Jordan AE, Perlman DC, Neurer J, et al. Prevalence of hepatitis C virus infection among HIV+ men who have sex with men: a systematic review and meta-analysis. Int J STD AIDS 2017;28(2):145–59.

92. Gamage DG, Read TRH, Bradshaw CS, et al. Incidence of hepatitis-C among HIV infected men who have sex with men (MSM) attending a sexual health service: a cohort study. BMC Infect Dis 2011;11:39.

93. Martin TCS, Martin NK, Hickman M, et al. Hepatitis C virus reinfection incidence and treatment outcome among HIV-positive MSM. AIDS Lond Engl 2013;27(16): 2551–7.

94. Sacks-Davis R, Aitken CK, Higgs P, et al. High rates of hepatitis C virus reinfection and spontaneous clearance of reinfection in people who inject drugs: a prospective cohort study. PLoS One 2013;8(11):e80216.
95. Martin NK, Thornton A, Hickman M, et al. Can hepatitis C virus (HCV) direct-acting antiviral treatment as prevention reverse the HCV epidemic among men who have sex with men in the United Kingdom? Epidemiological and modeling insights. Clin Infect Dis 2016;62(9):1072–80.
96. Martin NK, Hickman M, Hutchinson SJ, et al. Combination interventions to prevent HCV transmission among people who inject drugs: modeling the impact of antiviral treatment, needle and syringe programs, and opiate substitution therapy. Clin Infect Dis 2013;57(Suppl 2):S39–45.
97. Zahnd C, Salazar-Vizcaya L, Dufour J-F, et al. Modelling the impact of deferring HCV treatment on liver-related complications in HIV coinfected men who have sex with men. J Hepatol 2016;65(1):26–32.
98. Martin NK, Vickerman P, Dore GJ, et al. Prioritization of HCV treatment in the direct-acting antiviral era: an economic evaluation. J Hepatol 2016;65(1):17–25.
99. Scott N, McBryde ES, Thompson A, et al. Treatment scale-up to achieve global HCV incidence and mortality elimination targets: a cost-effectiveness model. Gut 2017;66(8):1507–15.
100. Turner KME, Hutchinson S, Vickerman P, et al. The impact of needle and syringe provision and opiate substitution therapy on the incidence of hepatitis C virus in injecting drug users: pooling of UK evidence. Addict Abingdon Engl 2011; 106(11):1978–88.
101. Coffin PO, Rowe C, Santos G-M. Novel interventions to prevent HIV and HCV among persons who inject drugs. Curr Hiv/aids Rep 2015;12(1):145–63.
102. Ingiliz P, Christensen S, Schewe K, et al. High incidence of HCV reinfection in HIV-positive MSM in the DAA era. 16th European AIDS Conference, October 25–27, 2017, Milan, Italy.
103. Chaillon A, Sun X, Cachay ER, et al. Incidence of hepatitis C among HIV-infected men who have sex with men in San Diego, 2000-2015. Washington, DC: AASLD; 2017.
104. Young J, Rossi C, Gill J, et al. Risk factors for hepatitis C virus reinfection after sustained virologic response in patients coinfected with HIV. Clin Infect Dis 2017;64(9):1154–62.
105. UNAIDS_15by15_en.pdf. Available at: http://www.unaids.org/sites/default/files/media_asset/UNAIDS_15by15_en.pdf. Accessed September 5, 2017.

Hepatitis C Virus Diagnosis and the Holy Grail

Tanya L. Applegate, B.App Sc (Hons), PhD[a],*, Emmanuel Fajardo, BSc (Hons), MSc[b],
Jilian A. Sacks, PhD[c]

KEYWORDS

- HCV • Diagnostics • Simplified • Rapid • Point-of-care • Test and treat
- Models of care • HCV elimination

KEY POINTS

- Innovative strategies to provide access to existing HCV diagnostic assays are an immediate priority.
- Decentralized models of care to diagnose HCV infection and confirm cure within community health care settings are critical to achieve HCV elimination by 2030.
- High quality, simple, affordable and rapid diagnosis of active infection at the point-of-care will be central to achievement of HCV elimination.
- Global partnerships and funding mechanisms are required to stimulate investment in the development of the holy grail - the ideal point-of-care diagnostic test.

HEPATITIS C VIRUS DIAGNOSTICS ARE ESSENTIAL TO ACHIEVE GLOBAL ELIMINATION

It is not often the world has the opportunity to turn a public health crisis into a good news story.[1,2] The development of oral, highly effective, pangenotypic direct-acting antivirals (DAAs) has now paved the way to cure the 71 million people estimated to be living with chronic hepatitis C virus (HCV) infection globally.[3–6] Unfortunately, fewer than 20% of those living with HCV are aware of their infection, and the challenge now is to engage, screen, and diagnose everyone in need of treatment.[7,8] While the world has focused its attention on the final steps within the cascade of care to develop and increase access to DAAs over the last decade,[9–11] considerably less investment has been made to ensure accurate and affordable diagnostic tools[10] are available to make wide-scale global treatment a reality (**Fig. 1**). Ironically, in many settings,

[a] The Kirby Institute, UNSW Sydney, High Street, Sydney, New South Wales 2052, Australia;
[b] Médecins Sans Frontières Access Campaign, Rue de Lausanne 78 P.O Box 1016, Geneva CH-1211, Switzerland; [c] Clinton Health Access Initiative, 383 Dorchester Avenue Suite 400, Boston, MA 02127, USA
* Corresponding author.
E-mail address: tapplegate@kirby.unsw.edu.au

Infect Dis Clin N Am 32 (2018) 425–445
https://doi.org/10.1016/j.idc.2018.02.010
0891-5520/18/© 2018 The Authors. Published by Elsevier Inc. This is an open access article under the CC BY-NC-ND license (http://creativecommons.org/licenses/by-nc-nd/4.0/).
id.theclinics.com

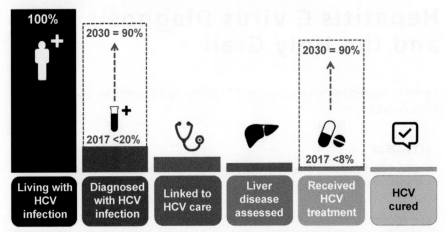

Fig. 1. Cascade of care for hepatitis C virus (HCV), indicating global gaps to reach World Health Organization 2030 elimination goals.[26] (*Adapted from* Grebely J, Bruggmann P, Treloar C, et al. Expanding access to prevention, care and treatment for hepatitis C virus infection among people who inject drugs. Int J Drug Pol 2015;26(10):893–8; with permission.)

prohibitively high costs of HCV diagnostics often now exceed the cost of curative therapy.[12] Improving access to rapid, simple, and affordable HCV diagnostics is critical to achieve global HCV elimination.[13–15]

The high efficacy and low toxicity of the new DAAs provide an exceptional opportunity to greatly simplify HCV diagnosis and care. Recently approved pangenotypic DAA regimens no longer depend on quantitative HCV RNA or genotype data to stratify the duration of treatment,[16–18] and many international clinical trials and demonstration studies are underway to generate evidence of the efficacy of a simplified approach to diagnosis and treatment monitoring (eg, in Cambodia, India, Iran, Rwanda, Nigeria, Mozambique, Myanmar, Pakistan, and Uzbekistan[19]). Likewise, excellent safety profiles, potent efficacy, and limited potential drug–drug interactions also negate the need for intensive on-treatment monitoring.[20,21]

From a public health perspective, HCV diagnosis and care could be simplified to just two visits: (1) diagnosis of active HCV infection and standardized treatment regardless of disease stage, and (2) confirmation of cure posttreatment completion (**Fig. 2**A). Considering the high rate of cure, experts in the field are currently debating if confirmation of cure may also be considered unnecessary in the near future. Although liver disease stage restrictions for treatment access are being removed globally,[22–24] liver assessment is important to inform treatment duration for some regimens and for monitoring patients with cirrhosis.[25–27] A lack of access to liver disease assessment, however, should not be considered a barrier and treatment should be provided to all. The integration of noninvasive liver assessment into a 30-minute visit in the primary care setting would require the development of an as yet unavailable, rapid, point-of-care (POC) test to measure aspartate aminotransferase and platelet count to calculate the aspartate aminotransferase to platelet ratio index[28–31] or a transient elastography machine, such as the Fibroscan,[32] that is markedly more affordable than current options (**Fig. 2**B). The integration of liver assessment into a single 2-hour visit in a tertiary health care setting and centralized laboratory, however, is entirely feasible using current laboratory-based technologies (**Fig. 2**C).

A POC HCV "test and treat" for all, without liver staging

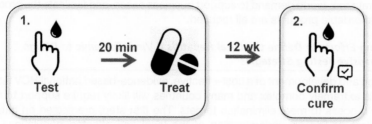

B POC HCV diagnosis and rapid liver staging, in primary care settings

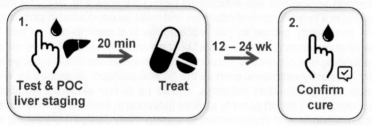

C POC HCV diagnosis and routine liver staging, in tertiary care settings

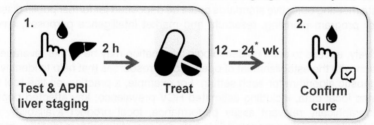

Fig. 2. "Test and treat models" for health care settings. (*A*) A simple point-of-care (POC) "test and treat" using standardized 12 week treatment for hepatitis C virus (HCV) infection, regardless of liver disease staging. (*B*) POC HCV diagnosis and rapid liver staging, and 12 to 24 weeks of treatment in primary care settings. (*C*) POC HCV diagnosis and routine liver testing, in tertiary care settings where (*asterisk*) the duration of treatment could be extended to 24 weeks, if required, when liver test results are available by the patient's next visit for drug refill.

INCREASING ACCESS TO EXISTING HEPATITIS C VIRUS DIAGNOSTICS IS A PUBLIC HEALTH PRIORITY

The world now eagerly awaits the "holy grail" for HCV POC diagnosis—an accurate, simple, rapid, and affordable diagnosis of active HCV infection in a single visit. In the meantime, national programs should develop and prioritize new approaches to scale-up access to existing diagnostic assays, particularly in low- and middle-income countries (LMICs), which account for approximately 80% of the global burden.[7] Many opportunities exist that may provide solutions to optimize diagnostic and treatment networks and increase the market attractiveness of existing HCV diagnostic technologies to make testing more affordable. Efforts to accurately define the local epidemic, provide access to globally representative validation data for quality assured diagnostics, streamline national regulatory and registration processes, demonstrate real-world demand to support business cases, and facilitate the procurement of affordable products are all required.

Supporting Efforts to Define the Local Hepatitis C Virus Epidemic to Design Comprehensive Testing Strategies

The design and development of a cost-effective, evidence-based national HCV testing strategy is extremely complex and many countries will likely require support to navigate this process to meet elimination targets. The first step, predicated on national stakeholders having an understanding of the local key affected populations and drivers of transmission, is of course impossible without access to quality assured, high-performing assays and well-established testing services (**Fig. 3**A). This foundation is missing in a large number of countries and must be conducted in close consultation with community groups to gain acceptance and participation as well as a comprehensive understanding of the local context and the needs of those affected. Innovative funding mechanisms to support national surveillance studies that generate preliminary in-country estimates, such as the generic protocol developed by WHO[33] and develop strong laboratory networks, should be further explored. Additionally, the development of an expert panel to provide guidance to local nongovernmental organizations, ministries, and implementers to appropriately design and interpret small epidemiologic studies could help to build local capacity and expedite the generation of this needed data. Such input could also be linked to an open access database where survey data meeting objective standards could be deposited for further public dissemination, for program planning, research, and market intelligence purposes, among others.

Collectively, access to such epidemiologic information may be further leveraged in combination with the establishment of open access resources that help to identify the ideal diagnostic algorithm for each setting. For example, a practical on-line tool that incorporates local data, including estimated HCV prevalence, key affected populations, geographically relevant assay performance, local product availability, and cost, could build on existing models[34,35] to help national stakeholders identify optimal, cost-effective diagnostic algorithms.[36] Such a model could assess whether there are

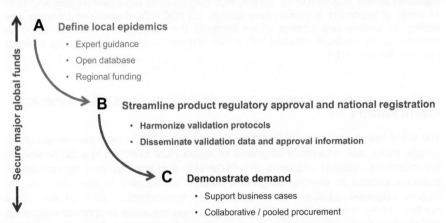

Fig. 3. Opportunities to help increase the market attractiveness of existing diagnostics including (*A*) providing support to define local epidemics and harmonizing validation data, (*B*) streamlining approval and registration, and (*C*) demonstrating real-world demand.

settings in which 1-step diagnosis of active infection, using a particular product, would be a more feasible and impactful approach to reduce transmissions or decrease the burden of disease among a key population.

Streamlining Transparent Processes to Expedite and Encourage Assay Approval and Registration

As a high-risk in vitro diagnostic (IVD), meaning that inaccurate results pose a high risk to public safety, an HCV screening or diagnostic assay undergoes rigorous assessment during review by stringent regulatory authorities (SRA), including members and observers of the International Medical Device Regulators Forum (IMRDF) ICH, or regulatory bodies associated with an ICH member of the International Council for Harmonization (ICH),[37] present in Australia, Canada, Europe, Japan, Iceland, Leichtenstien, Norway, and the United States. Comprehensive assessment includes a review of a significant body of evidence of diagnostic performance in clinical samples from the population in which the IVD is intended to be used, independent laboratory evaluation of the product, as well as a site inspection to assess compliance with good manufacturing practice, in some jurisdictions. Although data supporting US Food and Drug Administration registration[38] and World Health Organization (WHO) prequalification[39] is available through their websites, access to the European Databank on Medical Devices is currently restricted to competent national authorities, creating an unintended barrier to rapid identification of CE-IVD marked assays. It is, therefore, important that validation data from these SRAs be made widely available. It should be noted, however, that the studies supporting the SRAs are generally restricted to laboratory settings and may have limited applicability to other populations, particularly with respect to genotypes 4, 5, and 6[40] and coinfection with human immunodeficiency virus (HIV), or real-world field use.

Therefore, to facilitate the uptake of quality-assured and accurate testing products in all countries, collaborative efforts are needed to not only undertake regionally representative clinical validation studies, and share validation data through novel mechanisms and systematic reviews,[41–43] but also to establish cohesive international standards[44] (**Fig. 3**B). Although significant inroads have been made through the WHO Prequalification Programme,[45] which assesses the quality of IVDs specifically for use in more resource-limited settings, and the likely inclusion of HCV assays on the Essential Diagnostics List[46] is laudable, additional mechanisms to expedite and harmonize national assay approval and registration are required. Initiatives such as the POC Early Infant Diagnosis Consortium, in which multicountry data are pooled to accelerate evaluations, may have wider applicability to fill this need.[47,48] The WHO technical Guidance Series,[49] intended for manufacturers, provide a framework for national laboratories to design and conduct local validation studies and are valuable resources. However, simple guidance documents on how to generate reliable population-specific in-country HCV diagnostic validation data, similar to the generic protocols produced by the International Diagnostic Centre (London School of Hygiene and Tropical Medicine[50]) for CD4, HIV viral load, and so on, would also be valuable. Additionally, the development of an open access database of existing real-world performance data collected from peer-reviewed publications, as well as unpublished and government-led studies could increase access to existing validation data. Although this approach would require significant engagement with each country and a large investment of time to ensure data quality, it could be an important step toward improving transparency and increasing access to known high-performing tests. Greater visibility into clinical accuracy might help to consolidate the market around a handful of high-performing HCV screening and diagnostic tests, more akin to the scenario for HIV, rather than the current situation for HCV in which dozens of different tests can be found within an individual country and even greater variability may be seen across a region. Furthermore, the generation of and access to more diverse local performance data may also help to inform the selection of products that are not yet SRA approved, but perform well. When combined, these collaborative, open access processes may provide new opportunities to increase education and awareness of the significant risks associated with purchasing cheaper products of unassured quality and performance from manufacturers other than those indicated on a list of approved assays.

Last, for those companies interested in marketing their product in geographies with an SRA, the approval pathway may be relatively clear, albeit associated with significant costs. However, if a country with an SRA does not mandate that a test, or a sample type for that test, be approved before clinical implementation, this may further reduce the incentive for companies to pursue SRA review and inadvertently lead to the restricted use of key diagnostics. For instance, dried blood spots (DBS) could be an important method of collecting, storing, and transporting samples to centralized facilities. The expedited approval of DBS as an alternative sample type to diagnose and manage HCV infection using existing approved assays that already have DBS-adapted protocols, such as the Abbott RealTime HCV Viral Load assay (Abbott Diagnostics, Abbott Park, IL), Aptima HCV Quant Dx assay (Hologic Inc, Danbury, CT), and COBAS Ampli-Prep/COBAS TaqManHCV Test (Roche Molecular Diagnostics, Basel, Switzerland), would be likely to make significant global impact on rates of HCV diagnosis in both higher income countries and LMICs.[43,51] For companies whose target HCV testing market is restricted to LMICs, the need for SRA approval is often less clear and country-specific validation, registration, and approval processes may be vague.[52] Unfortunately, national registration in many LMIC may depend on existing and often unreliable package insert data as the sole source of test performance information. Alternatively, countries may require duplicative local assay validation, adding further costs and delays in implementation. Although products that have not pursued SRA approval or WHO prequalification may be considerably less expensive than products that have, their performance often cannot be guaranteed. Because inaccurate diagnostic results can significantly compromise both public health outcomes and individual patient management, the temptation to procure unapproved or unqualified tests by LMIC must be avoided. LMICs could consider requiring SRA approval or meeting diagnostic accuracy specifications through independent externally generated data as part of the national registration or tendering process to ensure implementation of high-quality products.

Demonstrating Real-World Demand to Support Business Cases to Pursue Approval and Registration of Existing Assays

A greater understanding of the demand for HCV diagnostics among LMICs and higher income countries is urgently required to develop strong business cases that justify the investment in the approval, registration, and marketing of existing assays (**Fig. 3C**). Further clarity around the real-world market could be developed through strong partnerships between community, academics, clinicians, national stakeholders, nongovernmental organizations, and industry. As countries develop national strategic plans and individual stakeholders, such as ministries of health, nongovernmental organizations, and community groups, embark on testing and treatment programs, a forum to share indicative volumes with industry may be helpful. The cost of testing continues to be a key barrier to designing optimal testing programs and opportunities for more transparent and deconstructed pricing structures from manufacturers and service providers are clearly needed.[53]

A range of local and collaborative regional testing efforts that may lead to higher volume and more predictable demand estimates for specific HCV diagnostic assays should be explored to achieve more competitive pricing. Pricing currently varies greatly between countries, so increased transparency could also enable individual countries to have stronger negotiation power. One approach is to use a coordinated regional forecast that allows suppliers to provide more indicative pricing linked to volumes, while still allowing procurement to be managed through each individual country. Alternatively, more regionally collaborative approaches could be considered to leverage increased volumes for improved bargaining power to achieve lower pricing: (1) pooled procurement among multiple countries is an option, but would need to balance country sovereignty during the process, or (2) external pooled purchasing through a third party is a possibility for negotiation of a more comprehensive volume guarantee based on regional estimates from multiple stakeholders, such as the not-for-profit Global Procurement Fund.[54] Last, LMICs should also consider negotiating with diagnostic companies that already offer testing across multiple diseases to provide options for bundle pricing across the test menu to reach threshold volumes for discount pricing, as well as to negotiate alternative procurement models for equipment acquisition, for example, reagent rental.

Each of these mechanisms can be further enhanced by strong patient advocacy to convince companies of the value of investment and to urge governments, funders, and stakeholders to ensure public HCV services are routinely available, accessible, and affordable. For patients, peers and communities to be empowered to have sustainable impact, support materials and education are needed.[55]

COMPLEMENTARY, CENTRALIZED LABORATORIES AND POINT-OF-CARE TESTING SERVICES ARE NEEDED TO INCREASE ACCESS TO CARE FOR ALL

In addition to addressing barriers of limited education, awareness, and health equity, as well as the high stigma and discrimination in ensuring access to HCV care, well-designed testing networks of existing HCV diagnostic tools are needed.[56-58] The elimination of HCV will likely require both centralized laboratories and decentralized POC testing services at community clinics. No single product or testing mechanism is likely to reach all populations affected (**Fig. 4**A). In addition to patient management, centralized testing is critical for regional surveillance programs to monitor progress toward elimination goals.[7] Likewise, as decentralized testing is expanded, countries should also prospectively ensure that data are linked centrally for both surveillance and quality control purposes. Centralized testing also clearly provides advantages in economies of scale, oversight for quality assurance, and data management. Systematic assessment of existing national laboratory testing services (eg, WHO Global Laboratory Initiative and African Society for Laboratory Medicine[59]), provides countries the opportunity to design improved diagnostic networks and data connectivity. The existing investment in centralized facilities can and should be leveraged to provide efficient and affordable multidisease services.[60-62] New mechanisms to invest in integrated health care systems that address the practical constraints of vertical, disease-specific funding, which can inadvertently limit access to existing infrastructure and equipment, requires strong collaborative commitment from national stakeholders and global funders.[60]

Decentralized Testing Strategies Are Required to Improve Equitable Access to Hepatitis C Virus Diagnostics for Many Communities

Although providing distinct advantages, centralized testing depends heavily on strong sample transport and result delivery networks, and can delay the time to result. This

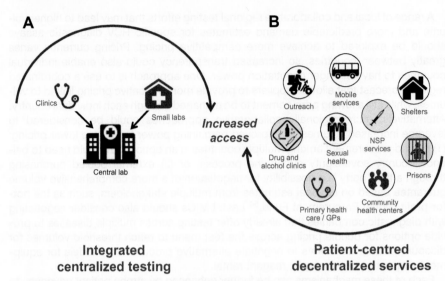

Fig. 4. hepatitis C virus (HCV) testing models at both (*A*) integrated centralized, tertiary or district laboratories and (*B*) patient-centered decentralized primary health care services are required for global elimination. GPs, general practitioners; NSP, needle/syringe program.

increase in time consequently increases the number of patient visits and likewise the risk of patient loss along the care cascade. Patient-centered, decentralized testing strategies that empower the patient to control their health care are likely to further reduce the health disparity among communities disproportionately affected by HCV and increase access to HCV diagnosis and care. Decentralized testing services must be adapted to suit a broad range of key affected communities living in urban, regional, rural, and remote settings (**Fig. 4**B). Task-shifting in these services that allows health care and peer support workers to expand the availability of testing will be critical to scale-up HCV diagnosis.[63–66] Patient-centered approaches embedded within existing services, such as primary care clinics,[67–69] services for the homeless community,[70] men who have sex with men,[71] sex workers,[72] correctional facilities,[73,74] specialist drug services,[75–77] and needle and syringe programs,[78,79] among others, have clearly demonstrated improved access to key populations who may otherwise not be reachable by centralized services.

Several sampling techniques, including oral fluid or fingerstick capillary blood, can facilitate the decentralization of diagnostics.[80–82] Fingerstick capillary blood provides a particularly important sample collection method among many people who inject drugs, for whom poor past health care experiences when accessing veins for standard phlebotomy can remain a huge barrier.[83] Capillary blood from a fingerstick can be also collected onto filter paper as a DBS, as a strategy to increase access to centralized HCV testing among people who inject drugs or those in rural or remote populations.[51,84–86] Studies are underway in the Netherlands[87] and Australia (NCT02102451) to assess the potential for self-collected DBS samples as a tool to increase screening, confirm cure, and help monitor reinfection[88] among those at risk. Sample collection by finger prick in these settings also provides a unique opportunity for POC HCV RNA testing to provide an immediate result and treatment to the patient.[89,90] Existing near-POC/POC platforms, for example, the CE-marked GeneXpert or Genedrive HCV RNA assays, currently require plasma or serum, but their rational placement and availability could assist to make faster diagnosis more widely available to ensure better testing coverage and promote improved linkage to follow-up services.

GLOBAL EFFORTS TO FIND THE HOLY GRAIL: THE SEARCH FOR A POINT-OF-CARE HEPATITIS C VIRUS DIAGNOSTIC FOR ACTIVE HEPATITIS C VIRUS INFECTION MUST CONTINUE

Detection of the Hepatitis C Virus Is the Only Test Required to Confirm Active Infection

HCV diagnosis of active infection through direct detection of the HCV virus is the only test required for patient treatment and care. Despite this, HCV is currently diagnosed in 2 steps: first through the detection of HCV antibodies (anti-HCV) using either centralized laboratory tests or rapid diagnostic tests to determine exposure to the virus[25–27]; and, second, among those who are anti-HCV positive, active HCV infection is confirmed by nucleic acid testing (NAT) or HCV core antigen (HCVcAg) detection.[91] The need for anti-HCV screening followed by HCV RNA and/or HCVcAg testing is entirely driven by the relative costs of each test. As a result, this 2-step diagnostic algorithm is likely to continue until the costs of HCV RNA or HCVcAg tests are significantly reduced. Although anti-HCV rapid diagnostic tests are easy to use and currently provide an affordable screening strategy in many settings,[78,82,92] multiple studies have demonstrated that up to 25% to 50% of people who are anti-HCV positive fail to return for follow-up NAT to diagnose active infection.[93–95] Concerns also remain around the sensitivity of the anti-HCV assays, particularly in the presence of HIV or hepatitis B coinfection, in other immunocompromised patients, or owing to other poorly understood regional differences in assay performance, although current data remain limited.[96,97] Although reflex testing, in which anti–HCV antibody-positive samples are automatically referred to undergo HCV RNA testing without the need for a separate sample collection visit, has been rolled out in the United States and the UK, limited data are available to demonstrate an impact on improving the retention of people in care and increasing cure in the era of DAA therapy.[98,99] Furthermore, this strategy still relies on centralized testing and, therefore, diagnosis cannot be accomplished in a single visit. Modeling data clearly demonstrate that a shift to a 1-step diagnosis of active HCV infection, without HCV antibody screening, is central to achieving HCV elimination goals.[100]

The Holy Grail Point-of-Care Diagnostic Assay for Active Hepatitis C Virus Infection That Links All People with Hepatitis C Infection to Immediate Care Is Essential to Achieve Global Elimination

To eliminate HCV by 2030 as a public health concern, HCV care will need to be simplified to "test and treat" for all. In the perfect world, simple "test and treat" facilities would be embedded within existing decentralized community services to enable the diagnosis of millions of people with HCV infection and link them immediately into care. The holy grail diagnostic assay would enable a person to walk into a local community health care center without stigma, provide a simple sample, receive their diagnosis of active HCV infection, and start treatment immediately—all in a single visit in under 30 minutes (**Fig. 5**). Patients would then return to the center to confirm cure. Those with advanced liver disease and/or those who are at risk of reexposure would revisit the center for continued monitoring and care. Alternatively, more regular self-testing could occur at home to screen for reinfection. In this ideal setting, the diagnostic assay would test for active infection and require only a finger prick capillary blood sample or self-collected oral fluid to be loaded directly onto the platform by

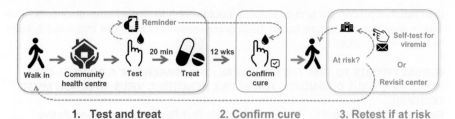

1. Test and treat   2. Confirm cure   3. Retest if at risk

Fig. 5. The holy grail: a point-of-care test for active hepatitis C virus (HCV) infection. (1) Walk into a community health care center to complete a rapid test to diagnose active HCV infection and received standard duration treatment. (2) Receive a reminder to return to the center for a second test to confirm cure. (3) If patient feels at risk of reexposure to the virus, they either return to the center to retest for HCV infection, or complete a self-test for viremia (eg, via a rapid home test for active infection or a self-collected dried blood spot posted to a central laboratory).

any health care worker or the patient themselves. The results would be available in 20 minutes and be simple to interpret accurately. Although the platform would ideally be instrument free, a small handheld device or a small, portable instrument may also be fit for this purpose. Any power required by the device would be provided by a long-life, solar-powered, rechargeable battery. If performed using a smart phone or small instrument, the platform would have the capacity to capture and, where connectivity was available, automatically transmit data to facilitate data collection and surveillance reporting. For platforms with this connectivity, the assay could automatically link the patient to their preferred notification tool as a reminder to complete a posttreatment follow-up visit to confirm cure and assist continuity of care. This follow-up visit could occur either at the clinic or through a self-testing option as preferred. Although likely unachievable, the perfect assay that would allow global scale access to POC diagnosis of active infection would cost less than $US5 per test (includes reagent cost only, at scale, ex-works), although consensus on this remains controversial.[101]

Several Existing Assays and Point-of-Care Platforms Could Be Readily Adapted to Diagnose Active Hepatitis C Virus Infection

Unlike the saturated market for anti-HCV rapid diagnostic tests,[102,103] the GeneXpert HCV Viral Load test (Cepheid, Sunnyvale, CA) and the Genedrive HCV IVD kit (Genedrive Diagnostics, Manchester, UK) are the only SRA-approved near-POC, plasma-based assays that detect active HCV infection. Cepheid is currently the only supplier in LMIC of a multianalyte, integrated platform that uses single-use cartridges to extract, amplify, and detect the presence of HCV by fluorescent reverse transcriptase polymerase chain reaction (PCR).[89,104,105] However, there are several similar nucleic acid platforms that also use PCR amplification and fluorescent detection that are in development, for example, the TrueNAT Chip-based Real-Time micro PCR test (Diagnostics Molbio Pvt Ltf, Goa, India), or could be adapted to diagnose HCV from existing systems, such as the Enigma Minilab (Enigma Diagnostics Ltd., San Diego, CA)[106] and DxNA GeneSTAT System (DxNA LLC, St George, UT). Likewise, several simplified platforms that use alternative amplification technologies, such as reverse transcriptase loop-mediated isothermal amplification, also have commercially-available assays for other viral infections including the Alere i and Alere q for HIV 1/2 Early Infant Diagnosis (Abbott Diagnostics).[107-109] The isothermal reaction within reverse transcriptase loop-mediated isothermal amplification reduces time to result, minimizes platform complexity, and is amenable to a visual result.[110] The addition of HCV assays to already approved molecular POC platforms would greatly improve competition in the field and help to reduce prices, likely in a more expedient fashion than the launch of a new product platform. In addition, the development of a true POC NAT that diagnoses active HCV infection from finger stick whole blood outside of a laboratory setting is still yet to be realized.

In addition to NAT, a considerable amount of evidence has been generated to support the clinical utility of the HCVcAg in plasma as a marker of active infection. HCVcAg is a viral protein released into the circulation during viral assembly and offers a potentially more stable, alternative marker to HCV RNA for diagnosis of active infection. Currently, there is only 1 CE-IVD marked test for the quantification of HCVcAg in plasma samples for HCV diagnosis and treatment monitoring: the Architect HCV Ag performed on the ARCHITECT Immunoassay Analyser (Abbott Diagnostics) is suitable for centralized testing facilities. Unfortunately, access to the ARCHITECT remains limited in many settings. Therefore, because the instrument footprint for PCR often already exists and the bundled pricing of HCV RNA tests continues to be reduced in LMIC (US$14–$25), NAT is likely to continue to be a more affordable option for LMIC, at least in the short term. However, centralized HCVcAg testing may provide a more affordable option for middle-income countries where platforms are already in use and upfront investment is not required.[42,111–114] More recent efforts, including by the Center for Innovation in Global Health Technologies (Northwestern University), Abbott Diagnostics, and Qoo Labs (San Diego, CA) have focused on adapting the immunoassay detection of the HCVcAg into a rapid diagnostic lateral flow test, although these platforms are often challenging[115] and are still in early stages of prototype development.[116]

New Classes of Technologies May Transform the Hepatitis C Virus Point-of-Care Landscape in the Next Decade

Although very few new classes of POC diagnostics have come to the market in recent years,[117] the world can expect the arrival of transformational technologies in the next few years. Fundamental advances in each diagnostic assay component are underway, including new assay chemistries and nanotechnologies to improve sample capture and detection, and novel materials and microfluidics to allow miniaturization.[118–120] Smart phone–assisted diagnosis of infection, through either the adaptation of reading devices or addition of biosensing platforms to a mobile device, are also on the horizon and promise to improve access to testing, including in rural and remote communities.[121,122] Investments to maximize smart phone diagnostic innovations may provide opportunities to improve health care more broadly, including improved surveillance data collection in remote and resource-limited settings, increased telehealth capacity, and the ability to more easily implement interventions to enhance linkage to care.[123] The availability of new materials and innovative solutions such as 3-dimensional printing are also likely to further reduce costs and facilitate the scale-up of many of these technologies.[124,125] Although many of these new classes of diagnostic tools have been developed for other viral infections, such as HIV or Zika, these advances can undoubtedly be quickly translated to HCV diagnosis and management if there is commitment.

Mechanisms to Further Stimulate Investment in the Development of Novel Diagnostics Suitable for Resource Limited Settings Are Essential

Although promising new, transformational diagnostic technologies are on the horizon, novel mechanisms to decrease costs and risks to further stimulate investment in research and development are needed.[126,127] Although the diagnostic development pathway is relatively low cost and low risk when compared with drug development, the successful penetration of a new diagnostic assay into the market can take at least 7 years and needs to overcome 2 "valleys of death" before launch.[128,129] There can also be an overwhelming lack of interest to develop diagnostic assays suitable for LMIC where the market has not been strongly developed, despite potentially high volumes. Considering that 80% of those with chronic HCV infection live in LMIC, it is imperative to find new funding models to accelerate the development of commercially viable, fit-for-purpose assays for LMIC if elimination goals of HCV are to be achieved.

Several approaches may be considered to decrease the cost and risk associated with investing in a diagnostic product (**Fig. 6**). Diagnostic companies could reassess the unmet need and business advantages of focusing on the development of assays for multiple diseases on integrated, single platforms to improve efficiencies and increase profits. Another strategy may be to implement differential pricing that allows the sale of premium priced assays within high-income countries to support the sale of reduced priced assays in LMICs. Although there are not many examples of this previously being successful, the fact that POC/1-step diagnosis of HCV is applicable in both higher income countries and LMIC settings may present a unique situation where the same product can be viable in both markets. Another possibility would be for drug and diagnostic companies to find synergy: although, at least in theory, it would seem to be in the interests of drug companies to invest in companion diagnostics that identify those in need of their treatment, unfortunately, the profit margins remain concentrated in high-income countries so there is currently little incentive for originator drug companies to invest in affordable diagnostics suitable for LMICs. More recently, generic drug companies are exploring partnerships with diagnostic suppliers or developing companion diagnostics to offer bundled pricing and bridge the diagnosis-to-treatment gap in LMICs.[55] However, considering the potential for this approach to introduce product monopolies where a diagnosis may only be offered in concert with a single drug supplier, this strategy would need to be assessed, regulated, and

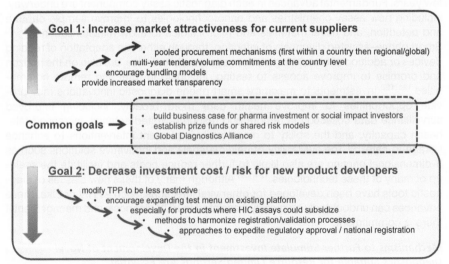

Fig. 6. Approaches to decrease investment cost and risks to stimulate investment in research and development of diagnostics suitable for low- to middle-income countries. HIC, higher income countries; TPP, target product profile.

monitored carefully. Diagnostic companies can also be constrained by current treatment guidelines,[25,27,130] which define strict lower limits of quantitation to guide patient management. These guidelines are based on currently available analytical thresholds for HCV RNA assays rather than the real-world clinical sensitivity required for effective patient management.[131] Because analytical HCV RNA thresholds are likely considerably lower than clinically relevant thresholds, a global systematic review of the distribution of HCV RNA among real-world cohorts has been commissioned by FIND and WHO to help define the lower qualitative HCV RNA thresholds required for effective patient management and update current target product profiles for new qualitative nucleic acid diagnostics.[101] Although ensuring testing guidelines keep pace in a rapidly changing therapeutic environment can be challenging, this strategy to review analytical and clinical requirements may help to further encourage industry to invest in the development of simple and affordable diagnostic solutions.

Last, innovative funding mechanisms to drive program scale up are needed. Proposals such as the Global Alliance for Medical Diagnostics Initiative could prove valuable, but will require significant funding commitments and careful management around governance, independence and conflict of interests.[132] Recent initiatives such as the Stop TB Partnership "Venture Lab" (vLab) provide examples of how private–public partnerships may be able to accelerate and scale up diagnostics.[133] Innovative approaches to provide needed initial funding to galvanize large-scale national public health HCV programs as well advocacy to global donors, such as PEPFAR and the Global Fund, to support diagnosis and treatment of HCV will be key. Commitments from these funders would send very powerful signals to suppliers that a viable market is achievable.

SUMMARY: REMAINING CHALLENGES FOR GLOBAL ACCESS TO HEPATITIS C VIRUS DIAGNOSTICS

It is time the world took HCV diagnostics seriously. Wide-spread diagnosis of HCV is essential to achieve global elimination and increasing access is now a public health priority. The global community must come together to collectively support efforts to develop testing strategies that are patient-centric, expedite assay registration, reduce costs, and generate the demand required for businesses to invest in wide-scale roll out of existing products. No one diagnostic solution will fit all purposes, but the global community must invest in partnerships that facilitate the development and introduction of the holy grail POC HCV diagnostic test to ensure finding the missing millions in need of curative treatment.

REFERENCES

1. World Health Organization (WHO). Global health sector strategy, 2016-2021. Available at: http://www.who.int/hepatitis/strategy2016-2021/ghss-hep/en/. Accessed November 20, 2016.
2. D'Ambrosio R, Degasperi E, Colombo M, et al. Direct-acting antivirals: the endgame for hepatitis C? Curr Opin Virol 2017;24:31–7.
3. Polaris Observatory Collaborators. Global prevalence and genotype distribution of hepatitis C virus infection in 2015: a modelling study. Lancet Gastroenterol Hepatol 2017;2(3):161–76.
4. Manns MP, Buti M, Gane E, et al. Hepatitis C virus infection. Nat Rev Dis Primers 2017;3:17006.
5. Lanini S, Easterbrook PJ, Zumla A, et al. Global epidemiology and strategies for control. Clin Microbiol Infect 2016;22(10):833–8.

6. Stanaway JD, Flaxman AD, Naghavi M, et al. The global burden of viral hepatitis from 1990 to 2013: findings from the Global Burden of Disease Study 2013. Lancet 2016;388(10049):1081–8.

7. World Health Organization (WHO). Global Hepatitis Report 2017. Available at: http://www.who.int/hepatitis/publications/global-hepatitis-report2017/en/. Accessed June 14, 2017.

8. Easterbrook PJ. Who to test and how to test for chronic hepatitis C infection - 2016 WHO testing guidance for low- and middle-income countries. J Hepatol 2016;65(1 Suppl):S46–66.

9. Dore GJ, Feld JJ. Hepatitis C virus therapeutic development: in pursuit of "perfectovir". Clin Infect Dis 2015;60(12):1829–36.

10. UNITAID. Technology and market landscape: hepatitis C medicines August 2017. Available at: https://unitaid.eu/assets/HCV-Medicines-Landscape_Aug-2017.pdf. Accessed September 16, 2017.

11. Jakobsen JC, Nielsen EE, Feinberg J, et al. Direct-acting antivirals for chronic hepatitis C. Cochrane Database Syst Rev 2017;(9):CD012143.

12. MSF. MSF Access campaign. Putting HIV and HCV to the test: a product guide for point-of-care CD4 and laboratory-based and point-of-care virological HIV and HCV tests. 2017. Available at: https://www.msfaccess.org/PHHT2017. Accessed August 25, 2017.

13. Grebely J, Applegate TL, Cunningham P, et al. Hepatitis C point-of-care diagnostics: in search of a single visit diagnosis. Expert Rev Mol Diagn 2017; 17(12):1109–15.

14. Ford N, Swan T, Beyer P, et al. Simplification of antiviral hepatitis C virus therapy to support expanded access in resource-limited settings. J Hepatol 2014; 61(1 Suppl):S132–8.

15. Cohn J, Roberts T, Amorosa V, et al. Simplified diagnostic monitoring for hepatitis C, in the new era of direct-acting antiviral treatment. Curr Opin HIV AIDS 2015;10(5):369–73.

16. Wiesmann F, Braun P. Significance of HCV RNA monitoring in the era of new potent therapies. Expert Rev Anti Infect Ther 2016;14(9):837–44.

17. Hezode C. Pan-genotypic treatment regimens for hepatitis C virus: advantages and disadvantages in high- and low-income regions. J Viral Hepat 2017;24(2): 92–101.

18. Maasoumy B, Vermehren J. Diagnostics in hepatitis C: the end of response-guided therapy? J Hepatol 2016;65(1 Suppl):S67–81.

19. MSF. MSF Access Campaign. Not even close. Issue brief 2017. 2017. Available at: https://www.msfaccess.org/hep-c-not-even-close. Accessed January 27, 2018.

20. Juanbeltz R, Goni Esarte S, Uriz-Otano JI, et al. Safety of oral direct acting antiviral regimens for chronic hepatitis C in real life conditions. Postgrad Med 2017; 129(4):476–83.

21. University of Liverpool. HEP drug interactions. Available at: http://www.hep-druginteractions.org. Accessed October 14, 2017.

22. Kondili LA, Romano F, Rolli FR, et al. Modelling cost-effectiveness and health gains of a "universal" vs. "prioritized" HCV treatment policy in a real-life cohort. Hepatology 2017;66(6):1814–25.

23. Ooka K, Connolly JJ, Lim JK. Medicaid reimbursement for oral direct antiviral agents for the treatment of chronic hepatitis C. Am J Gastroenterol 2017; 112(6):828–32.

24. Marshall AD, Cunningham EB, Nielsen S, et al. Restrictions for reimbursement of interferon-free direct-acting antiviral drugs for HCV infection in Europe. Lancet Gastroenterol Hepatol 2018;3(2):125–33.
25. American Association for the Study of Liver Diseases (AASLD)/Infectious Diseases Society of America (IDSA). HCV guidance: recommendations for testing, managing and treating hepatitis C. 2017. Available at: www.hcvguidelines.org. Accessed September 27, 2017.
26. World Health Organization (WHO). WHO guidelines on hepatitis B and C testing. 2016. Available at: http://apps.who.int/iris/handle/10665/251330. Accessed May 20, 2017.
27. European Association for the Study of the Liver. EASL Recommendations on Treatment of Hepatitis C 2016. J Hepatol 2016;66(1):153–94.
28. Lin ZH, Xin YN, Dong QJ, et al. Performance of the aspartate aminotransferase-to-platelet ratio index for the staging of hepatitis C-related fibrosis: an updated meta-analysis. Hepatology 2011;53(3):726–36.
29. Chou R, Wasson N. Blood tests to diagnose fibrosis or cirrhosis in patients with chronic hepatitis C virus infection. Ann Intern Med 2013;159(5):372.
30. Houot M, Ngo Y, Munteanu M, et al. Systematic review with meta-analysis: direct comparisons of biomarkers for the diagnosis of fibrosis in chronic hepatitis C and B. Aliment Pharmacol Ther 2016;43(1):16–29.
31. Shiha G, Seif S, Eldesoky A, et al. A simple bedside blood test (Fibrofast; FIB-5) is superior to FIB-4 index for the differentiation between non-significant and significant fibrosis in patients with chronic hepatitis C. Hepatol Int 2017;11(3): 286–91.
32. Canadian Agency for Drugs and Technology in Health. Acoustic radiation force impulse imaging for diagnosis and monitoring of liver fibrosis in patients with hepatitis C: a review of diagnostic accuracy, clinical effectiveness, cost-effectiveness, and guidelines. Available at: https://www.ncbi.nlm.nih.gov/pubmedhealth/PMH0087797/pdf/PubMedHealth_PMH0087797.pdf. Accessed May 21, 2017.
33. Hutin Y, Low-Beer D, Bergeri I, et al. Viral Hepatitis Strategic Information to Achieve Elimination by 2030: Key Elements for HIV Program Managers. JMIR Public Health Surveill 2017;3(4):e91.
34. Parry JV, Easterbrook P, Sands AR. One or two serological assay testing strategy for diagnosis of HBV and HCV infection? The use of predictive modelling. BMC Infect Dis 2017;17(Suppl 1):705.
35. Unitaid. Global cost-effectiveness of Hepatitis C treatment. Available at: http://tool.hepccalculator.org/. Accessed February 8, 2018.
36. Morgan JR, Servidone M, Easterbrook P, et al. Economic evaluation of HCV testing approaches in low and middle income countries. BMC Infect Dis 2017; 17(Suppl 1):697.
37. World Health Organization (WHO)/PQT: medicines. Clarification with respect to a stringent regulatory organization as applicable to the stringent regulatory authority (SRA) guideline. 2017. Available at: https://extranet.who.int/prequal/sites/default/files/documents/75%20SRA%20clarification_February2017_0.pdf. Accessed February 2, 2018.
38. US Food and Drug Administration (FDA). Medical device database. 2018. Available at: https://www.fda.gov/MedicalDevices/DeviceRegulationandGuidance/Databases/default.htm Accessed January 27, 2018.
39. World Health Organization (WHO). Public reports of WHO prequalified IVDs. 2017. Available at: http://www.who.int/diagnostics_laboratory/evaluations/pq-list/hcv/public_report/en/. Accessed December 12 2017.

40. Asselah T, Hassanein T, Waked I, et al. Eliminating hepatitis C within low-income countries - the need to cure genotypes 4, 5, 6. J Hepatol 2018;68(4):814–26.

41. Khan H, Hill A, Main J, et al. Can hepatitis C virus antigen testing replace ribonucleic acid polymearse chain reaction analysis for detecting hepatitis C virus? A systematic review. Open Forum Infect Dis 2017;4(2):ofw252.

42. Freiman JM, Tran TM, Schumacher SG, et al. Hepatitis C core antigen testing for diagnosis of hepatitis C virus infection: a systematic review and meta-analysis. Ann Intern Med 2016;165(5):345–55.

43. Lange B, Cohn J, Roberts T, et al. Diagnostic accuracy of serological diagnosis of hepatitis C and B using dried blood spot samples (DBS): two systematic reviews and meta-analyses. BMC Infect Dis 2017;17(Suppl 1):700.

44. McNerney R, Sollis K, Peeling RW. Improving access to new diagnostics through harmonised regulation: priorities for action. Afr J Lab Med 2014;3(1): 123.

45. World Health Organization (WHO). Prequalification of in vitro diagnostics. Available at: http://www.who.int/diagnostics_laboratory/evaluations/en/. Accessed November 18, 2017.

46. Schroeder LF, Guarner J, Elbireer A, et al. Time for a model list of essential diagnostics. N Engl J Med 2016;374(26):2511–4.

47. Carmona P. Field performance of point-of-care HIV testing for early infant diagnosis: pooled analysis from six countries from the EID consortium. Poster presentation at the 21st International AIDS Conference, Durban, South Africa, July 18–22, 2016.

48. Turunga E. Tracking manufacturer performance to ensure the uninterrupted provision of timely, high quality early infant HIV diagnosis test results. International AIDS Society (IAS) meeting satellite session. Paris, France, July 25, 2017.

49. World Health Organization (WHO). WHO technical guidance series. 2017. Available at: http://www.who.int/diagnostics_laboratory/guidance/technical-specifications-series/en/. Accessed October 20, 2017.

50. London School of Health and Tropical Medicine. International Diagnostic Centre. London School of Hygiene and Tropical Medicine. 2018. Available at: http://www.idc-dx.org/resources?keys=Generic+Protocol. Accessed January 27, 2018.

51. Soulier A, Poiteau L, Rosa I, et al. Dried blood spots: a tool to ensure broad access to hepatitis C screening, diagnosis, and treatment monitoring. J Infect Dis 2016;213(7):1087–95.

52. Morin S, Bazarova N, Jacon P, et al. The manufacturers' perspective on world health organization prequalification of in vitro diagnostics. Clin Infect Dis 2018;66(2):301–5.

53. Easterbrook PJ, Roberts T, Sands A, et al. Diagnosis of viral hepatitis. Curr Opin HIV AIDS 2017;12(3):302–14.

54. CDA Foundation. Global procurement fund. Available at: http://gprofund.org/. Accessed July 16, 2017.

55. World Community Advisory Board. Forging a path to elimination: simpler tests and affordable generics. Report of the World Community Advisory Board on HCV Generics and Diagnostics. Available http://www.treatmentactiongroup.org/sites/default/files/HCV%20World%20CAB%20Report_2017.pdf. Accessed December 15, 2017.

56. Dowsett LE, Coward S, Lorenzetti DL, et al. Living with hepatitis C virus: a systematic review and narrative synthesis of qualitative literature. Can J Gastroenterol Hepatol 2017;2017:3268650.

57. Treloar C, Rance J, Backmund M. Understanding barriers to hepatitis C virus care and stigmatization from a social perspective. Clin Infect Dis 2013; 57(Suppl 2):S51–5.

58. Nitsche B, Miller SC, Giorgio M, et al. Improving hepatitis C identification: technology alone is not the answer. Health Promot Pract 2017. [Epub ahead of print].

59. World Health Organization (WHO). Global Laboratory Initiative. 2017. Available at: http://www.who.int/tb/areas-of-work/laboratory/gli/en/. Accessed December 12, 2017.

60. World Health Organization (WHO). Considerations for adoption and use of multidisease testing devices in integrated laboratory networks. Available at: http://apps.who.int/iris/bitstream/10665/255693/1/WHO-HTM-TB-2017.06-eng.pdf?ua51. Accessed October 17, 2017.

61. The Economist Intelligence Unit Limited, 2017. Technology offers creative strategies to prevent and treat HCV at scale. The Economy Newspaper Limited, 2017. London, United Kingdom. Available at: http://pathtozero.eiu.com/wp-content/uploads/sites/19/2017/07/Abbvie-Article-3-Technology-DV3.pdf. Accessed March 20, 2018.

62. Unitaid. Multi-disease diagnostic landscape for integrated management of HIV, HCV, TB and other coinfections. Available at: https://www.ghdonline.org/uploads/multi-disease-diagnostics-landscape-for-integrated-management-of-HIV-HCV-TB-and-other-coinfections-january-2018.pdf. Accessed January 7, 2018.

63. Kattakuzhy S, Gross C, Emmanuel B, et al. Expansion of treatment for hepatitis C virus infection by task shifting to community-based nonspecialist providers: a nonrandomized clinical trial. Ann Intern Med 2017;167(5):311–8.

64. Mathur P, Comstock E, McSweegan E, et al. A pilot study to expand treatment of chronic hepatitis C in resource-limited settings. Antiviral Res 2017;146:184–90.

65. Henderson C, Madden A, Kelsall J. 'Beyond the willing & the waiting' - The role of peer-based approaches in hepatitis C diagnosis & treatment. Int J Drug Pol 2017;50:111–5.

66. Yoo ER, Perumpail RB, Cholankeril G, et al. Expanding treatment access for chronic hepatitis C with task-shifting in the era of direct-acting antivirals. J Clin Transl Hepatol 2017;5(2):130–3.

67. Bajis S, Dore GJ, Hajarizadeh B, et al. Interventions to enhance testing, linkage to care and treatment uptake for hepatitis C virus infection among people who inject drugs: a systematic review. Int J Drug Pol 2017;47:34–46.

68. Wong K, Abdelqader A, Camire L, et al. A resident initiative improves hepatitis C screening rates in primary care clinics. J Grad Med Educ 2017;9(6):768–70.

69. Al-Hihi E, Shankweiler C, Stricklen D, et al. Electronic medical record alert improves HCV testing for baby boomers in primary care setting: adults born during 1945-1965. BMJ Open Qual 2017;6(2):e000084.

70. Morano JP, Zelenev A, Lombard A, et al. Strategies for hepatitis C testing and linkage to care for vulnerable populations: point-of-care and standard HCV testing in a mobile medical clinic. J Community Health 2014;39(5):922–34.

71. van Rooijen M, Heijman T, de Vrieze N, et al. Earlier detection of hepatitis C virus infection through routine hepatitis C virus antibody screening of human immunodeficiency virus-positive men who have sex with men attending a sexually transmitted infection outpatient clinic: a longitudinal study. Sex Transm Dis 2016; 43(9):560–5.

72. Saludes V, Folch C, Morales-Carmona A, et al. Community-based screening of hepatitis C with a one-step RNA detection algorithm from dried-blood spots:

analysis of key populations in Barcelona, Spain. J Viral Hepat 2018;25(3): 236–44.

73. Beckwith CG, Kurth AE, Bazerman LB, et al. A pilot study of rapid hepatitis C virus testing in the Rhode Island Department of Corrections. J Public Health (Oxf) 2016;38(1):130–7.

74. Schoenbachler BT, Smith BD, Sena AC, et al. Hepatitis C virus testing and linkage to care in North Carolina and South Carolina Jails, 2012-2014. Public Health Rep 2016;131(Suppl 2):98–104.

75. McAllister G, Innes H, McLeod A, et al. Uptake of hepatitis C specialist services and treatment following diagnosis by dried blood spot in Scotland. J Clin Virol 2014;61(3):359–64.

76. Read P, Lothian R, Chronister K, et al. Delivering direct acting antiviral therapy for hepatitis C to highly marginalised and current drug injecting populations in a targeted primary health care setting. Int J Drug Pol 2017;47:209–15.

77. Bregenzer A, Conen A, Knuchel J, et al. Management of hepatitis C in decentralised versus centralised drug substitution programmes and minimally invasive point-of-care tests to close gaps in the HCV cascade. Swiss Med Wkly 2017;147:w14544.

78. Fernandez-Lopez L, Folch C, Majo X, et al. Implementation of rapid HIV and HCV testing within harm reduction programmes for people who inject drugs: a pilot study. AIDS Care 2016;28(6):712–6.

79. Kaberg M, Hammarberg A, Lidman C, et al. Prevalence of hepatitis C and pretesting awareness of hepatitis C status in 1500 consecutive PWID participants at the Stockholm needle exchange program. Infect Dis (Lond) 2017;49(10): 728–36.

80. Drobnik A, Judd C, Banach D, et al. Public health implications of rapid hepatitis C screening with an oral swab for community-based organizations serving high-risk populations. Am J Public Health 2011;101(11):2151–5.

81. Comanescu C, Arama V, Grancea C, et al. The performance of a rapid test for anti-HCV screening in oral fluids. Roum Arch Microbiol Immunol 2015;74(1–2): 40–5.

82. Candfield S, Samuel MI, Ritchie D, et al. Use and acceptability of salivary hepatitis C virus testing in an English Young Offender Institution. Int J STD AIDS 2017;28(12):1234–8.

83. Bajis S, Lamoury F, Applegate T, et al. Acceptability of point of care finger-stick and venipuncture hepatitis C virus testing among people who inject drugs and homeless people. Poster presentation at the Australasian Viral Hepatitis Elimination Conference (AVHEC), Cairns, Australia, August 10–11, 2017.

84. Coats JT, Dillon JF. The effect of introducing point-of-care or dried blood spot analysis on the uptake of hepatitis C virus testing in high-risk populations: a systematic review of the literature. Int J Drug Pol 2015;26(11):1050–5.

85. Greenman J, Roberts T, Cohn J, et al. Dried blood spot in the genotyping, quantification and storage of HCV RNA: a systematic literature review. J Viral Hepat 2015;22(4):353–61.

86. Radley A, Melville K, Tait J, et al. A quasi-experimental evaluation of dried blood spot testing through community pharmacies in the Tayside region of Scotland. Frontline Gastroenterol 2017;8(3):221–8.

87. Zurre F. Online-mediated HCV-RNA home-based testing to reduce incidence of hepatitis C virus infection among men who have sex with men in Amsterdam, The Netherlands – an initiative of the MC Free project. Poster 17A World Hepatitis

Summit 2017. Available at: http://www.worldhepatitissummit.org/docs/default-source/posters/17a_frekezuure.pdf?sfvrsn=2. Accessed January 29, 2018.

88. Falade-Nwulia O, Sulkowski MS, Merkow A, et al. Understanding and addressing hepatitis C reinfection in the oral direct acting antiviral era. J Viral Hepat 2018;25(3):220–7.

89. Grebely JL, Lamoury FMJ, Hajarizadeh B, et al. Evaluation of the Xpert HCV Viral Load point-of-care assay from venipuncture-collected and finger-stick capillary whole-blood samples: a cohort study. Lancet Gastroenterol Hepatol 2017;2(7):514–20.

90. Lamoury FMJ, Bajis S, Hajarizadeh B, et al. Evaluation of the Xpert® HCV Viral Load Fingerstick point-of-care assay. The Journal of infectious diseases 2018, in Press

91. Peeling RW, Boeras DI, Marinucci F, et al. The future of viral hepatitis testing: innovations in testing technologies and approaches. BMC Infect Dis 2017; 17(Suppl 1):699.

92. Parisi MR, Soldini L, Vidoni G, et al. Point-of-care testing for HCV infection: recent advances and implications for alternative screening. New Microbiol 2014;37(4):449–57.

93. Yehia BR, Schranz AJ, Umscheid CA, et al. The treatment cascade for chronic hepatitis C virus infection in the United States: a systematic review and meta-analysis. PLoS One 2014;9(7):e101554.

94. Patel RC, Vellozzi C, Smith BD. Results of hepatitis C birth-cohort testing and linkage to care in selected U.S. Sites, 2012-2014. Public Health Rep 2016; 131(Suppl 2):12–9.

95. Spradling PR, Tong X, Rupp LB, et al. Trends in HCV RNA testing among HCV antibody-positive persons in care, 2003-2010. Clin Infect Dis 2014;59(7): 976–81.

96. Kosack CS, Nick S. Evaluation of two rapid screening assays for detecting hepatitis C antibodies in resource-constrained settings. Trop Med Int Health 2016; 21(5):603–9.

97. Barbosa JR, Colares JKB, Flores GL, et al. Performance of rapid diagnostic tests for detection of Hepatitis B and C markers in HIV infected patients. J Virol Methods 2017;248:244–9.

98. Viner K, Kuncio D, Newbern EC, et al. The continuum of hepatitis C testing and care. Hepatology 2015;61(3):783–9.

99. Ireland G. Reflex RNA testing on hepatitis C antibody positive samples: is it being adopted? HepHIV 2017 abstract. 2017. Available at: https://www.researchgate.net/publication/313529792_Reflex_RNA_testing_on_hepatitis_C_antibody_positive_samples_is_it_being_adopted. Accessed November 12, 2017.

100. Scott N, Doyle JS, Wilson DP, et al. Reaching hepatitis C virus elimination targets requires health system interventions to enhance the care cascade. Int J Drug Pol 2017;47:107–16.

101. Ivanova Reipold E, Easterbrook P, Trianni A, et al. Optimising diagnosis of viraemic hepatitis C infection: the development of a target product profile. BMC Infect Dis 2017;17(Suppl 1):707.

102. Khuroo MS, Khuroo NS, Khuroo MS. Diagnostic accuracy of point-of-care tests for hepatitis C virus infection: a systematic review and meta-analysis. PLoS One 2015;10(3):e0121450.

103. Tang W, Chen W, Amini A, et al. Diagnostic accuracy of tests to detect Hepatitis C antibody: a meta-analysis and review of the literature. BMC Infect Dis 2017; 17(Suppl 1):695.

104. McHugh MP, Wu AHB, Chevaliez S, et al. Multicenter evaluation of the Cepheid Xpert hepatitis C virus viral load assay. J Clin Microbiol 2017;55(5):1550–6.

105. Gupta E, Agarwala P, Kumar G, et al. Point -of -care testing (POCT) in molecular diagnostics: performance evaluation of GeneXpert HCV RNA test in diagnosing and monitoring of HCV infection. J Clin Virol 2017;88:46–51.

106. Douthwaite ST, Walker C, Adams EJ, et al. Performance of a novel point-of-care molecular assay for detection of influenza A and B viruses and respiratory syncytial virus (Enigma Minilab) in children with acute respiratory infection. J Clin Microbiol 2016;54(1):212–5.

107. Hsiao NY, Dunning L, Kroon M, et al. Laboratory evaluation of the Alere q point-of-care system for early infant HIV diagnosis. PLoS One 2016;11(3):e0152672.

108. Dunning L, Kroon M, Hsiao NY, et al. Field evaluation of HIV point-of-care testing for early infant diagnosis in Cape Town, South Africa. PLoS One 2017;12(12): e0189226.

109. Chang M, Steinmetzer K, Raugi DN, et al. Detection and differentiation of HIV-2 using the point-of-care Alere q HIV-1/2 Detect nucleic acid test. J Clin Virol 2017; 97:22–5.

110. Tanner NA, Zhang Y, Evans TC Jr. Simultaneous multiple target detection in real-time loop-mediated isothermal amplification. Biotechniques 2012;53(2):81–9.

111. Lamoury FMJ, Soker A, Martinez D, et al. Hepatitis C virus core antigen: a simplified treatment monitoring tool, including for post-treatment relapse. J Clin Virol 2017;92:32–8.

112. Rockstroh JK, Feld JJ, Chevaliez S, et al. HCV core antigen as an alternate test to HCV RNA for assessment of virologic responses to all-oral, interferon-free treatment in HCV genotype 1 infected patients. J Virol Methods 2017;245:14–8.

113. Duchesne L, Njouom R, Lissock F, et al. HCV Ag quantification as a one-step procedure in diagnosing chronic hepatitis C infection in Cameroon: the ANRS 12336 study. J Int AIDS Soc 2017;20(1):1–8.

114. Mohamed Z, Mbwambo J, Shimakawa Y, et al. Clinical utility of HCV core antigen detection and quantification using serum samples and dried blood spots in people who inject drugs in Dar-es-Salaam, Tanzania. J Int AIDS Soc 2017; 20(1):21856.

115. Mohd Hanafiah K, Arifin N, Bustami Y, et al. Development of multiplexed infectious disease lateral flow assays: challenges and opportunities. Diagnostics (Basel) 2017;7(3) [pii:E51].

116. Centers for Disease Control and Prevention (CDC). Hepatitis C diagnostic summit. Atlanta (GA): 2016. Available at: https://www.cdc.gov/hepatitis/resources/ mtgsconf/hepcdiagsummit2016.htm. Accessed January 28, 2018.

117. Nayak S, Blumenfeld NR, Laksanasopin T, et al. Point-of-care diagnostics: recent developments in a connected age. Anal Chem 2017;89(1):102–23.

118. Zarei M. Advances in point-of-care technologies for molecular diagnostics. Biosens Bioelectron 2017;98:494–506.

119. Radin JM, Topol EJ, Andersen KG, et al. A laboratory in your pocket. Lancet 2016;388(10054):1875.

120. Romao VC, Martins SAM, Germano J, et al. Lab-on-chip devices: gaining ground losing size. ACS Nano 2017;11(11):10659–64.

121. Ganguli A, Ornob A, Yu H, et al. Hands-free smartphone-based diagnostics for simultaneous detection of Zika, Chikungunya, and Dengue at point-of-care. Biomed Microdevices 2017;19(4):73.

122. Chen W, Yu H, Sun F, et al. Mobile platform for multiplexed detection and differentiation of disease-specific nucleic acid sequences, using microfluidic loop-

mediated isothermal amplification and smartphone detection. Anal Chem 2017; 89(21):11219–26.

123. Zhu H, Sencan I, Wong J, et al. Cost-effective and rapid blood analysis on a cell-phone. Lab A Chip 2013;13(7):1282–8.

124. Mulberry G, White KA, Vaidya M, et al. 3D printing and milling a real-time PCR device for infectious disease diagnostics. PLoS One 2017;12(6):e0179133.

125. Chan K, Wong PY, Parikh C, et al. Moving toward rapid and low-cost point-of-care molecular diagnostics with a repurposed 3D printer and RPA. Anal Biochem 2018;545:4–12.

126. Engel N, Wachter K, Pai M, et al. Addressing the challenges of diagnostics demand and supply: insights from an online global health discussion platform. BMJ Glob Health 2016;1(4):e000132.

127. Pai NP, Vadnais C, Denkinger C, et al. Point-of-care testing for infectious diseases: diversity, complexity, and barriers in low- and middle-income countries. PLoS Med 2012;9(9):e1001306.

128. GBCHealth. Crossing the valleys of death in TB: from development to roll-out. 2017. Available at: http://gbchealth.org/crossing-the-valleys-of-death-in-tb-from-development-to-roll-out/. Accessed January 29, 2018.

129. FIND. Turning complex diagnostic challenges into simple solutions. Strategy 2015-2020. 2014. Available at: https://www.finddx.org/wp-content/uploads/2016/01/FIND_Strategy.pdf. Accessed December 12, 2017.

130. World Health Organization (WHO). Guidelines for the screening, care and treatment of persons with chronic hepatitis C infection. 2016. Available at: http://apps.who.int/iris/bitstream/10665/205035/1/9789241549615_eng.pdf?ua=1. Accessed December 12, 2017.

131. Chou R, Easterbrook P, Hellard M. Methodological challenges in appraising evidence on diagnostic testing for WHO guidelines on hepatitis B and hepatitis C virus infection. BMC Infect Dis 2017;17(Suppl 1):694.

132. Mugambi ML, Palamountain KM, Gallarda J, et al. Exploring the case for a global alliance for medical diagnostics initiative. Diagnostics (Basel) 2017;7(1) [pii:E8].

133. Stop TB Partnership. Stop TB Partnership and its partners "Unite to end TB" by launching a social impact fund and an accelerator for impact. 2016. Available at: http://www.stoptb.org/news/stories/2016/ns16_052.asp. Accessed October 17, 2017.

A Guide to the Economics of Hepatitis C Virus Cure in 2017

Benjamin P. Linas, MD, MPH[a,b,c,]*, Shayla Nolen, MPH[a]

KEYWORDS

- Hepatitis C Virus • Cost-effectiveness • Health care economics

KEY POINTS

- This commentary reviews the core principals of cost-effectiveness and applies them to the rapidly evolving context of hepatitis C virus treatment in the United States.
- The article provides a foundation of evidence that treatment provides good economic value, even though it is expensive, and even when treating people who inject drugs who are at high risk for reinfection.
- The price of medications has decreased, but the high price continues to limit access to care.
- This wedge between cost effectiveness and affordability stands front and center as one of the leading obstacles to elimination.

The availability of effective, oral treatments for hepatitis C virus (HCV) has transformed HCV infection from a chronic disease with few treatment options to a curable condition with as little as 8 weeks of oral therapy. The tremendous potential for HCV cure has generated enthusiasm for using new treatments to eliminate HCV transmission in the United States. The National Academies of Sciences, Engineering, and Medicine calls for this goal, as does the Centers for Disease Control and Prevention and the US Department of Health and Human Services.[1] With effective treatment in hand, and the explicit goal of eliminating transmission, the challenge shifts from one of biology—how to cure a virus—to public health—how to identify and treat the more than 4 million people in the United States who are HCV infected.

The HCV elimination challenge is difficult when one considers that eliminating HCV transmission requires that we identify and treat the infection among those who are actively transmitting. Therefore, eliminating HCV transmission requires strategies to identify and treat HCV among people who inject drugs (PWID).[1–3] Working with current

Disclosure and Funding: Supported in part by the National Institutes of Drug Abuse (P30DA040500) and Allergy and Infectious Diseases (P30AI042853). No commercial funding to any of the authors.

[a] Section of Infectious Diseases, Boston Medical Center, Boston, MA, USA; [b] Department of Medicine, Boston University School of Medicine, Boston, MA, USA; [c] Department of Epidemiology, Boston University School of Public Health, Boston, MA, USA
* Corresponding author. Boston Medical Center, Crosstown Center Second Floor #2007, 801 Massachusetts Avenue, Boston, MA 02118.
E-mail address: Benjamin.Linas@bmc.org

Infect Dis Clin N Am 32 (2018) 447–459
https://doi.org/10.1016/j.idc.2018.02.013
0891-5520/18/© 2018 Elsevier Inc. All rights reserved.

id.theclinics.com

PWID is not always easy. There is concern that active PWID who achieve cure of their HCV infection might be reinfected if they continue to use injection drugs or relapse to use in the future.[4,5] There is also concern that patients identified with HCV infection will not link to HCV care, or will not complete the treatment course.[6]

Adding to this challenge is the reality that HCV treatments are expensive. When first released, a typical course of sofosbuvir, one of the most effective and commonly used agents for HCV treatment, cost approximately $84,000.[7] Since that time, multiple regimens have been approved by the US Food and Drug Administration. There is competition in the market for HCV treatments, and prices have decreased significantly. Even at the best price available on the market, however, a course of HCV treatment costs tens of thousands of dollars. Many of the PWID who transmit HCV rely on public payers, such as Medicaid or Departments of Corrections for their health care.[8] The high cost of HCV treatment places substantial stress on health care budgets.

This combination of factors—a prevalent disease that has an expensive, but curative treatment, the potential for reinfection among those who achieve cure, and the burden of curing patients falling primarily on public payers—has generated significant economic barriers to HCV care.[8–11] Payers are worried about the cost of treating HCV, especially if they are forced to pay for cure more than 1 time for those who are reinfected. Even when PWID with HCV are identified and linked to care, many payers restrict access to curative HCV treatments to those who have evidence of more advanced liver fibrosis and/or those who have been abstinent from drug use for 6 to 12 months.[12–14]

There are many social determinants of health, such as poverty, lack of education, and drug use, that create barriers to HCV care among PWID,[8–10] but at this time there can be no debate that the economic barriers are substantial.[14] HCV treatment is expensive.

Yet, many treatments and health care technologies that we routinely use in the United States are expensive, and many of them are not as effective as HCV treatment. Cost is not the only axis by which to prioritize health care interventions. There is a need for some outcome measure that considers both the cost of a treatment, and the benefit it provides to assess its value. How much benefit will we get for every dollar spent on HCV treatment? How does that ratio of cost to benefit compare to other treatments that we use in the United States? In other words, is HCV therapy worth it? What is its value?

Cost effectiveness is the field of research that focuses on defining the value of health care technologies.[15] Cost effectiveness seeks to estimate the cost of using a new therapy, as well as the additional health benefits that therapy will provide, and ultimately to define a ratio of cost–benefit that one can compare with other possible interventions and make priorities.[16–18] This article reviews the core concepts of cost-effectiveness research, clarifies the difference between cost effectiveness and affordability, and then reviews the tension between cost effectiveness and affordability when seeking to improve HCV care.

WHAT IS COST EFFECTIVENESS?

Cost-effectiveness analysis seeks to maximize public health benefits given the resources that are available for health care.[19] The central question that cost-effectiveness analysis asks is, "Should we invest our limited health care dollars in a new treatment? Or should we instead use that money to invest in another health care intervention that would provide better outcomes for the same money invested?" Cost-effectiveness analysis is not interested in reducing cost or saving money. Rather, cost-effectiveness analysis seeks to spend all of the available money, but to spend it well. Cost-effectiveness analysis assumes that all available resources will be spent and provides a framework for prioritizing available treatment options.

The cost-effectiveness of a treatment is typically expressed as an incremental cost-effectiveness ratio (ICER)[15,20]:

$$\frac{\text{cost new treatment} - \text{cost current treatment}}{\text{benefit new treatment} - \text{benefit current treatment}}$$

Estimating and interpreting the ICER requires that we answer 3 questions.

1. What are the costs with new and with old treatment and how much more will we spend? The additional cost of HCV treatments includes that of new medications, as well as the costs of staging and evaluation, and the costs that are avoided by preventing future complications of disease. Considering the prevention of long-term complications is especially important when analyzing the cost effectiveness of HCV treatments, because the costs of the therapy are immediate, whereas costs avoided by preventing end-stage liver disease often accrue years in the future.[21]
2. What are the benefits of the interventions? One valuable measure of benefit is life expectancy, but considering only mortality benefits fails to recognize the value of treatments that improve quality of life. The quality-adjusted life-year (QALY) provides a measure that integrates both longevity and quality of life and is the preferred outcome for cost-effectiveness analysis.[22]

How can we interpret the ICER? The ideal cost-effectiveness analysis would list every possible health care intervention, its lifetime medical cost, and QALYs lived. With such a list, we could theoretically prioritize spending perfectly to maximize QALY across the population. In reality, it is impossible to estimate lifetime costs and QALY for everything we do in health care. Instead, cost-effectiveness analysis compares the ICER for a specific treatment to a threshold value and rejects treatments that have an ICER great than the threshold as not cost effective. The threshold value to which we compare an ICER is referred to as the willingness-to-pay (WTP) threshold.[15] Importantly, the WTP threshold is not meant to be a valuation of how much we are "willing" to pay to save a life. WTP is not an ethical judgment or a valuation of how much life is worth. Rather, WTP is an attempt to quantify the opportunity cost of a new treatment. In other words, WTP is meant to reflect the return in QALY that we could expect if we did not use available budget to provide a new treatment and instead invested that money into the current health care system. For example, if I expect that a $100,000 investment into an existing health care intervention will provide 1 additional QALY ($100,000/QALY gained), but instead, I could invest the same $100,000 into a new treatment that results in an additional 1.25 QALY ($80,000/QALY), then investing in the new treatment makes sense. We would conclude that the new treatment is cost effective. If, in contrast, my $100,000 investment into a new treatment provides only 0.75 additional QALY ($133,333/QALY), then I probably should not make that investment. We would then conclude that the new treatment is not cost effective. In the United States, the WTP threshold is typically considered to be either $50,000 or $100,000/QALY gained, but there is good reason to use a WTP $100,000 to $200,000/QALY.[23] The WTP threshold is country specific and reflects the budgetary pressures and resources available in a given state.[15] In an effort to provide some rubric for making cost-effectiveness conclusions, the World Health Organization defines an ICER less than per-capita GDP for a country as being "very cost effective," and less than 3 times per capita GDP as "cost effective."[24] However, although the concept of the WTP is grounded in sound economic theory, the actual value of the appropriate WTP in a given country is somewhat arbitrary. Certainly, WTP cannot be interpreted strictly, and some leaders in the field of cost effectiveness feel that it is inappropriate to use WTP to label interventions as cost effective or not.[25]

What Do We Know About the Cost Effectiveness and Affordability of Treating Hepatitis C Virus?

In the last 5 years, several groups, working entirely independently, have been investigating the cost effectiveness and cost of HCV treatment. With few exceptions, treatment with DAAs has an ICER of less than $100,000/QALY gained, and therefore would typically be considered a good value in the United States.[26–43] Some of the earliest studies, which used the list price of the first treatment regimens available, determined that therapy was not cost effective for some patient types or genotypes, but those conclusions predated the availability of pangenotypic regimens, nor did they reflect the substantial price decreases that have characterized the HCV treatment market in the past 1 to 2 years.[28,30,44] Studies have compared treat all patients with various forms of treatment restrictions, and routinely determine that treat all is a cost-effective approach (**Table 1**).[26,27,44]

Why Is It Cost Effective to Treat Early Stage Hepatitis C Virus if Early Hepatitis C Virus Is a Silent Disease?

Studies that consider treat all versus treat advanced fibrosis only strategies typically find that treat all provides good value when compared with a cost control strategy that limits HCV therapy to those with more advanced liver fibrosis.[26,27,44] This finding may be counterintuitive, given that early stage HCV is deemed a silent disease.[45] If HCV has no impact on mortality, quality of life, or health care use until it has advanced to a more advanced stage of liver fibrosis, then why bother treating HCV in its early stages, especially if resources are limited?

Although many patients with HCV infection do not know that they have the disease, data consistently demonstrate that the quality of life of patients with early stage HCV is lower than similar patients who do not have HCV infection, even when controlling for known confounders.[46,47] Similarly, studies of health care use among patients with early stage HCV demonstrate significantly higher use and cost among those with HCV—even those without advanced liver fibrosis.[44,48] If curing early HCV prevents the accumulation of morbidity and cost while patients wait for cure, then it provides good value. In other words, if ultimately a patient will be treated for HCV at some point, then it is better to spend the money now and prevent disutility and health care costs that would have accumulated while waiting. In modeling studies, cost-effectiveness conclusions about treating early stage HCV are sensitive to assumptions about quality of life with early disease and the cost of early HCV infection.[26] If HCV were really a silent disease in its early stages—with no effect on quality of life or cost—then treating early disease would provide little value and it would be rational to defer treatment until HCV becomes a more active issue for the patient. However, empirical data suggest that HCV is not entirely silent.

Is It Cost Effective to Treat Hepatitis C Virus Among People Who Inject Drugs, Given the Risk of Reinfection After Hepatitis C Virus Cure?

Given that HCV treatments cost the same when used among PWID as the general population, those treatments might be expected to have similar cost-effectiveness ratios. Two factors, however, could reduce the cost effectiveness of HCV therapies

Table 1
Recent cost-effectiveness studies of HCV DAAs

Author, Year	Treatment Regiment	Comments
DAA regimens vs IFN-based treatments		
Chhatwal et al,[28] 2015	LDV/SOF to IFN-based treatment	ICER < $100,000 for all genotypes and fibrosis stage.
Najafzadeh et al,[29] 2015	Genotype-specific SOF regimens to IFN-based regimens	ICER < $100,000 for all genotypes but genotype 2. Predated current GT2 regimens.
Linas et al,[30] 2015	SOF-based regimens for GT 2 and 3 to IFN-based regimens	ICER < $100,000 for all patients when accounting for 2017 prices.
Younossi et al,[31] 2015	LDV/SOF compared with IFN-based treatment for GT1	LDV/SOF cost saving.
Chidi et al,[32] 2016	LDV/SOF compared with PROD and IFN-based in the VA system	PROD without restrictions is cost saving at VA prices for PROD.
Saab et al,[33] 2016	PROD, LDV/SOF, and SOF/SMV vs PEG/RBV for GT 1 and 4	ICER of DAA in all scenarios <$100,000.
Zhang et al,[34] 2015	Genotype appropriate DAA therapy compared with IFN-based treatment	ICER <$100,000 for DAA regimens.
Saint-Laurent Thibault et al,[35] 2017	SOF/DCV vs SOF/RBV for GT3 infection	SOF/DCV cost saving compared with SOF/RBV.
Chhatwal et al,[36] 2017	Metaanalysis of cost-effectiveness studies of DAA therapy; adjusted treatment prices to current market	At best estimate of current price, DAA treatment cost saving in 71% of studies and cost effective in 93%.
Costs and cost-effectiveness of HCV treatment restrictions		
Leidner et al,[26] 2015	DAA therapy prioritized by stage of liver fibrosis	ICER for treating all patients compared with limiting to more advanced fibrosis <$100,000.
Chahal et al,[44] 2016	LDV/SOF treatment prioritized by disease stage	Treating patients with F1 disease ICER <$100,000 compared with treating F2+.
Linas et al,[27] 2016	Cost control by treatment restrictions compared with cost control by price negotiation	Aggressive price negotiation in exchange for formulary preference better than fibrosis stage restrictions.
Cost-effectiveness of implementation models to increase HCV treatment capacity		
Jayasekera et al,[37] 2017	Expanding capacity for DAA by task shifting to specialized nurses compared with treating fewer patients with MD provider	Treating more patients with specialized nurses cost-saving and better outcomes.
Cost-effectiveness of HCV treatment in key populations		
Martin et al,[57] 2012	Treatment for PWID with and without advanced fibrosis; included impact of HCV cure on future transmission	Treating PWID with moderate or mild HCV cost-effective compared with delay until cirrhosis, except when reinfection risk is very high.
Elbasha et al,[38] 2017	EBR/GZR vs PEG/RBV among patients with chronic kidney disease	ICER < $100,000 for treatment with EBR/GZR

(continued on next page)

Table 1
(continued)

Author, Year	Treatment Regiment	Comments
Saab et al,[33] 2016	PROD and LDV/SOF vs PEG/RBV/SOF in HIV/HCV coinfected	ICER for both PROD and LDV/SOF <$100,000/QALY
Assoumou et al,[43] 2017	Screening of young PWID based on the type of screening method; targeted vs routine; rapid vs standard testing; and physician vs counselor	ICER <$100,000 for routine rapid testing by a counselor. Routine rapid screening of young PWID was cost effective when prevalence >0.59%.
Cost-effectiveness of HCV therapy in liver transplant recipients		
Ahmed et al,[39] 2017	DAA therapy on wait list vs treating after liver transplant	ICER for treatment before transplant of <$50,000
Salazar et al,[40] 2017	DAA therapy on wait list vs treating after liver transplant Allows for availability of HCV⁺ livers in deferred treatment strategy	Deferring to treat posttransplant provides best outcomes and is cost saving.
Njei et al,[41] 2016	DAA therapy on wait list vs treating after liver transplant considered by MELD category	MELD <25, treatment pretransplant best outcomes and is cost saving. MELD ≥25, treating posttransplant best outcomes and cost saving.
Tapper et al,[42] 2017	DAA therapy on wait list vs treating after liver transplant considered by MELD category	Treatment before transplantation provides best outcomes and is cost saving in all but MELD <10

Abbreviations: DAA, direct acting antivirals; EBR/GZR, elbasvir/grazoprevir; GT, genotype; HCV, hepatitis C virus; HIV, human immunodeficiency virus; ICER, incremental cost-effectiveness ratio; IFN, interferon; LDV/SOF, ledipasvir/sofosbuvir; MD, physician; MELD, Model for End-stage Liver Disease; PEG/RBV, peginterferon/ribavirin; PEG/RBV/SOF, peginterferon/ribavirin/sofosbuvir; PROD, paritaprevir/ritonavir/ombitasvir/dasabuvir; PWID, people who inject drugs; QALY, quality-adjusted life-year; SOF, sofosbuvir; SOF/DCV, sofosbuvir/daclatasvir/; SOF/RBV, sofosbuvir/ribavirin; SOF/SMV, sofosbuvir/simeprevir; VA, Veterans Health Administration.

in PWID: (1) if treatment default and poor retention result in poor cure rates, or (2) if reinfection mitigates the benefit of cure. Several randomized, controlled trials of direct-acting antivirals among PWID, as well as real-world observational cohorts, demonstrate that PWID can be treated with direct-acting antivirals and have treatment completion and cure rates similar to those among people who do not use drugs.[8,49–52] In addition, providers are beginning to develop and evaluate effective models for delivering HCV treatment to PWID that both improve treatment completion, and are cost effective.[53] Although not all PWID are prepared for HCV treatment, it is increasingly clear that drug use itself should not be a categorical exclusion from HCV treatment.[54]

Reinfection rates among PWID are relatively high, ranging between approximately 2 and 4 infections per 100 person-years observed after cure.[55,56] Further, an honest discussion should acknowledge that, as we become more aggressive treating HCV among PWID, reinfection rates will likely increase as we begin treating individuals with more recent histories of current drug use. Reinfection, however, has relatively little impact on cost-effectiveness conclusions.[43,57] Although perhaps counterintuitive, the reality is that every course of HCV treatment provides good economic value and is, by itself, cost effective.[57] Thus, although reinfection increases the ICER of HCV treatment and there is some hypothetical number of reinfections that would ultimately drive the ICER of treatment of more than $100,000/QALY gained, HCV treatment remains cost effective, even when it is assumed that more than 90% of the cohort will be reinfected at least once in their lifetime.[43]

Does Reducing Hepatitis C Virus Transmission Improve the Cost Effectiveness of Treatment?

Certainly, if every HCV cure actually provides more than 1 cure (because curing HCV in an index case prevents a future infection), then HCV treatment will seem to be even more cost effective than it does when considering only the benefits in the index case. It is important to realize, however, that, although cure as prevention it is an appealing concept, there are no data to prove that HCV cure as prevention works in the real world. Several simulation modeling studies consider HCV cure as prevention and conclude that the approach is cost effective, but the effectiveness of such an approach is not certain.[28,57] Treating PWID who are currently or recently using drugs could have 2 effects: (1) it could prevent future transmissions by eliminating the infection, or (2) it could generate future opportunities for reinfection by increasing the pool of susceptible PWID. The real-world balance of these potential dynamics is not known.

Importantly, however, the cost effectiveness of HCV treatments does not depend on transmission benefits. Preventing future infections is important to elimination goals, but it is not actually very important to economic conclusions about HCV therapy. Treating a person for HCV, even if that person has very early disease and is a current PWID, provides benefit to the individual being treated today and is cost effective. Advocacy for HCV treatment need not depend on claims to prevention.

If Hepatitis C Virus Treatment Is Cost Effective, Why Are More People Not Being Treated?

The short answer to this question is that payers in the United States do not make their coverage decisions based on economic value; they make decisions based on budgetary impact, or cost. An intervention that is cost effective is not necessarily affordable.[28,57] Affordability refers to whether a payer has sufficient resources in its annual budget to pay for an HCV treatment for all who might need or want it within that year. Several characteristics of cost-effectiveness analysis limit its ability to speak to the budget impact of interventions being implemented in the real world.

Perspective on cost

Cost-effectiveness analysis seeks to inform decisions about how society should prioritize health care spending and, therefore, typically assumes a societal perspective on cost. When making coverage decisions for therapy, however, an insurer considers only its own revenues and expenses. Costs and savings that are routinely incorporated into cost-effectiveness analyses are appropriately omitted from assessments of budgetary impact. One example of how the cost perspective fundamentally changes economic conclusions about HCV therapy is in departments of corrections. In many states, the department of corrections budget is responsible for paying for HCV treatments for those living behind bars, but it does not cover the cost of hospitalizations in the community, and certainly does not cover those costs after a person completes his or her sentence and is released to the community.[58] As a result, the department of corrections sees all of the cost of HCV medicines, but little of the savings that accrue from curing HCV. As a result, a department of corrections might rationally conclude that, although HCV therapy is cost effective, it is not affordable.

Time horizon

Cost-effectiveness analysis uses a lifetime time horizon, meaning that it considers lifetime costs and benefits, including those that occur in the distant future. Businesses however, typically assume a 1- to 5-year perspective on budgets. Savings that accrue 30 years from now have no impact on spending decisions today, because they have little bearing on the solvency of the budget today. An example of how time horizon directly impacts decision making about HCV treatment is in Medicaid programs. When Medicaid provides HCV treatment, the costs of the therapy accrue immediately. The benefits, however, may not be apparent for decades. As a result, those future savings have very little meaning for budgeting today.[59,60]

Weak association between willingness-to-pay and the real-world bottom line

Societal WTP thresholds in cost-effectiveness analyses are not based on actual budget calculations and have little relationship to a payer's bottom line. WTP is meant to be an estimate of the opportunity cost of investing in a new therapy. When payers make decision about coverage, the calculation is more straightforward and relates to the cost of medications and the amount of money in the budget. Given the rapid development of new technologies, funding all of them, even if they all fell below the societal WTP threshold, would likely lead to uncontrolled growth in demand and would likely exceed the limited health care budget.[61]

This is not to say that payers ignore data comparing the economic value of alternative treatments. All things being equal, any rational payer would rather cover the treatment that provides the best bang for the buck. But demonstrating that HCV therapy has an ICER of less than $100,000/QALY does not address the reality that treatment is expensive and that any given payer is likely responsible for treatment for tens or even hundreds of thousands of HCV-infected people covered by their plans. The simple arithmetic of (number infected) × (cost of treatment) adds up to numbers in the hundreds of billions of dollars across the United States.[58]

What Is the Budgetary Impact of Treating Hepatitis C Virus?

There is no single budgetary impact of treating HCV. As discussed, budgetary impact is entirely specific to the budget being analyzed. All of this being said, the budgetary impact of HCV treatment is not as high as it once was. The cost of HCV treatment has decreased substantially in the United States. Whereas the 2014 list price of a 12-week treatment course of ledipasvir/sofosbuvir was approximately $94,500, the cost of a complete 8-week course of glecaprevir/pibrentasvir is $26,400—without any price negotiation or discounting.[28] Still, many payers, the media, and even progressive advocacy groups seem to remain captivated by the $1000 per day narrative around HCV treatment.[62] HCV treatment is expensive, and the price point for such a prevalent disease creates barriers to care, but in 2017 some of those barriers are created by advocacy that is intended to pressure pharmaceutical companies to lower prices, but instead has had an unintended consequence of reinforcing payer concerns about cost.

Fortunately, many payers do see the changing cost landscape and have begun to loosen their treatment restrictions. In the fall of 2017, for example, both North Carolina and Vermont Medicaid lifted HCV treatment restrictions based on disease stage.[63,64] Importantly, however, neither state changed restrictions on HCV treatment that require abstinence from drugs. Indeed, even as states are loosening treatment restrictions based on liver fibrosis stage, they typically maintain restrictions based on recent or active drug use.[65] Although eliminating HCV requires treatment for PWID and treating current PWID is cost effective, the specter of paying for HCV treatment more than 1 time leads payers to restrict access.

How Can I Use These Data to Improve Care for My Patients?

The bottom line to all of this discussion and data is that, although HCV treatment is clearly cost effective and provides good economic value compared with other health care interventions that we routinely use in the United States, the combination of high cost, high prevalence, and need to treat a difficult-to-reach, stigmatized group clearly continues to limit access to HCV cure. At this point, the barriers are about cost, not effectiveness and not value. Based on sophisticated work from multiple independent investigative teams, HCV treatment is cost-effective—even with early stage disease, even with a high risk of HCV reinfection, and even if we ignore any potential benefit of cure on HCV transmission. But although it is true that HCV treatments continue to be expensive, it is important to ensure that when we are discussing those costs, we use the most up-to-date data. HCV treatment no longer costs $1000 per day, and any policy that is using the $1000 price tag to inform decision making is misguided and misleading.

The everyday role that HCV treatment providers and advocates can play to mitigate that barrier is being aware of price when choosing regimens. There are now multiple once-a-day treatment options for HCV.[14] Typically, for any combination of HCV geno-type, treatment experience, and disease stage it is possible to find several once daily options. Some are 1 tablet and some are multiple tablets. Some require extra testing for resistance, or extending therapy among some patient subgroups, but all have a greater than 95% cure rate in clinical trials. In such a context of choice, it is appropriate to think about the societal context of decision making and to choose a regimen that may not be the prescriber's favorite option, but that has the lowest price. This choice may require discussions with payers, who confidentially negotiate discounts and re-bates that lead to certain regimens being substantially less expensive than others. Doing so would limit the budgetary impact of treatment and make cure available to more people. Insisting that all patients have access to all regimens at all times may paradoxically limit the availability of therapy.[66]

Above all, providers should practice comfortably knowing that when they are aggressive about treating HCV—in patients with early disease and in those who have histories of current or recent drug use—they are using a high value intervention that provides cure and improves both quality of life and life expectancy. When thinking about the costs and the benefits of HCV treatment—from the perspective of the patient or that of society—HCV treatment provides excellent economic value and is worth the cost of treatment.

REFERENCES

1. Department of Health and Human Services. National viral hepatitis action plan 2017-2020. 2017.
2. Centers for Disease Control and Prevention (CDC). Surveillance for viral hepatitis—United States, 2015. 2017.
3. World Health Organization (WHO). Global health sector strategy on viral hepatitis 2016-2021 towards ending viral hepatitis. 2016.
4. Grady BP, Schinkel J, Thomas XV, et al. Hepatitis C virus reinfection following treatment among people who use drugs. Clin Infect Dis 2013;57(Suppl 2):S105–10.
5. Page K, Hahn JA, Evans J, et al. Acute hepatitis C virus infection in young adult injection drug users: a prospective study of incident infection, resolution, and reinfection. J Infect Dis 2009;200(8):1216–26.
6. Grebely J, Raffa JD, Lai C, et al. Low uptake of treatment for hepatitis C virus infection in a large community-based study of inner city residents. J Viral Hepat 2009;16(5):352–8.

7. Red Book online. Micromedex healthcare series. Greenwood Village (CO): Truven Health Analytics; 2014.

8. Edlin BR, Kresina TF, Raymond DB, et al. Overcoming barriers to prevention, care, and treatment of hepatitis C in illicit drug users. Clin Infect Dis 2005; 40(Suppl 5):S276–85.

9. Zeremski M, Zibbell JE, Martinez AD, et al. Hepatitis C virus control among persons who inject drugs requires overcoming barriers to care. World J Gastroenterol 2013;19(44):7846–51.

10. Morrill JA, Shrestha M, Grant RW. Barriers to the treatment of hepatitis C. J Gen Intern Med 2005;20(8):754–8.

11. Konerman MA, Lok AS. Hepatitis C treatment and barriers to eradication. Clin Transl Gastroenterol 2016;7(9):e193.

12. Tumber MB. Restricted access: state Medicaid coverage of sofosbuvir hepatitis C treatment. J Leg Med 2017;37(1–2):21–64.

13. Barua S, Greenwald R, Grebely J, et al. Restrictions for Medicaid reimbursement of sofosbuvir for the treatment of hepatitis C virus infection in the United States. Ann Intern Med 2015;163(3):215–23.

14. Wong RJ, Jain MK, Shiffman ML, et al. Disparate access based on insurance status to highly effective direct acting antivirals (DAA) for hepatitis C virus treatment in the post-DAA era persists: alarmingly impaired access in Medicaid recipients. Hepatology 2017;66:307a.

15. Neumann PJ, Russell LB, Sanders GD, et al. Cost effectiveness in health and medicine. 2nd edition. Oxford (NY): Oxford University Press; 2017.

16. Edejer TT-T, World Health Organization. Making choices in health: WHO guide to cost-effectiveness analysis. Geneva (Switzerland): World Health Organization; 2003.

17. Kamm FM. Cost effectiveness analysis and fairness. J Pract Ethics 2015;3(1):1–14.

18. Russell LB, Gold MR, Siegel JE, et al. The role of cost-effectiveness analysis in health and medicine. Panel on cost-effectiveness in health and medicine. JAMA 1996;276(14):1172–7.

19. Neumann PJ, Sanders GD. Cost-effectiveness analysis 2.0. N Engl J Med 2017; 376(3):203–5.

20. Cohen DJ, Reynolds MR. Interpreting the results of cost-effectiveness studies. J Am Coll Cardiol 2008;52(25):2119–26.

21. Thein HH, Yi Q, Dore GJ, et al. Estimation of stage-specific fibrosis progression rates in chronic hepatitis C virus infection: a meta-analysis and meta-regression. Hepatology 2008;48(2):418–31.

22. Weinstein MC, Torrance G, McGuire A. QALYs: the basics. Value Health 2009; 12(Suppl 1):S5–9.

23. Neumann PJ, Cohen JT, Weinstein MC. Updating cost-effectiveness–the curious resilience of the $50,000-per-QALY threshold. N Engl J Med 2014;371(9):796–7.

24. World Health Organization. Choosing interventions that are cost-effective. Geneva (Switzerland): World Health Organization; 2014. Available at: http://www.who.int/choice/en/. Accessed February 11, 2018.

25. Marseille E, Larson B, Kazi DS, et al. Thresholds for the cost-effectiveness of interventions: alternative approaches. Bull World Health Organ 2015;93(2):118–24.

26. Leidner AJ, Chesson HW, Xu F, et al. Cost-effectiveness of hepatitis C treatment for patients in early stages of liver disease. Hepatology 2015;61(6):1860–9.

27. Linas BP, Morgan JR, Pho MT, et al. Cost effectiveness and cost containment in the era of interferon-free therapies to treat hepatitis C virus genotype 1. Open Forum Infect Dis 2016;4(1):ofw266.

28. Chhatwal J, Kanwal F, Roberts MS, et al. Cost-effectiveness and budget impact of hepatitis C virus treatment with sofosbuvir and ledipasvir in the United States. Ann Intern Med 2015;162(6):397–406.
29. Najafzadeh M, Andersson K, Shrank WH, et al. Cost-effectiveness of novel regimens for the treatment of hepatitis C virus. Ann Intern Med 2015;162(6):407–19.
30. Linas BP, Barter DM, Morgan JR, et al. The cost-effectiveness of sofosbuvir-based regimens for treatment of hepatitis C virus genotype 2 or 3 infection. Ann Intern Med 2015;162(9):619–29.
31. Younossi ZM, Stepanova M, Afdhal N, et al. Improvement of health-related quality of life and work productivity in chronic hepatitis C patients with early and advanced fibrosis treated with ledipasvir and sofosbuvir. J Hepatol 2015;63(2): 337–45.
32. Chidi AP, Rogal S, Bryce CL, et al. Cost-effectiveness of new antiviral regimens for treatment-naive U.S. veterans with hepatitis C. Hepatology 2016;63(2): 428–36.
33. Saab S, Virabhak S, Parise H, et al. Cost-effectiveness of genotype 1 chronic hepatitis C virus treatments in patients coinfected with human immunodeficiency virus in the United States. Adv Ther 2016;33(8):1316–30.
34. Zhang S, Bastian ND, Griffin PM. Cost-effectiveness of sofosbuvir-based treatments for chronic hepatitis C in the US. BMC Gastroenterol 2015;15:98.
35. Saint-Laurent Thibault C, Moorjaney D, Ganz ML, et al. Cost-effectiveness of combination daclatasvir-sofosbuvir for treatment of genotype 3 chronic hepatitis C infection in the United States. J Med Econ 2017;20(7):692–702.
36. Chhatwal J, He T, Hur C, et al. Direct-acting antiviral agents for patients with hepatitis C virus genotype 1 infection are cost-saving. Clin Gastroenterol Hepatol 2017;15(6):827–37.e8.
37. Jayasekera CR, Beckerman R, Smith N, et al. Sofosbuvir-based regimens with task shifting is cost-effective in expanding hepatitis C treatment access in the United States. J Clin Transl Hepatol 2017;5(1):16–22.
38. Elbasha E, Greaves W, Roth D, et al. Cost-effectiveness of elbasvir/grazoprevir use in treatment-naive and treatment-experienced patients with hepatitis C virus genotype 1 infection and chronic kidney disease in the United States. J Viral Hepat 2017;24(4):268–79.
39. Ahmed A, Gonzalez SA, Cholankeril G, et al. Treatment of patients waitlisted for liver transplant with all-oral direct-acting antivirals is a cost-effective treatment strategy in the United States. Hepatology 2017;66(1):46–56.
40. Salazar J, Saxena V, Kahn JG, et al. Cost-effectiveness of direct-acting antiviral treatment in hepatitis C-infected liver transplant candidates with compensated cirrhosis and hepatocellular carcinoma. Transplantation 2017;101(5):1001–8.
41. Njei B, McCarty TR, Fortune BE, et al. Optimal timing for hepatitis C therapy in US patients eligible for liver transplantation: a cost-effectiveness analysis. Aliment Pharmacol Ther 2016;44(10):1090–101.
42. Tapper EB, Afdhal NH, Curry MP. Before or after transplantation? A review of the cost effectiveness of treating waitlisted patients with hepatitis C. Transplantation 2017;101(5):933–7.
43. Assoumou SA, Tasillo A, Leff JA, et al. Cost-effectiveness of one-time hepatitis C screening strategies among adolescents and young adults in primary care settings. Clin Infect Dis 2017;66(3):376–84.
44. Chahal HS, Marseille EA, Tice JA, et al. Cost-effectiveness of early treatment of hepatitis C virus genotype 1 by stage of liver fibrosis in a US treatment-naive population. JAMA Intern Med 2016;176(1):65–73.

45. World Health Organization (WHO). There's a reason viral hepatitis has been dubbed the "silent killer". Geneva: WHO; 2016.

46. Hsu PC, Federico CA, Krajden M, et al. Health utilities and psychometric quality of life in patients with early- and late-stage hepatitis C virus infection. J Gastroenterol Hepatol 2012;27(1):149–57.

47. Sullivan PW, Ghushchyan V. Preference-based EQ-5D index scores for chronic conditions in the United States. Med Decis Making 2006;26(4):410–20.

48. Davis KL, Mitra D, Medjedovic J, et al. Direct economic burden of chronic hepatitis C virus in a United States managed care population. J Clin Gastroenterol 2011;45(2):e17–24.

49. Hellard M, Sacks-Davis R, Gold J. Hepatitis C treatment for injection drug users: a review of the available evidence. Clin Infect Dis 2009;49(4):561–73.

50. Edlin BR, Seal KH, Lorvick J, et al. Is it justifiable to withhold treatment for hepatitis C from illicit-drug users? N Engl J Med 2001;345(3):211–5.

51. Dore GJ, Altice F, Litwin AH, et al. Elbasvir-grazoprevir to treat hepatitis C virus infection in persons receiving opioid agonist therapy: a randomized trial. Ann Intern Med 2016;165(9):625–34.

52. Norton BL, Fleming J, Bachhuber MA, et al. High HCV cure rates for people who use drugs treated with direct acting antiviral therapy at an urban primary care clinic. Int J Drug Policy 2017;47:196–201.

53. Litwin AH, Agyemang L, Akiyama MJ, et al. The PREVAIL study: intensive models of HCV care for people who inject drugs. J Hepatol 2017;66(1):S72.

54. Grebely J, Bruneau J, Lazarus JV, et al. Research priorities to achieve universal access to hepatitis C prevention, management and direct-acting antiviral treatment among people who inject drugs. Int J Drug Policy 2017;47:51–60.

55. Grebely J, Knight E, Ngai T, et al. Reinfection with hepatitis C virus following sustained virological response in injection drug users. J Gastroenterol Hepatol 2010; 25(7):1281–4.

56. Aspinall EJ, Corson S, Doyle JS, et al. Treatment of hepatitis C virus infection among people who are actively injecting drugs: a systematic review and meta-analysis. Clin Infect Dis 2013;57(Suppl 2):S80–9.

57. Martin NK, Vickerman P, Miners A, et al. Cost-effectiveness of hepatitis C virus antiviral treatment for injection drug user populations. Hepatology 2012;55(1):49–57.

58. Bilinski A, Neumann P, Cohen J, et al. When cost-effective interventions are unaffordable: integrating cost-effectiveness and budget impact in priority setting for global health programs. PLoS Med 2017;14(10):e1002397.

59. Spaulding AC, Weinbaum CM, Lau DT, et al. A framework for management of hepatitis C in prisons. Ann Intern Med 2006;144(10):762–9.

60. Spaulding AS, Kim AY, Harzke AJ, et al. Impact of new therapeutics for hepatitis C virus infection in incarcerated populations. Top Antivir Med 2013;21(1):27–35.

61. Rein DB, Zhang P, Wirth KE, et al. The economic burden of major adult visual disorders in the United States. Arch Ophthalmol 2006;124(12):1754–60.

62. Micromedex solutions. Drug topics red book online. 2017. Available at: http://www.micromedexsolutions.com/. Accessed September 13, 2017.

63. Waldman A. Big pharma quietly enlists leading professors to justify $1,000-Per-Day Drugs. HCV Advocate: Hepatitis C Support Project: News & Pipeline Blog 2017. Available at: http://hepatitisc.hcvadvocate.org/2017/02/big-pharma-quietly-enlists-leading-professors-justify-1000-per-day-drugs-annie-waldman.html.

64. Lewis C. Advocates urge New York Gov. Cuomo to address high-cost of hep C drugs. 2017. Available at: http://www.modernhealthcare.com/article/20170215/NEWS/170219934.

65. Fisher M. Medicaid review board lifts liver damage restriction on life-saving cures for Vermonters with hepatitis C. 2017. Available at: https://vtdigger.org/2017/11/01/medicaid-review-board-lifts-liver-damage-restriction-life-saving-cures-vermonters-hepatitis-c/#.WgtmTLbMy7D.
66. Morgan JR, Kim AY, Naggie S, et al. The effect of shorter treatment regimens for hepatitis C on population health and under fixed budgets. Open Forum Infect Dis 2017;5(1):ofx267.

Estimation of Hepatitis C Disease Burden and Budget Impact of Treatment Using Health Economic Modeling

Jagpreet Chhatwal, PhD[a],*, Qiushi Chen, PhD[b],
Rakesh Aggarwal, MD, DM[c]

KEYWORDS

- Markov modeling • Simulation • Health economics • Cost-effectiveness
- Direct-acting antivirals • Hepatitis C elimination • Public health

KEY POINTS

- Chronic hepatitis C is a major public health problem, affecting 71 million people worldwide and 2 to 4 million people in the United States.
- With the availability of oral direct-acting antivirals 2014 onward, hepatitis C elimination as a public health threat is feasible; however, several barriers need to be addressed to achieve this.
- Mathematical modeling provides a framework that integrates data from multiple sources, and projects future trends of disease burden and costs under different conditions and intervention strategies.
- Modeling analysis can assist policy makers and stakeholders with strategic decisions in a timely and economical way.
- In this article, we have described the key components of a mathematical model that projects disease burden and budget impact of different interventions to manage HCV in the United States, and discussed the types of data needed to develop a similar model for another country.

Disclosure: Dr J. Chhatwal has received research grants from Merck and Gilead and served on the scientific advisory panel of Merck and Gilead. Drs Q. Chen and R. Aggarwal have nothing to disclose.
[a] Massachusetts General Hospital Institute for Technology Assessment, Harvard Medical School, 101 Merrimac Street, Floor 10th, Boston, MA 02114, USA; [b] Harold and Inge Marcus Department of Industrial and Manufacturing Engineering, The Pennsylvania State University, 310 Leonhard Building, University Park, PA 16802, USA; [c] Department of Gastroenterology, Sanjay Gandhi Postgraduate Institute of Medical Sciences, Rae Bareli Road, Lucknow, Uttar Pradesh 226014, India
* Corresponding author.
E-mail address: jagchhatwal@mgh.harvard.edu

Infect Dis Clin N Am 32 (2018) 461–480
https://doi.org/10.1016/j.idc.2018.02.008
0891-5520/18/© 2018 Elsevier Inc. All rights reserved.

id.theclinics.com

INTRODUCTION

Chronic infection with hepatitis C virus (HCV) is a major public health problem, affecting 71 million worldwide and 2 to 4 million people in the United States.[1] HCV is associated with more deaths in the United States than 60 other infectious diseases combined, including human immunodeficiency virus and tuberculosis.[2] In 2015, an estimated 400,000 people died worldwide as the result of complications of HCV infection, including cirrhosis and hepatocellular carcinoma (HCC).

The availability of oral direct-acting antivirals (DAAs) from 2014 onward has revolutionized HCV treatment. These therapies are superior, with an efficacy greater than 95% in most patient groups, are safe, and have shorter treatment durations and fewer adverse effects than older therapies.[3] Because of this major advancement, the World Health Assembly has pledged itself to "elimination" of HCV as a public health threat, a term defined as 90% reduction in HCV incidence and 65% reduction in HCV-related mortality, by 2030.[4,5] It has been estimated that, to reach this goal, 90% of HCV-infected people need to be diagnosed, and 80% of eligible people need to be treated by 2030.

Nonetheless, several barriers need to be addressed before HCV can be eliminated; the most critical barriers are the low awareness rates,[6] and limited budgets, in developed and underdeveloped countries, to treat all HCV patients, causing some payers to impose restrictions on who can get treatment. To address such barriers to HCV elimination, data on disease burden and economic burden associated with this infection are needed. Elimination requires detection of HCV-infected persons who are currently undiagnosed, treatment of a large proportion of those diagnosed, and efforts at prevention of transmission of HCV and occurrence of new cases. For each of these steps, namely screening, treatment, and prevention, several different approaches are feasible, and there is a need for a better understanding of which of these is the most cost-effective and what are the effects of the combinations.

A recent systematic review found that cost-effectiveness of DAAs has been evaluated only for a few countries.[7] Such data are particularly lacking for low- and middle-income countries, where despite low incomes, HCV treatment may be more affordable, because of the availability of low-cost generic DAAs. This has meant that HCV treatment in these low- and middle-income countries may not be merely cost-effective but cost-saving, as has been shown for India.[8] Availability of such cost-effectiveness and economic data for different countries would, by informing politicians and health administrators of the value of investing resources in HCV screening and treatment, address a major barrier to the implementation of HCV elimination strategies.

Projections of disease burden, cost-effectiveness data, and budget impact are typically generated using decision-analytic modeling. In addition, modeling can help compare the outcomes of different intervention strategies even before these have been implemented in practice by simulating the expected life course of patients following each pathway. This article provides an overview of common types of decision-analytic models used in HCV, the scope of such models and how to create clinically valid models to project the burden of HCV in a country, what inputs are required and how to obtain those inputs, and how to calculate the budget impact and cost-effectiveness of HCV treatment.

SCOPE OF DECISION-ANALYTIC MODELING IN HEPATITIS C VIRUS MANAGEMENT

Mathematical modeling is increasingly recognized as a type of comparative effectiveness research that combines best-available evidence on several small components of a health care system or medical problem to better understand the system as a whole and to inform decisions.[9] These models can incorporate biologic disease representations, predict future disease trends, and capture many of the complex intricacies of health care delivery in the real world. The purpose of such models is to provide insights to aid in decision making.

Estimation of Hepatitis C Disease Burden

Population level measures of disease burden of hepatitis C, such as HCV prevalence, incidence of HCV-associated HCC, and HCV-related liver deaths, can be estimated using decision-analytic models.[1,10–12] These models have the advantage that they combine data from multiple sources, including national surveys of prevalence of HCV infection, longitudinal studies of persons with HCV infection, and death certificates, to predict the current and future disease burden. In addition, models can predict disease burden under different conditions, such as changes in screening policies or uptake of treatment with DAAs.

Identification of Cost-Effective Screening Policies for Hepatitis C Virus

A cost-effectiveness analysis can examine the incremental health benefits and costs of a new intervention in comparison with an old or existing intervention. The health benefits are typically measured in terms of quality-adjusted life years, which account for the quantity and quality of life lived. These long-term outcomes are typically estimated using decision-analytic models. The incremental cost-effectiveness ratio, which is the ratio of incremental costs to incremental benefits, is used to determine if a new intervention is cost-effective, that is, whether it provides good value for the money spent. The incremental cost-effectiveness ratio estimates how much more needs to be spent to gain one additional quality-adjusted life year, and an intervention is deemed cost-effective if the corresponding incremental cost-effectiveness ratio is below a predetermined willingness-to-pay threshold.

Most HCV patients remain unaware of their infection. Therefore, to reap the benefits of new DAAs, patients with HCV infection must be first diagnosed. Population-level screening programs are being used in many settings. For example, in the United States and Canada, people belonging to a specific birth cohort are recommended for one-time HCV testing. Similarly, HCV screening in high-risk groups, such as persons who inject drugs or persons with a history of incarceration, is recommended. To determine which groups should be tested for HCV, cost-effectiveness analysis is often conducted to estimate the value of providing such screening, that is, is it worth spending additional resources to provide screening to a specific group? Several decision-analytic models have been used to determine the cost-effectiveness of HCV testing in different groups including baby boomers,[13,14] people who inject drugs,[15] prison inmates,[16,17] and adolescents.[18]

Assessment of the Value and Budget Impact of Providing Hepatitis C Virus Treatment

The high price coupled with the high demand for oral DAAs have created concerns about their impact on health care budgets, delaying timely treatment to several groups of HCV patients. The high price of these drugs has led to a national debate about the cost-effectiveness and affordability of HCV treatment in the United States and elsewhere. Because of high costs, numerous health care payers have restricted these treatments to patients with advanced stages of hepatic fibrosis, that is, those that are likely to benefit most immediately.[19] Cost-effectiveness analysis can inform stakeholders regarding the value of HCV treatment and allow them to compare its value with other medical interventions. Such analyses usually use a decision-analytic modeling approach, and can project the long-term health benefits of HCV treatment and predict savings in long-term costs of treating HCV sequelae, and weigh these against the upfront cost of HCV treatment. Several such cost-effectiveness analyses have assessed the value of HCV treatment, and a systematic review of recent modeling studies found that DAAs are cost-effective/saving in more than 90% of the cases at current drug prices.[7,20] In addition, decision-analytic models can estimate the budget impact of providing HCV treatment[21] and future projections of the cost of managing HCV.[12]

COMMON TYPES OF DECISION-ANALYTIC MODELS

Several different types of decision-analytic models have been used for medical and health policy decision making. The choice of model type depends on the scope and purpose of the question being evaluated, time and resources available for the project, and expertise of the modeling team. The common modeling approaches used to inform HCV management are categorized in the following three categories: (1) state-transition-based models (including Markov models), (2) system dynamics or compartment models, and (3) agent-based simulation models.

Markov models are useful when the different stages of a disease can be described as a series of health states, with persons in one state transitioning to another state (or one of several other states) over time. The model schematic is represented concisely using a diagram with boxes representing various health states and arrows representing transitions among health states. At the end of each discrete time period (cycle length), some individuals make a transition from one state to another based on predetermined probability. Each health state can also be associated with a specified quality of life and cost (per cycle length). By running the model for a specified cohort (say of 10,000 persons) over a specified period of time (say for a particular number of years or for lifetime of the cohort), one can estimate average outcomes for the cohort, such as life expectancy, quality-adjusted life years, and total health care costs.

A key feature of Markov models is that the health states follow "Markovian" or "memory-less" property. This implies that a person in a given state (eg, a particular disease state) has no record of prior history. This property makes calculations easier but also adds limitations to the model when prior medical history is important (eg, persons having a history of injection drug use are more likely to use inject drugs in future). In addition, Markov models provide outcomes that are aggregated for the entire cohort. This limitation is overcome by individual-level state-transition models, also commonly known as microsimulation models. In these models, Individual characteristics of patients (eg, age, health condition, prior history) are incorporated, and each individual is followed over time. Thus, in contrast to Markov models, microsimulation can keep track of a particular patient's history and determine future events based on prior history.

Besides Markov models, two other types of modeling approaches have been commonly used in HCV: system dynamics (or compartment) models and agent-based models. The compartment models are primarily used in situations where interaction between individuals is important (eg, simulation of transmission of an infectious disease to evaluate the effectiveness of preventive/control interventions). In this approach, different population pools/cohorts (eg, uninfected and susceptible, infected, treated but susceptible to reinfection, immune) are represented by separate compartments and transition between compartments is represented by differential equations.[22] A unique advantage of system dynamics models over state-transition models is that the former can capture indirect benefits of interventions.[23] For example, screening for hepatitis C followed by treatment can, by reducing the pool of infectious persons, cut the rate of transmission of virus to uninfected people (ie, prevention by treatment).

Agent-based models provide one of the most flexible frameworks and can overcome some common limitations of state-transition and system dynamics models by capturing heterogeneity, prior history, and interaction among individuals.[24] They consist of agents that interact with each other and their environment. These agents can be people who have certain individual-level characteristics, such as age, sex, risk behavior, disease status, which can change with time. An advantage of agent-based models is their ability to capture relationship networks among individuals.[25] The network structure determines which individuals can possibly interact with which individuals and potentially transmit disease.[26]

COMPONENTS OF A DECISION ANALYTICAL MODEL: A CASE STUDY OF HEPATITIS C DISEASE BURDEN SIMULATION MODEL

Below we describe different steps in construction of a decision-analytic model to estimate HCV disease and economic burden, types and potential sources of inputs are needed and the outcomes of interest that the outputs from such a model can provide. For illustration, we use a previously developed model, Hepatitis C Disease Burden Simulation model (HEP-SIM),[10,27] HEP-SIM is an individual-level state-transition model (microsimulation model) that simulates the natural history of HCV of individuals under different conditions. The HEP-SIM model has been used to project the changing prevalence and various outcomes of HCV infection in the United States from 2001 onward. The model has been validated with multiple clinical studies and national surveys including data from the National Health and Nutrition Examination Survey (NHANES) 1999 to 2002 and 2003 to 2009 studies and reports from the US Centers for Disease Control and Prevention (CDC).[6,28–30] **Fig. 1** describes the key components of HEP-SIM that include patient demographics, HCV disease progression, HCV screening, therapeutic advancement, access to health care including insurance status, and the cost of care and treatment.

Initial Cohort (Patient Demographics)

Construction of a state-transition model begins with definition of an initial cohort, or the baseline population as it exists at the start of the model. For the HEP-SIM model, we first generated this population, that is, people who were infected with HCV in the United States in 2001 (the year when the model starts), based on the NHANES studies that estimated HCV prevalence.[28] For this cohort, we defined distribution of HCV genotype, age, gender, stages of chronic HCV, and prior antiviral treatment history based on published studies (**Table 1**).

Insurance status of each individual was based on NHANES data.[31,32] We assumed that all patients age 65 and older were covered by Medicare, and 90% of them had drug coverage through Medicare Part D or some other sources.[33] Among non-Medicare patients, we estimated the percentage of patients who have private, Medicaid, and other public insurance, and uninsured as 49.8%, 9.2%, 14.3%, and 26.7%, respectively.[10] We also incorporated changes in the insurance pool because of the implementation of the Affordable Care Act using a report by the Congressional Budget Office and the staff of the Joint Committee on Taxation.[34,35]

Model Structure Using Health States and Transition Rates (Natural History of Hepatitis C Virus)

State-transition models simulate the natural history of individual patients. In these models, the disease course is presented as a series of steps, beginning with initial stages to subsequent, more advanced stages, and possible movements between

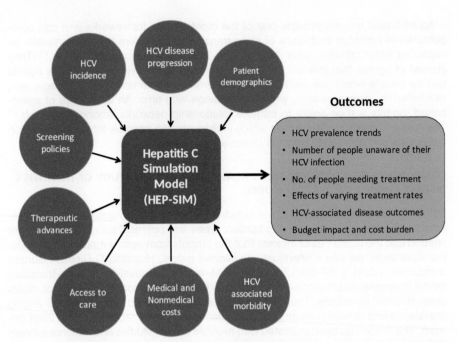

Fig. 1. Schematic showing the key components and outcomes of HEP-SIM model. HEP-SIM model included patient demographics, HCV disease progression, HCV screening, therapeutic advancement, access to health care including insurance status, and the cost of care and treatment. Outcomes of HEP-SIM include temporal trends in HCV prevalence, awareness rate of HCV-infection, HCV-associated advanced sequelae, and budget impact of different interventions.

these stages. These various stages of disease are referred to in the modeling parlance as "disease states" and the movements from one stage to another as "transitions." Each individual patient in the model must at any time be in one (and only one) of these health states.

Specifically, we defined the natural history of HCV in HEP-SIM using several health states that represented acute and chronic phases of HCV (**Fig. 2**, adapted from Kabiri and colleagues[27]). Chronic HCV was represented by five health states defined using METAVIR fibrosis scores (no fibrosis [F0], portal fibrosis without septa [F1], portal fibrosis with few septa [F2], numerous septa without fibrosis [F3], or cirrhosis [F4]), and additional states based on clinical features, namely decompensated cirrhosis, HCC, liver transplantation, liver-related death, and death from other causes. To allow the use of this model for studying the effect of HCV treatment, a separate state F4-SVR was created to capture individuals with HCV cirrhosis who had achieved a sustained virologic response (SVR) following treatment and hence had different rates of clinical progression than untreated patients with HCV cirrhosis.

We used data from a published meta-analysis to specify the transition rates from F0 through F1-F3 to F4 (**Table 2**).[36] The disease progression rates from cirrhosis to decompensated cirrhosis were estimated from published observational studies.[37,38] Patients developing decompensated cirrhosis or HCC had higher mortality rates.[39] A patient could transition to a death state from any of the previously mentioned states from background mortality (not shown in the figure), the estimates for which are publicly available from the US lifetable.[40]

Table 1		
Population characteristics of HCV-infected patients in the United States		
HCV-Infected Population Characteristics	**Value**	**Reference**
Total HCV-infected population in 2001 (million)	4.2	Armstrong et al,[28] 2006
Chronic infection ratio (%)	78	Armstrong et al,[28] 2006
Contraindicated for treatment (%)[a]	34.6	Rein et al,[13] 2012
Sex (%)		
Male	64.22	Armstrong et al,[28] 2006
Female	35.78	
HCV genotype (%)		
1	73	Blatt et al,[48] 2000
2	14	
3	8	
Other	5	
Stage distribution of HCV-infected population in 2001 (%)		
F0	27.20	Davis et al,[49] 2010
F1	33.39	
F2	17.11	
F3	11.08	
F4	9.61	
DC	1.43	
HCC	0.18	
Age distribution for HCV-infected population in 2001 (%)		
18–19	1.78	Armstrong et al,[28] 2006
20–29	10.67	
30–39	22.67	
40–49	28.89	
50–59	20.44	
60–69	9.33	
70–100	6.22	
Proportion of treatment-experienced patients in 2001 (%)	1.78	HEP-SIM
Distribution of types of treatment-experienced patients (%)		
Genotype 1		
Relapse	53	Zeuzem et al,[50] 2011
Partial	19	Zeuzem et al,[50] 2011
Null response	28	Zeuzem et al,[50] 2011
Genotype 2–6		
Relapse	47	Poynard et al,[51] 2009
Partial	16	Poynard et al,[51] 2009
Null response	37	Poynard et al,[51] 2009

Abbreviations: F0, no fibrosis; F1, portal fibrosis without septa; F2, portal fibrosis with few septa; F3, numerous septa without cirrhosis; F4, cirrhosis.

[a] The ratio of patients with contraindication (with modifiable and nonmodifiable reasons) among chronically infected patients.

New Cases (Incidence) of Hepatitis C Virus Infection

In addition to the initially generated base-case population, the model takes into account the new (incident) cases of HCV infection. Estimates of new HCV incidence by year were obtained from CDC reports for the years 2001 to 2014 (**Tables 3**

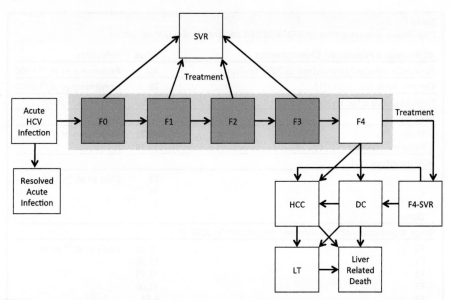

Fig. 2. State-transition model of the natural history of HCV. At any given time, a patient is represented by one of the health states, which are shown by squares. Arrows between states represent possible transitions based on annual probabilities. Patients whose disease is successfully treated transition to the SVR state. Patients who achieve SVR from F0 to F3 states are assumed to be cured; however, patients in an F4 state who are successfully treated transition to an F4-SVR state and may develop further complications. Patients in HCC, DC, and LT states have a higher mortality rate than the general population. All other patients have the same risk for death as the general population. The probability of death from other causes exists in every state, but deaths from other causes are not shown. According to the Meta-analysis of Histologic Data in Viral Hepatitis (METAVIR) scoring system, F0 indicates no fibrosis of the liver, F1 indicates portal fibrosis without septa, F2 indicates portal fibrosis with few septa, F3 indicates many septa without cirrhosis, and F4 indicates cirrhosis. DC, decompensated cirrhosis; LT, liver transplantation; SVR, sustained virologic response. *Adapted from* Kabiri M, Jazwinski AB, Roberts MS, et al. The changing burden of hepatitis C in the United States: Model-based predictions. Annals of Internal Medicine 2014;161(3):170–80. Copyright © 2016. American College of Physicians. All Rights Reserved. Reprinted with the permission of American College of Physicians, Inc.)

and **4**). For incidence projection in future years, we assumed that the HCV incidence remained constant beyond 2014 in the base case analysis.

One of the main difficulties in HCV modeling relates to lack of reliable data, particularly on HCV incidence, in many countries. In such a situation, one could use expert opinion and conduct sensitivity analysis using rates in the range within which the value is expected to lie. Alternatively, one could estimate age-specific incidence rates using age-specific prevalence rates, an approach used in previously published modeling study.[12] A third possible approach is to model HCV transmission using a dynamic model that takes into account the proportion of infectious and susceptible people in the population and their effective contact rate (ie, the number of contacts that can lead to HCV transmission occurring between an average infectious person and an average susceptible person per unit time)[16,41]; however, such modeling is quite difficult at a large scale (eg, at the level of a country), because of difficulties in estimating the input variables, and heterogeneities in the population. A simpler approach may be to use data from another country with a similar epidemiologic situation for HCV infection.

Table 2		
State transition probabilities used in HEP-SIM		
Transition Probabilities	**Value**	**Reference**
F0 to F1	0.117	Thein et al,[36] 2008
F1 to F2	0.085	Thein et al,[36] 2008
F2 to F3	0.120	Thein et al,[36] 2008
F3 to F4	0.116	Thein et al,[36] 2008
F4 to DC	0.039	Fattovich et al,[37] 1997
F4 to HCC	0.014	Fattovich et al,[37] 1997
F4-SVR to DC	0.008	Cardoso et al,[52] 2010
F4-SVR to HCC	0.005	Cardoso et al,[52] 2010
DC to HCC	0.068	Planas et al,[38] 2004
DC to LT	0.023	Davis et al,[49] 2010; Thuluvath et al,[53] 2010
DC (first year) to death from liver disease	0.182	Planas et al,[38] 2004
DC (subsequent years) to death from liver disease	0.112	Planas et al,[38] 2004
HCC to LT	0.040	Lang et al,[46] 2009; Saab et al,[54] 2010
HCC to death from liver disease	0.427	Fattovich et al,[37] 1997
LT (first year) to death from liver disease	0.116	Wolfe et al,[39] 2010
PLT to death from liver disease	0.044	Wolfe et al,[39] 2010

Abbreviations: DC, decompensated cirrhosis; F0, no fibrosis; F1, portal fibrosis without septa; F2, portal fibrosis with few septa; F3, numerous septa without cirrhosis; F4, cirrhosis; LT, liver transplantation (first year); PLT, post liver transplantation (>1 year).

Table 3	
Annual incidence of hepatitis C patients from 2001 to 2040	
Year	**Estimated Incident Cases**
2001	24,000
2002	29,000
2003	28,000
2004	26,000
2005	21,000
2006	19,000
2007	17,000
2008	18,000
2009	16,000
2010	17,000
2011	16,500
2012	24,700
2013	29,700
2014	30,500
2015–2020	33,900

Annual HCV incidence in 2001–2015 were based on the reports by the Centers for Disease Control and Prevention.[55] In addition, we assumed that the annual HCV infection was constant beyond 2015 at 33,900 cases.

Table 4
Age distribution of new hepatitis C incidence

Age Group	Distribution (%)
18–19	2.7
20–29	41.8
30–39	28.3
40–49	15.6
50–59	9.6
60+	2.0

Hepatitis C Virus Awareness and Screening

The likelihood of HCV-infected persons to be aware of their infection depends on their age and insurance status. This information was extracted from published studies that evaluated NHANES data. For instance, in 2008, a total of 49.7% of all HCV-infected persons, including 57.0% of those insured and 23.7% of those uninsured, were aware of their HCV status.[32] We also accounted for differences in the awareness rates by age: 29% for age less than 40 years, 57.6% for ages 40 to 49 years, 56% for ages 50 to 59 years, and 44.8% for ages older than 60 years. **Table 5** presents the HCV awareness rate by age and insurance used in HEP-SIM.

People unaware of their HCV infection could become aware over time either by birth-cohort screening or during usual health care encounters, which includes risk-based testing. Birth-cohort screening was defined as one-time screening of anyone born between 1945 and 1965, recommended by the CDC and the US Preventive Services Task Force. Our model assumed that, overall, 90% of those covered by insurance and 10% of those not covered were offered screening, and that such screening was distributed evenly over time. Thus, we estimated that 66,572 persons/year were offered screening from 2013 to 2019; and 81.9% of them would accept screening and receive correct results.[13] Once diagnosed, if they had an insurance to cover the treatment costs, they could receive treatment. We implemented the usual care strategy by assigning probability of getting diagnosed with HCV depending on person's age and fibrosis level (more details are found elsewhere).[10]

To obtain such estimates of screening or awareness rates for another country, one would need to carefully study the testing policies followed there, and then develop an estimate. Surveys at national or subnational levels are used to obtain this information. In cases where such estimates vary across different subgroups in the population, it is reasonable to assume that the country has two (or more) subpopulations, obtain estimates as described previously for each subgroup, and summate these.

Table 5
Percentage of HCV-infected people aware of their disease status

Age	Awareness Rate by Insurance Status (%)	
	Insured	Uninsured
<40	17.63	5.81
40–49	60.45	19.50
50–59	54.59	16.29
>60	34.94	5.77

Hepatitis C Virus Treatment Waves

We modeled HCV treatment in different waves reflecting clinical practice starting with a combined therapy of peginterferon and ribavirin until 2011, followed by the launch of first-generation protease inhibitors, boceprevir and telaprevir, in 2011 (**Fig. 3**). From 2014, we simulated the availability of non-NS5A inhibitors sofosbuvir and simeprevir (denoted as DAA1 non-NS5A wave). From 2015, we simulated all-oral DAA combinations including both non-NS5A and NS5A inhibitors (denoted by DAA1 non-NS5A and DAA1 NS5A), followed by the availability of next wave of NS5A inhibitors (denoted by DAA2 NS5A) from 2018 onward. We obtained SVR rates from multiple clinical trials and real-world data from the TRIO and TARGET studies (see Chhatwal and colleagues,[42] for details).

Treatment Uptake Rate and Capacity

If patients were aware of their disease and had access to insurance, they were considered candidates for receiving treatments. Previous studies showed that 8.5% of the treatment candidates declined therapy.[13] Therefore, we assumed that 91.5% (ie, 100%–8.5%) of those candidates initiated HCV treatment. The number of patients who received treatment between 2001 and 2007 were estimated from published sources, and we assumed that the treatment rates remained steady between 2008 and 2013 (**Table 6**). From 2014 onward, we used drug sales data to estimate the number of persons who received treatment. We assumed that the maximum treatment uptake rate would remain at 280,000/year beyond 2015.

Often, such detailed data may not be available. In such situations, one needs to look for other data sources. For instance, the pharmaceutical industry may be able to provide information on the number of treatment regimens sold. Alternatively, in a small country, one could contact the limited number of hospitals or physicians that provide

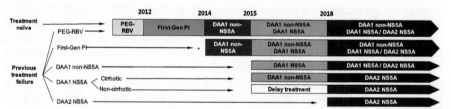

Fig. 3. Hepatitis C treatment landscape from 2001 onward showing treatment with peginterferon-ribavirin, first-generation protease inhibitors, multiple waves of oral DAAs (non-NS5A inhibitors and NS5A inhibitors) by treatment history (naive or type of prior experience), and the year treatment is offered. First-generation PI (BOC/TEL + PEG + RBV) used for HCV genotype 1 only. Note that the timing of treatment waves is positioned such that the HCV patients will complete treatment in the given year (not necessarily initiate treatment in that year). DAA1 non-NS5A includes the following drug combinations: SOF + PEG ± RBV, SOF ± RBV, SOF + SMV ± RBV, and SMV + PEG ± RBV. DAA1 NS5A includes the following drug combinations: LDV/SOF ± RBV, SOF + DCV, DCV + PEG ± RBV, OBV/PTV/r + DSV ± RBV, OBV/PTV/r ± RBV, EBR/GZR, and SOF/VEL. DAA2 NS5A includes the next wave of potential drug combinations, such as SOF/VEL/VOX, and glecaprevir/pibrentasivr for selected subgroups. Although these drugs became available in mid-2017, the SVR status of patients receiving them would become available from 2018 onward; therefore, we noted 2018 as the year for this wave of DAAs. BOC, boceprevir; DCV, daclatasvir; DSV, dasabuvir; EBR, elbasvir; GZR, grazoprevir; LDV, ledipasvir; NS5A, nonstructural protein 5A; OBV, ombitasvir; PEG, peginterferon; PI, protease inhibitor; PTV, paritaprevir; r, ritonavir; RBV, ribavirin; SMV, simeprevir; TEL, telaprevir; VEL, velpatasvir; VOX, voxilaprevir.

Year	Treatment Capacity	Reference
Table 6		
Annual uptake of hepatitis C treatment in the United States in the era of DAAs		
2001	126,040	Volk et al,[56] 2009
2002	126,040	Volk et al,[56] 2009
2003	107,131	Volk et al,[56] 2009
2004	144,276	Volk et al,[56] 2009
2005	114,197	Volk et al,[56] 2009
2006	88,083	Volk et al,[56] 2009
2007	83,270	Volk et al,[56] 2009
2008–2013	83,270	[a]
2014	150,000	Silverman,[57] 2015
2015	280,000	Gilead sciences earnings report,[58] 2015
2016–2020[b]	280,000	Assumption

[a] Assumption: treatment capacity in 2008–2013 same as 2007.
[b] Maximum treatment uptake rate implies that in a given year no more than 280,000 patients would receive treatment. The effective number of patients who receive treatment in a year could be lower than the maximum capacity, which would depend on the awareness and insurance status of HCV patients.

facilities for HCV treatment. Information could also be obtained from nonmedical data sources, such as governmental records for import of a particular drug or from documents that the manufacturers/importers may file with drug regulators.

Medical Costs

To evaluate the economic impact of interventions, such as screening and treatment to the disease population, the model incorporates cost components including cost for health states and costs of HCV testing and treatment from a third-party payer perspective. Each health state in the model was associated with the cost of managing that state. For instance, a person in cirrhosis state for 2 years could consume more resources compared with another patient in earlier fibrosis stage (eg, F1) for the same period. We estimated the annual cost for each health state from previously published studies.[43,44]

The cost of testing represented the efforts for identifying and diagnosing one HCV-infected patient, which varied by the type of screening strategy used: universal screening, risk-based screening/usual care, or birth-cohort screening. To estimate the per-person testing cost, one can further differentiate the cost of screening (eg, antibody testing for screening) and cost of confirmation test (eg, RNA testing for diagnosis). In the following demonstrative analysis, we used the estimate of $2874 per case identified via birth-cohort screening from the literature.[13]

Treatment cost, or drug cost, was determined by the drug regimen, the duration of treatment, and the discount provided by the manufacturer. Note that the exact discounted price of drugs usually varies by payer and is not publicly available information. It is also difficult to estimate the exact market share of each regimen in a given year. Thus, we made simplifying assumptions by coupling the treatment cost with the treatment waves and year, to reflect the temporal changes in treatment cost caused by the major shifts of treatment paradigm (**Table 7**). All costs were converted to 2016 baseline US dollar values using the Consumer Price Index.

Table 7	
Cost of hepatitis C treatment	
Year	Treatment Cost ($)
2010–2011 (PEG-RBV based treatment)	30,000
2012–2014 (First-gen PI and DAA1)	53,900[a]
2015 onward (DAA2)	20,328[b]

Abbreviations: PEG, peginterferon; PI, protease inhibitor; RBV, ribavirin.
[a] 23% discount applied to $70,000 listing price.
[b] 23% discount applied to $26,400 listing price.

Model Validation

One of the important steps in model development is validation of the model with observed or known outcomes. Validation assesses whether the model is consistent with a real-world system and thus provides decision makers with trust and confidence in the model results.[45]

We validated our model with several published studies: the predicted average prevalence of HCV infection with data from NHANES 2003 to 2010,[6] liver-related deaths in 2010 with the CDC report, and HCC incidence in 2005 with published studies.[46,47] Our model projected that the average number of chronic HCV cases in 2003 to 2010 would be 2.73 million, which was within 1.2% of the reported value; that liver-related deaths in 2010 would be 17,100, within 3%; and that the incidence of HCC would be 7600, within 17%.

We also validated the natural history of HEP-SIM with the results of a 10-year multicenter observation study.[30] For patients who failed to achieve SVR, the predicted 10-year cumulative incidence rates of decompensated cirrhosis, HCC, and liver-related deaths or liver transplants closely matched the reported values; but for those who achieved SVR, our predicted incidence rates for these complications were slightly higher. Because van der Meer and colleagues[30] used the Ishak scoring system and our study used the METAVIR scoring system, a direct comparison of results was not possible.

MODEL OUTCOMES

We simulated the current management of HCV in the United States, which was defined by the changing screening practice over time (risk-based/usual care until 2011 followed by introduction of birth-cohort testing in 2012), the standard of care of treatment (as it evolved over time), and the annual treatment uptake. The model was run to estimate projected temporal trends in HCV disease burden between 2015 and 2030, which included the number of persons with viremia, decompensated cirrhosis and HCC cases, number of liver transplants, and HCV-associate deaths at the end of each year. In addition, we estimated a 5-year budget impact resulting from uptake of HCV screening and treatment with DAAs. As a reference for budget impact analysis, we simulated a "no treatment" scenario that projected the cost burden if no treatment was provided.

Hepatitis C Virus Prevalence

Our model predicted that the number of patients with viremia in the United States will decrease over time. At the end of 2010, a total of 2.45 million noninstitutionalized people had viremia, which dropped to 1.84 million in 2015 (**Fig. 4**). Under current HCV

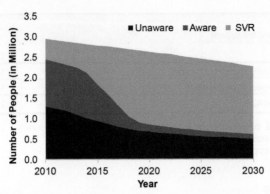

Fig. 4. Number of hepatitis C–infected patients aware and unaware of their disease status, and those who achieved SVR from 2010 to 2030. The results provide a snapshot of number of noninstitutionalized patients with viremia in the United States by taking into account the launch of oral direct-acting antivirals, updates in hepatitis C screening policy, disease progression, and expansion of insurance pool.

management practice, the number of people with viremia is projected to drop further to 0.61 million by the end of 2030. Of note, these trends did not include institutionalized HCV-infected groups, such as homeless and incarcerated.

Among infected people, 1.30 million (53% of all people with viremia) were unaware of their HCV status in 2010, which dropped to 933,000 people (50% of all people with viremia) in 2015 and 0.50 million people (82% of all people with viremia remaining) by 2030. The percentage of patients unaware of their HCV status increased over time, paradoxically, because most patients aware of their infection would have been successfully treated by then.

Hepatitis C Virus Disease Burden

Fig. 5 shows HCV disease burden by the stage of HCV—METAVIR fibrosis scores F0 to F4 and advanced sequelae consisting of decompensated cirrhosis and HCC.

In the DAA era, the prevalence of HCV-associated decompensated cirrhosis and HCC are expected to decrease from 2015 onward (**Fig. 6**). Under current HCV management, we projected that 220,000 people would die because of HCV between 2015 and 2030. During the same period, 112,000 people are expected to develop

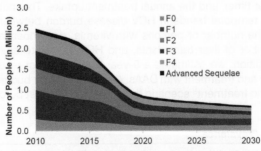

Fig. 5. Number of noninstitutionalized hepatitis C–infected patients by disease stage from 2010 to 2030. Advanced sequelae included patients who developed decompensated or hepatocellular carcinoma.

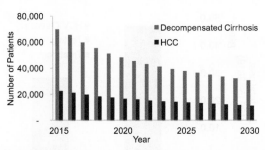

Fig. 6. Prevalence of hepatitis C–associated decompensated cirrhosis and hepatocellular carcinoma from 2010 to 2030 in noninstitutionalized population in the United States.

HCC and 131,000 people would develop decompensated cirrhosis (**Fig. 7**). Most of these cases will occur among people who remain unaware of their infection and therefore unable to receive DAA treatment.

Budget Impact Analysis

To estimate the budget impact of treatment, we estimated the total cost of managing HCV under no treatment scenario and compared it with the corresponding cost of care under current practice with DAA treatment. We found that the 5-year cost of HCV management under no treatment scenario was $28.5 billion between 2015 and 2019 (**Fig. 8**). The total cost consisted of two components: cost of testing and cost of managing HCV disease (eg, cirrhosis, HCC). To estimate the corresponding cost of HCV care under current practice where treatment with DAAs is the standard, we first estimated the number of people who will receive treatment between 2015 and 2019, by accounting for awareness status, insurance, and access to health care. We found that 1,288,000 patients would receive treatment with DAAs during those 5 years, and corresponding cost treatment was estimated at $26.2 billion. The cost of HCV disease and testing in comparison with no treatment scenario was lower at $21 billion. The net budget impact, calculated as the difference in the cost of the two strategies, was $18.7 billion over 5 years. Treatment with DAAs (compared with no treatment) would result in a budget impact of $3.7 billion per year at the national level in the United States.

DISCUSSION

The availability of oral DAAs from 2014 onward has changed the treatment paradigm for HCV infection, and has opened the prospect of a major reduction in disease burden

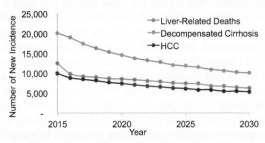

Fig. 7. Hepatitis C–associated deaths and incidence of new cases of decompensated cirrhosis and HCC from 2015 to 2030 in noninstitutionalized population in the United States.

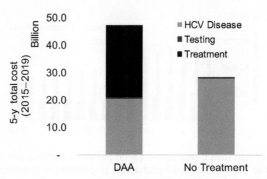

Fig. 8. Five-year budget impact of treating hepatitis C with DAAs compared with no treatment from 2015 to 2019.

of this condition through expansion of screening and treatment programs. This has led the World Health Assembly and several other stakeholders to pledge elimination of HCV as a public health threat by the year 2030. Notwithstanding the resolve of several governmental and nongovernmental organizations, several barriers exist that need to be addressed if the elimination target is to be met.

Mathematical modeling can help analyze these barriers and assess the effectiveness of potential solutions by simulating the HCV epidemic over time under different conditions, with and without each intervention. Furthermore, mathematical modeling provides a way to compare the effectiveness of various alternative intervention strategies that may be proposed. Importantly, although the usual research techniques to directly compare different interventions require that each intervention be in place for some time, modeling does not impose such a precondition. Thus, by providing answers to relevant questions before a demonstration project for a new strategy is put in place, modeling can save precious time, effort, and money. In addition, such models can play a major role in advocacy, by helping answer questions from politicians, health administrators, and decision makers about the short- and long-term impact of implementation of the proposed interventions on HCV disease burden and about the resources required. The modeling approach can also be used to maximize the impact of health care interventions, while keeping the costs within permissible limits.

In this article, we have discussed the steps involved in developing a mathematical model that can be used to calculate the burden of HCV in a country, the required inputs and their possible sources, and potential outcomes of interest. A particular advantage of mathematical modeling techniques is the ability to combine several unrelated pieces of information to better define the real-world situation. For instance, in the illustrative case used in this article, we were able to use data from various unrelated sources to characterize the HCV-infected cohort in the United States and project future disease trends under different conditions using our hepatitis C simulation model. Modeling techniques also permit us to draw reasonable conclusions, even when all the required pieces of information are not available. Furthermore, these allow us to look into the future with a reasonable degree of accuracy. Thus, using the model that we have described here, we found that the HCV prevalence and the number of people needing treatment would drop substantially in the next 10 years.

Results from such modeling study could provide policymakers with important data to inform the management of existing and future resources to maximize the benefits of oral DAAs. For instance, results emphasize the need to diagnose HCV patients who otherwise would remain unaware even in the era of DAAs, progress to advanced stages of HCV, and could die. Under the current management practice, 0.5 million noninstitutionalized patients would still remain unaware of their HCV status in 2020; therefore, more aggressive screening policies are needed that could detect HCV patients outside the birth-cohort. In addition, we will need to continue regular surveillance for HCC in people who have achieved SVR, because many will remain at risk of developing HCC.

We acknowledge that not all data needed for constructing such models are available in many countries. However, modeling tools can often work with imperfect data. Thus, in such cases, one could make reasonable assumptions, based either on one's opinion, or preferably based on expert opinion, such as using a Delphi process. If experts specify a range rather than a specific value, one can undertake a sensitivity analysis, that is, run the model using different values within this range; a similar result in all or most of the iterations would suggest that the conclusion is likely to be robust. Also, mathematical modeling can help identify the variables whose values have the maximum influence on the outcomes of interest (eg, on cost-effectiveness of an intervention). Such identification can then help prioritize which studies to undertake in a particular field to better characterize these critical variables. Availability of this information would in turn drive the model toward greater fidelity.

As with most of the published modeling studies, the HEP-SIM model used as an illustration in this article has several limitations. First, it only included noninstitutionalized HCV-infected persons as estimated by the NHANES studies, which resulted in underestimation of the disease burden associated with HCV in the era of DAAs. Second, because of lack of robust HCV surveillance programs, the estimates of HCV incidence have high uncertainty. Moreover, HCV incidence is increasing over time because of the opioid epidemic, therefore, the results from HEP-SIM did not consider future trends in the incidence rate. Third, it incorporated changes in the insurance pool as a result of the Affordable Care Act based on the available reports from the Congressional Budget Office; however, it did not model any future changes in the implementation of the Affordable Care Act that could either increase or decrease the insurance pool. Fourth, the model did not explicitly incorporate the benefits of HCV treatment in reducing HCV transmission. Such projections are beyond the scope of the modeling methodology used in this study and could be estimated using dynamic models. Lastly, it did not include human immunodeficiency virus–HCV coinfection and other comorbidities.

In conclusion, mathematical modeling can inform policymakers and other stakeholders about the impact of various proposed interventions on future HCV disease burden before they are implemented in practice. Use of mathematical models can identify barriers to HCV elimination and can help assess how to best address those barriers.

REFERENCES

1. Blach S, Zeuzem S, Manns M, et al. Global prevalence and genotype distribution of hepatitis C virus infection in 2015: a modelling study. Lancet Gastroenterol Hepatol 2017;2(3):161–76.

2. Campbell CA, Canary L, Smith N, et al. State HCV incidence and policies related to HCV preventive and treatment services for persons who inject drugs—United States, 2015-2016. MMWR Morb Mortal Wkly Rep 2017;66(18):465–9.

3. Afdhal N, Reddy KR, Nelson DR, et al. Ledipasvir and sofosbuvir for previously treated HCV genotype 1 infection. N Engl J Med 2014;370(16):1483–93.

4. World Health Organization. Global health sector strategy on viral hepatitis 2016-2021. 2016. Available from: http://www.who.int/hepatitis/strategy2016-2021/ghss-hep/en/. Accessed January 3, 2017.

5. National Academies of Sciences, Engineering, and Medicine. A national strategy for the elimination of hepatitis B and C. Washington, DC: The National Academies Press; 2017.

6. Denniston MM, Jiles RB, Drobeniuc J, et al. Chronic Hepatitis C virus infection in the United States, National Health and Nutrition Examination Survey 2003 to 2010. Ann Intern Med 2014;160(5):293–300.

7. He T, Lopez-Olivo MA, Hur C, et al. Systematic review: cost-effectiveness of direct-acting antivirals for treatment of hepatitis C genotypes 2-6. Aliment Pharmacol Ther 2017;2017(00):1–11.

8. Aggarwal R, Chen Q, Goel A, et al. Cost-effectiveness of hepatitis C treatment using generic direct-acting antivirals available in India. PLoS One 2017;12(5): e0176503.

9. Roberts MS, Smith KJ, Chhatwal J. Mathematical modeling. In: Gatsonis C, Morton SC, editors. Methods in comparative effectiveness research. Boca Raton (FL): CRC Press; 2017. p. 409–46.

10. Chhatwal J, Wang X, Ayer T, et al. Hepatitis C disease burden in the United States in the era of oral direct-acting antivirals. Hepatology 2016;64(5):1442–50.

11. Kabiri M, Chhatwal J, Donohue JM, et al. Long-term disease and economic outcomes of prior authorization criteria for hepatitis C treatment in Pennsylvania Medicaid. Healthc (Amst) 2017;5(3):105–11.

12. Razavi H, Elkhoury AC, Elbasha E, et al. Chronic hepatitis C virus (HCV) disease burden and cost in the United States. Hepatology 2013;57(6):2164–70.

13. Rein DB, Smith BD, Wittenborn JS, et al. The cost-effectiveness of birth-cohort screening for hepatitis C antibody in U.S. primary care settings. Ann Intern Med 2012;156(4):263–70.

14. Liu S, Cipriano LE, Holodniy M, et al. Cost-effectiveness analysis of risk-factor guided and birth-cohort screening for chronic hepatitis C Infection in the United States. PLoS One 2013;8(3):e58975.

15. Martin NK, Hickman M, Miners A, et al. Cost-effectiveness of HCV case-finding for people who inject drugs via dried blood spot testing in specialist addiction services and prisons. BMJ Open 2013;3(8) [pii: e003153].

16. He T, Li K, Roberts MS, et al. Prevention of hepatitis C by screening and treatment in U.S. prisons. Ann Intern Med 2016;164(2):84–92.

17. Stone J, Martin NK, Hickman M, et al. Modelling the impact of incarceration and prison-based hepatitis C virus (HCV) treatment on HCV transmission among people who inject drugs in Scotland. Addiction 2017;112(7):1302–14.

18. Assoumou SA, Tasillo A, Leff JA, et al. Cost-effectiveness of one-time hepatitis C screening strategies among adolescents and young adults in primary care settings. Clin Infect Dis 2018;66(3):376–84.

19. Canary LA, Klevens RM, Holmberg SD. Limited access to new hepatitis C virus treatment under state Medicaid programs. Ann Intern Med 2015;163(3):226–8.

20. Chhatwal J, He T, Hur C, et al. Direct-acting antiviral agents for patients with hepatitis C virus genotype 1 infection are cost-saving. Clin Gastroenterol Hepatol 2017;15(6):827–37.e8.

21. Chhatwal J, Kanwal F, Roberts MS, et al. Cost-effectiveness and budget impact of hepatitis C virus treatment with sofosbuvir and ledipasvir in the United States. Ann Intern Med 2015;162(6):397–406.

22. Keeling MJ, Rohani P. Modeling infectious diseases in humans and animals. Princeton (NJ): Princeton University Press; 2008.
23. Kim S-Y, Goldie SJ. Cost-effectiveness analyses of vaccination programmes. Pharmacoeconomics 2008;26(3):191–215.
24. Chhatwal J, He T. Economic evaluations with agent-based modelling: an introduction. Pharmacoeconomics 2015;33(5):423–33.
25. Koopman J. Controlling smallpox. Science 2002;298(5597):1342–4.
26. Rahmandad H, Sterman J. Heterogeneity and network structure in the dynamics of diffusion: comparing agent-based and differential equation models. Manage Sci 2008;54(5):998–1014.
27. Kabiri M, Jazwinski AB, Roberts MS, et al. The changing burden of hepatitis C in the United States: model-based predictions. Ann Intern Med 2014;161(3):170–80.
28. Armstrong G, Wasley A, Simard E, et al. The prevalence of hepatitis C virus infection in the United States, 1999 through 2002. Ann Intern Med 2006;144(10):705.
29. Surveillance for Viral Hepatitis—United States, 2013. 2016. Centers for Disease Control and Prevention. Available at: http://www.cdc.gov/HEPATITIS/Statistics/index.htm.
30. van der Meer AJ, Veldt BJ, Feld JJ, et al. Association between sustained virological response and all-cause mortality among patients with chronic hepatitis C and advanced hepatic fibrosis. JAMA 2012;308(24):2584–93.
31. Stepanova M, Kanwal F, El-Serag HB, et al. Insurance status and treatment candidacy of hepatitis C patients: analysis of population-based data from the United States. Hepatology 2011;53(3):737–45.
32. Denniston MM, Klevens RM, McQuillan GM, et al. Awareness of infection, knowledge of hepatitis C, and medical follow-up among individuals testing positive for hepatitis C: National Health and Nutrition Examination Survey 2001-2008. Hepatology 2012;55(6):1652–61.
33. Donohue JM. The impact and evolution of Medicare Part D. N Engl J Med 2014; 371(8):693–5.
34. Congressional Budget Office. Updated budget projections: 2014 to 2024. Pub. No. 4928. 2014. Available at: http://www.cbo.gov/publication/45229. Accessed September 28, 2015.
35. Long SK, Kenney GM, Zuckerman S, et al. Taking stock at mid-year: health insurance coverage under the ACA as of June 2014. Urban Institute Health Policy Center; 2014. Available at: http://hrms.urban.org/briefs/taking-stock-at-mid-year.html. Accessed March 15, 2018.
36. Thein H, Yi Q, Dore G, et al. Estimation of stage specific fibrosis progression rates in chronic hepatitis C virus infection: a meta analysis and meta regression. Hepatology (Baltimore, Md) 2008;48(2):418–31.
37. Fattovich G, Giustina G, Degos F, et al. Morbidity and mortality in compensated cirrhosis type C: a retrospective follow-up study of 384 patients. Gastroenterology 1997;112(2):463–72.
38. Planas R, Ballesté B, Antonio Álvarez M, et al. Natural history of decompensated hepatitis C virus-related cirrhosis. A study of 200 patients. J Hepatol 2004;40(5): 823–30.
39. Wolfe R, Roys E, Merion R. Trends in organ donation and transplantation in the United States, 1999–2008. Am J Transplant 2010;10(4p2):961–72.
40. Arias E, Heron M, Xu JQ. United States life tables, 2013. National vital statistics reports; vol 66 no 3. Hyattsville (MD): National Center for Health Statistics; 2017.
41. Martin NK, Vickerman P, Brew IF, et al. Is increased hepatitis C virus case-finding combined with current or 8-week to 12-week direct-acting antiviral

therapy cost-effective in UK prisons? A prevention benefit analysis. Hepatology (Baltimore, Md) 2016;63(6):1796–808.

42. Chhatwal J, Chen Q, Ayer T, et al. Hepatitis C virus re-treatment in the era of direct–acting antivirals: projections in the USA. Aliment Pharmacol Ther 2018; 47:1023–31.

43. Chhatwal J, Ferrante SA, Brass C, et al. Cost-effectiveness of boceprevir in patients previously treated for chronic hepatitis C genotype 1 infection in the United States. Value Health 2013;16(6):973–86.

44. McAdam-Marx C, McGarry LJ, Hane CA, et al. All-cause and incremental per patient per year cost associated with chronic hepatitis C virus and associated liver complications in the United States: a managed care perspective. J Manag Care Pharm 2011;17(7):531–46.

45. Eddy DM, Hollingworth W, Caro JJ, et al. Report of the ISPOR-SMDM modeling good research practices task force–7. Med Decis Making 2012;32(5):733–43.

46. Lang K, Danchenko N, Gondek K, et al. The burden of illness associated with hepatocellular carcinoma in the United States. J Hepatol 2009;50(1):89–99.

47. El-Serag HB. Hepatocellular carcinoma: recent trends in the United States. Gastroenterology 2004;127(5):S27–34.

48. Blatt LM, Mutchnick MG, Tong MJ, et al. Assessment of hepatitis C virus RNA and genotype from 6807 patients with chronic hepatitis C in the United States. J Viral Hepat 2000;7(3):196–202.

49. Davis G, Alter M, El-Serag H, et al. Aging of hepatitis C virus (HCV)-infected persons in the United States: a multiple cohort model of HCV prevalence and disease progression. Gastroenterology 2010;138(2):513–21.

50. Zeuzem S, Andreone P, Pol S, et al. Telaprevir for retreatment of HCV infection. N Engl J Med 2011;364(25):2417–28.

51. Poynard T, Colombo M, Bruix J, et al. Peginterferon alfa-2b and ribavirin: effective in patients with hepatitis C who failed interferon alfa/ribavirin therapy. Gastroenterology 2009;136(5):1618–28.

52. Cardoso AC, Moucari R, Figueiredo-Mendes C, et al. Impact of peginterferon and ribavirin therapy on hepatocellular carcinoma: incidence and survival in hepatitis C patients with advanced fibrosis. J Hepatol 2010;52(5):652–7.

53. Thuluvath P, Guidinger M, Fung J, et al. Liver transplantation in the United States, 1999–2008. Am J Transplant 2010;10(4p2):1003–19.

54. Saab S, Hunt DR, Stone MA, et al. Timing of hepatitis C antiviral therapy in patients with advanced liver disease: a decision analysis model. Liver Transplant 2010;16(6):748–59.

55. Surveillance for viral hepatitis—United States. Section: estimated actual new cases of HCV. 2013. Available at: http://www.cdc.gov/hepatitis/hcv/statistics hcv.htm - section1. Accessed February 2, 2016.

56. Volk ML, Tocco R, Saini S, et al. Public health impact of antiviral therapy for hepatitis C in the United States. Hepatology (Baltimore, Md) 2009;50(6):1750–5.

57. Silverman E. What the 'shocking' Gilead discounts on its hepatitis C drugs will mean. Wall Street Journal. 2015. Available at: http://blogs.wsj.com/pharmalot/2015/02/04/what-the-shocking-gilead-discounts-on-its-hepatitis-c-drugs-will-mean/. Accessed April 9, 2015.

58. Gilead sciences earnings report: Q2 2015 conference call transcript. 2015. Available at: https://seekingalpha.com/article/3366825-gilead-sciences-gild-ceo-john-martin-on-q2-2015-results-earnings-call-transcript. Accessed: September 28, 2015.

The Road to Hepatitis C Virus Cure
Practical Considerations from a Health System's Perspective

M. Cabell Jonas, PhD[a],*, Bernadette Loftus, MD[a],
Michael A. Horberg, MD, MAS[b]

KEYWORDS

- Hepatitis C virus • Viral hepatitis • Cascade of care • Clinical pathway
- Infectious disease screening

KEY POINTS

- Curative treatments offer promise for disease eradication, but gaps in patient identification, comprehensive screening, and treatment for hepatitis C virus persist.
- An integrated program of hepatitis C virus diagnosis, staging, and treatment will help more hepatitis C virus-infected adults achieve cure.
- Innovations to close gaps along the hepatitis C virus cascade of care will contribute to progress in disease eradication.

BACKGROUND ON HEPATITIS C CARE

As an integrated delivery and financing system, Kaiser Permanente is uniquely positioned to pilot innovations in clinical care pathways and share learnings with other organizations. Kaiser Permanente Mid-Atlantic States (KPMAS), which is composed of the Kaiser Foundation Health Plan of the Mid-Atlantic States and the Mid-Atlantic Permanente Medical Group (MAPMG), provides care to more than 750,000 individuals in the District of Columbia, Maryland, and Virginia area, including the major urban centers of Baltimore, Maryland, and Washington, DC. In 2013, MAPMG leadership identified hepatitis C care as a quality improvement opportunity for several reasons. First, reducing the transmission of infectious diseases is an ongoing priority. An estimated 54% of individuals infected with hepatitis C virus (HCV) are not aware of their infection

Disclosures: All authors report no potential conflicts of interest.
[a] Mid-Atlantic Permanente Medical Group, PC, 2101 East Jefferson Street, Rockville, MD 20852, USA; [b] Mid-Atlantic Permanente Medical Group, PC, Mid-Atlantic Permanente Research Institute, 2101 East Jefferson Street, Rockville, MD 20852, USA
* Corresponding author.
E-mail address: Cabell.Jonas@kp.org

Infect Dis Clin N Am 32 (2018) 481–493
https://doi.org/10.1016/j.idc.2018.02.007
0891-5520/18/© 2018 Elsevier Inc. All rights reserved.

id.theclinics.com

and the disease can remain asymptomatic for years.[1–3] As a result, individuals risk infecting others, including sexual partners and others who may come in close contact with infected blood. MAPMG has been a leader in transforming human immunodeficiency virus (HIV) care over many years; this work has served as a model for improving care for other infectious diseases.[4,5] Second, the US Preventive Services Task Force released B-grade recommendations that all individuals born from 1945 to 1965 (the Baby Boomer generation) undergo 1-time HCV Ab testing to detect HCV exposure (this recommendation is in addition to screening persons at high risk).[6–8] The Baby Boomer age population is 5 times more likely to have HCV infection when compared with the general US population.[6,9,10] From the health plan perspective, USPSTF services with a grade A or B must be provided without cost sharing to patients who purchased health plans on the Affordable Care Act health insurance exchanges, so improving HCV screening was more relevant.[11] Additionally, for a large integrated system it is more efficient to apply improved screening to all members (not to differ screening approaches by business line). This approach also improves screening and care generally.

Third, a new noninvasive technology (vibration-controlled transient elastography [VCTE; FibroScan®]) provided an alternative to liver biopsy for assessing liver fibrosis, with good sensitivity and specificity.[12,13] This innovation was attractive for easily and safely staging patients for liver fibrosis and engaging them in care.[12,14,15]

Last, curative direct-acting antiviral agents (DAA) became available to treat HCV infected patients.[16] These 8- to 24-weeks' duration, well-tolerated, oral medications are highly effective for select genotypes and increasingly for all genotypes and with less regard to degree of renal dysfunction.[17,18] Specifically for genotype 1, which accounts for 70% of chronic HCV in the United States, cure was achieved for greater than 95% of patients treated (with cure defined as a sustained virologic response [SVR] for at least 12 weeks after treatment completion). SVR attainment among other genotypes has also been trending in a positive direction.[17,19,20]

The decision to improve hepatitis C care in KPMAS was timely, because the program implementation coincided with the opioid epidemic, which is now a nationwide problem. In the United States, the majority of incident HCV infections are due to current or former injection drug use, a trend impacting both urban and rural communities.[21–26]

OPPORTUNITIES AND CHALLENGES

In late 2014 KPMAS, spearheaded by MAPMG leadership, began piloting a new HCV cascade of care (**Fig. 1**) designed to improve clinical care quality while providing value to the organization by streamlining screening access, optimizing staffing, reducing the burden on primary care physicians, and reducing unnecessary steps for the patient.[27] This pathway addressed known barriers to optimal HCV screening and care.

For example, Baby Boomer age patients should be screened one time for HCV antibodies (HCV Ab). In many clinical practices, insufficient documentation of prior HCV Ab testing may result in retesting of previously screened patients, which increases costs unnecessarily. In addition, a well-known gap in HCV screening is obtaining the initial HCV Ab test result, but failing to obtain a confirmatory HCV RNA test result, resulting in an incomplete diagnosis.[28] Regardless of the reason for failure, completing the diagnosis would require an additional laboratory order by the clinician and an additional blood draw visit from the patient, adding cost, complexity, time, and workload to health care delivery systems.

An examination of gaps in screening beyond patient identification and testing reveals opportunities to optimize clinical staffing—matching specific tasks to the staff

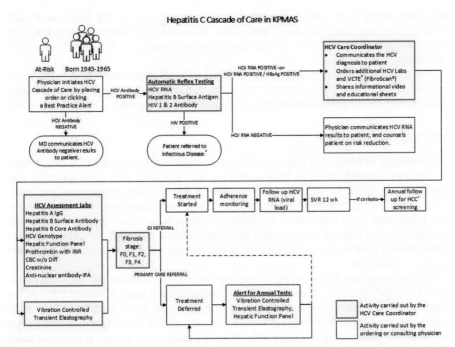

Fig. 1. Hepatitis C virus (HCV) cascade of care at Kaiser Permanente Mid-Atlantic States (KPMAS). [a] Infectious Disease physician completes HCV workup concurrent with HIV treatment. [b] Vibration Controlled Transient Elastography. [c] Hepatocellular Carcinoma. CBC, complete blood count; GI, gastrointestinal; HBsAg, hepatitis B surface antigen; HCC, hepatocellular carcinoma; HIV, human immunodeficiency virus; IFA, immunofluorescence assay; INR, International Normalized Ratio; SVR, sustained virologic response; VCTE, vibration-controlled transient elastography. (*Adapted from* Jonas MC, Rodriguez CV, Redd J, et al. Streamlining screening to treatment: the Hepatitis C cascade of care at Kaiser Permanente Mid-Atlantic States. Clin Infect Dis 2016;62(10):1292; with permission.)

member best equipped to handle them along the cascade of care, without burdening primary care physicians. The bulk of the responsibility for HCV screening has historically rested with primary care—a team already overstretched. Without support, it is infeasible for primary care teams to handle population wide screening that includes multistep laboratory testing processes, extensive patient education, and hand-off to another department (often gastroenterology or infectious disease). When tasks are thoughtfully distributed to the right staff member at the right time, the patient experience is enhanced, unnecessary clinical costs may be avoided (as well as the potential avoidance of disease escalation and downstream costs), and the opportunity to close care gaps is improved.

From a health plan and care delivery perspective, breakthrough treatments for HCV offer new opportunities for cure, but also introduce additional challenges—including high patient demand and extremely high cost. DAA treatments ranged from $80 to $100,000 or more per patient per treatment course when initially released, stressing the finances of various payers nationwide; even as prices decrease, the total cost for population wide HCV treatment remains high.[29–33] However, health plans, particularly those with strong year-over-year patient retention, must take a longitudinal view on the value of HCV screening and proactive care. Improving diagnosis rates and intervening early can potentially adjust the trajectory of the disease—ideally avoiding the morbidity, mortality, and costs associated with disease progression to liver cirrhosis, development of hepatocellular carcinoma, or the need for a liver transplant.[34,35]

The following section outlines the MAPMG/KPMAS experience and highlights a subset of promising improvements in at-risk patient identification, comprehensive testing, and value considerations that contribute to reducing the HCV disease burden.

INNOVATIONS IN CARE

The MAPMG/KPMAS HCV cascade of care uses technology and an HCV coordinator to advance patients through HCV screening and triage to care. The cascade was mindfully designed to reduce the workload of primary care physicians and close care gaps. The HCV cascade of care includes screening, detection, HCV infection status notification (and notification of common coinfections), liver fibrosis staging and monitoring, and linkage to care via a physician referral (see **Fig. 1**).[27] The physician then advises best treatment and a clinical pharmacist helps to monitor the treatment and potential cure.

This pathway was piloted in 2014 and implemented throughout the Mid-Atlantic region in 2015.[27] To date, more than 100,000 patients have been screened through the pathway, and more than 1000 chronic HCV cases have been identified. Total HCV screening doubled in 2015 when the new cascade of care was expanded throughout KPMAS. KPMAS' progress with HCV care transformation offers a practical case example of how improved screening and diagnostic approaches can be effectively deployed to advance HCV elimination goals. Details of the approach are outlined herein.

At-Risk and Baby Boomer Patient Identification

Identifying at-risk populations using provider-centric electronic medical record (EMR) alerts supports timely and comprehensive screening of the right patients, while avoiding duplicate testing of previously screened patients. This solution addresses the operational challenges that contribute to low screening rates and duplicate screening—including a limited ability for providers to easily identify at-risk patients within a brief clinical encounter, difficulty in confirming prior HCV Ab screening within the medical record (for the Baby Boomer age population), or a lack of knowledge among primary care providers about patient screening eligibility.[36–38] Using EMR-based prompts enables providers to take advantage of every medical encounter for HCV screening. This step is critical because at-risk populations (such as persons who inject drugs) may have very low engagement with the health care delivery system.[39]

KPMAS implemented EMR alerts for 3 patient subgroups: Baby Boomer age patients (but programmed to exclude patients with a prior HCV Ab test documented), patients with a social history documentation of prior or current injection drug use, and men who have sex with men (documented in the EMR social history).[27] These alerts were initially activated within primary care, gastroenterology, infectious disease, and OB/GYN, but are now active in nearly all medical specialty departments, because any health care encounter is an opportunity to intervene and improve patient care. After the implementation of the new HCV cascade of care and associated best practice alerts, Baby Boomer patients were being screened at a higher rate than in the comparison time period.[40] Of the total patients screened through the new HCV cascade of care, 77% were Baby Boomer age. Patients were screened in response to the best practice alerts as well as by physicians ordering the new HCV cascade of care independent of an alert.

Owing to the low cost of best practice alert implementation and minimal disruption to the clinical care delivery process, alerts are a simple mechanism for providers to easily identify HCV screening eligible patients within the limited timeframe of a medical encounter.[41] This care improvement is particularly actionable by clinicians because it only requires the data within the medical record to implement. Alerts have been used across health systems and provider groups, within different types of EMRs.[42–45] Within UCLA Health, a health maintenance EMR alert increased HCV Ab screening 145% in the year after alert implementation.[44] Although challenges remain with the social history documentation practices that drive certain alerts (including the persons who inject drugs and men who have sex with men alerts), the alerts still offer the opportunity to identify at-risk patients and will identify more at-risk patients as social history data capture improves.

Closing Gaps in Comprehensive Hepatitis C Virus Testing

The gaps along the HCV testing and linkage to care cascade have been consistently noted in the literature—and the gap between obtaining a positive HCV Ab test and confirming current HCV infection with the HCV RNA test is the most significant.[46–52] The gap between HCV Ab and HCV RNA testing persists in part owing to patient failure to return for a second blood draw after the initial positive HCV Ab result, incomplete communication with patients, or incomplete ordering of HCV tests by providers.[53–55] This gap represents wasted time and resources for the patient and the health care delivery system.

The use of laboratory reflex testing for HCV Ab to HCV RNA closes this gap. Within a reflex testing pathway, sufficient blood specimens are collected at a single patient visit to cover both HCV Ab and HCV RNA tests. Reflex testing eliminates a return patient visit and enables providers to order multiple laboratory tests together, instead of selecting 2 tests independently. Reflex testing has been shown to be effective across a broad array of health care delivery settings, including the Veterans Health Administration.[56,57]

In KPMAS at the first blood draw, the patient provides 2 tubes of blood. One tube is immediately tested for HCV Ab and, if positive, the remaining specimen is tested for common coinfections (hepatitis B surface antigen and HIV antibody); the second tube is tested for HCV RNA level (quantitative). In an analysis comparing HCV cascade of care screening with traditional screening, when MAPMG providers used the combined reflex test order, more than 99% of patients with a positive HCV Ab were tested for HCV RNA; when providers ordered the 2 tests independently, only 78% of HCV Ab positive patients received the HCV RNA confirmatory test.[40] This intervention requires laboratory partnership to set up the mechanics of reflex testing (or access to a laboratory vendor providing reflex testing).

As noted, KPMAS expanded the reflex testing strategy to address another gap in HCV care—screening for commonly occurring coinfections.[58] Hepatitis B virus (HBV), HCV, and HIV share modes of transmission; patients unaware of their HCV infection may be undiagnosed for HBV or HIV coinfections.[59,60] HCV/HIV coinfected patients have increased mortality compared with monoinfected individuals and treatment strategies for coinfected patients can differ owing to drug–drug interactions, making coinfection detection extremely important for patient care.[61,62] The KPMAS HCV cascade of care successfully uses reflex testing to identify patients with chronic HCV coinfected with either HIV or HBV and, to date, has triaged coinfected patients into infectious disease (if HIV/HCV coinfected) or gastroenterology care (if HBV/HCV coinfected).[27] Developing these referral pathways required collaboration and continuous engagement with the infectious disease and gastroenterology departments, who agreed to take on the responsibility of caring for these coinfected patients. When replicating similar approaches, organizations must account for the time and effort involved in meaningfully engaging clinicians around developing the optimal patient referral and management pathways.

Closing Gaps in Liver Assessment and Engagement in Care

Gaps also occur at the point of assessing liver fibrosis, which is important for determining a disease management and treatment strategy. Only 22.3% of the HCV-positive patients followed within 1 large cohort obtained a liver biopsy.[47] Within the Veterans Health Administration the percentage of patients with chronic HCV with a liver biopsy result were similarly low—estimated between 5% and 18%.[63] Noninvasive technologies such as VCTE or serum markers provide an alternative option for assessing liver fibrosis, with good sensitivity and specificity.[12,13] Assessment is particularly important for patients unaware of their chronic HCV infection; 1 study showed that 27% of Baby Boomers (and 23% of newly diagnosed HCV patients overall) had advanced fibrosis or cirrhosis.[64]

In the KPMAS HCV cascade of care, an HCV coordinator (LPN level nursing) conducts telephone outreach to newly diagnosed patients with chronic HCV to engage/link the patient into care, provide essential patient education and answer questions, and schedule VCTE and other pertinent laboratory tests for accurate staging of disease (including HCV genotype and liver function testing).[27] As a result, more than 86% of chronic HCV patients diagnosed through the coordinator-supported cascade of care complete the VCTE and obtain a fibrosis or cirrhosis assessment; outside of the HCV cascade of care, this number decreases to 72%.[40] To date, KPMAS has successfully scanned more than 4110 unique patients using VCTE. However, there is a portion of patients who are ineligible for VCTE owing to weight, ascites, an implantable electronic device (pacemaker, defibrillator, cochlear implant), or pregnancy.[15] The HCV cascade of care includes the laboratory testing needed to calculate the FIB-4 score as an alternative fibrosis measurement if VCTE is not possible. Preliminary results show a slightly higher percent of F3 and F4 fibrosis scores among Baby Boomer age patients, when compared with all patients receiving VCTE within KPMAS, further underscoring the importance of closing the gap in liver fibrosis staging for patients with chronic HCV. Implementing VCTE required health plan and medical group partnership around technology purchase, patient copay, and operator training. In KPMAS, medical assistants conduct the VCTE scan (instead of higher cost staff such as physician assistants or registered nurses) in a procedure-only visit within the gastroenterology clinic that does not include physician time.[27] The VCTE encounter was mindfully designed to judiciously use the right staff for the right tasks, and reduce financial barriers for patients.

In addition to closing the specific gaps as discussed, the use of HCV coordinators has closed other gaps in HCV care. Because at-risk patients are known to have difficulties completing comprehensive HCV screening and being linked to care, the coordinator is responsible for contacting the patient via phone and mail until all tests are complete. The use of telephone-based care delivered by HCV coordinators has increased the percent of patients who complete each step of the pathway, which is similar to results seen within other care delivery settings (including public health settings) and with similar staff members (such as navigators).[40,44,57,65] Because KPMAS is an integrated delivery system, the cost of hiring the HCV coordinators was projected to be covered by the longer term financial savings from identifying HCV-positive patients sooner and triaging patients to needed care—thereby avoiding or delaying downstream costs. For systems seeking to replicate this model, a more detailed discussion of patient ratios per coordinator and coordinator activities can be found in the supplementary information of our article that has been published elsewhere.[27]

Management and Treatment

The extremely high cost of HCV medication is a significant barrier to treatment access. Various models have explored the cost effectiveness of HCV treatment, the potential opportunity for avoided costs, and quality-of-life benefits.[29,66,67] Additional studies have examined the impact of initiating versus delaying treatments based on fibrosis score.[68] Although there is clear medical merit in treatment, costs are a barrier for some health plans. Furthermore, the costs are magnified when considered on a population-level scale (as a health system or payer must do), and when the associated costs of care, including professional fees, are included.

Before the availability of DAAs, Kaiser Permanente Northern California examined whether 5-year health care use and costs differed between patients with chronic HCV who achieved SVR on the currently available treatment (pegylated interferon and ribavirin) versus those patients who did not achieve SVR.[69] Results demonstrated liver-related hospitalization rates were 2.45 times higher and clinic visit rates were 1.39 times higher for patients who did not achieve SVR. Although this experience differs from the current situation of high cost DAAs, it demonstrates the potential downstream impact untreated (or unsuccessfully treated) HCV can have on the care delivery and payment system. Of particular note is the fact that, within Kaiser Permanente nationally, the average tenure of a health plan member is more than a decade, meaning that the organization is more likely to incur the downstream costs of untreated HCV. This article highlighted the clear clinical burden and financial challenges associated with unmanaged HCV, which underscored the need for a proactive, patient focused HCV cascade of care. For KPMAS, which has an organizational focus on clinical excellence and high patient loyalty, the decision to transform care was clear. For insurance plans with higher rates of year-over-year membership churn, the fiscal tradeoffs could be murkier.

KPMAS has 2 program features—financial and staff support—to help DAA-treated patients have the best opportunity to compete the treatment course. Our health plan partner offers a financial assistance program that patients with HCV can access. As a result, early data showed that access to DAAs did not differ by gender or by race/ethnicity.[70] Regional clinical pharmacists support adherence, monitor HCV RNA and laboratory tests, and manage potential side effects for patients on HCV medication. Of the population of patients who are active members of Kaiser Permanente, and who have been diagnosed with chronic HCV within the KPMAS delivery system, 52% have been treated with DAAs (includes first- and second-generation DAA treatment).

Within other communities, access to staff who can manage HCV treatment has been a barrier, whether owing to advanced knowledge of the disease, competing priorities, or perceived challenges in HCV care; task shifting between providers has shown to be an effective solution to this problem. By using specialists to educate primary care providers through a telemedicine ("telementoring") program, Project ECHO has expanded the number and type of physicians capable of managing care and treatment for a variety of clinical issues, including HCV.[71–73] The Project ECHO model has been particularly useful in expanding access in rural communities, where teams can contribute to improving upstream issues related to HCV, including opioid addiction treatment.[74] Task shifting between providers in the same community may also expand patient access to treatment. An urban federally qualified health care center–based program in Washington, DC, demonstrated that DAA treatment response rates were similar when treatment was administered by a specialist, primary care provider, or nurse practitioner, offering a promising model for expanding the scope of providers available to facilitate HCV treatment.[75]

Although newer DAAs are creating downward price pressure (most recently, 2 new therapies were priced at roughly $74,000 per treatment course and $39,000 per treatment course), the cost remains high.[76,77] The additional costs of screening, staging, monitoring, treatment, and potential success of treatment cannot be ignored when considered on a population-wide scale.[78] For health care providers with limited resources to treat, predictive risk models may inform which patients are most at risk for clinical escalation, therefore offering the ability make informed choices about treatment prioritization.[79,80] A University of Michigan team used longitudinal data from the HALT-C trial (Hepatitis C Antiviral Long-term Treatment against Cirrhosis) to develop a predictive model for chronic HCV disease progression.[81,82] Iterations of this type of tool, available to a broad array of providers, could inform patient prioritization to ensure those most at risk are accessing treatment. In KPMAS, we also use HCV provider reports to remind providers about untreated patients and patients who potentially could be lost to follow-up. We are using a graphic user interface program (Tableau) to produce actionable reports tailored to the physician's data needs. We originally developed these actionable reports for HIV and had positive response from our providers in closing care gaps.[83–85] Although challenges remain, the outlook on a financially sustainable screening to treatment cascade is more hopeful as medication prices have decreased.

SUMMARY

There are many competing priorities in health care today—for example, obesity, diabetes, hypertension, flu shot campaigns—and all require resources and attention. But making HCV elimination a priority sets in motion the needed deliberate actions to improve care. Ongoing deficiencies in HCV screening and comprehensive testing will limit disease elimination, even if DAAs are readily available.[86] The old truism of "we cannot treat what we have not diagnosed" (and in this case confirmed, staged, and engaged the patient in care) holds. Thus, a comprehensive pathway for screening, staging, and treatment is required by health systems and payers alike to realize the potential of HCV cure and elimination. We would be remiss if we did not emphasize the role of leadership in the success of any clinical program, especially within an integrated health system. By making HCV a priority, staff and technology resources are prioritized for this program.

For these complex issues, health plans and providers must collaborate effectively to meet the needs of patients in an equitable and sustainable manner. In the end, the desire to cure and prevent transmission of disease remains the primary motivator. By working in collaboration, clinical providers and health plans can advance the goals of increased treatment and potential for cure.

ACKNOWLEDGMENTS

The authors would like to acknowledge the HCV Coordinators (Linda Steeby, LPN and Halina Williams, LPN), the Gastroenterology Chiefs (Dr Jacquelyn Redd, Dr Dana Sloane, Dr Eric Wollins), and technology team (Dr Frank Genova, Theresa McHugh, Tirna Singh) for contributions to this pathway. The authors thank Kevin Foley, Haihong Hu, Kevin Rubenstein, Yan Sun, and Michelle Turner for assistance in preparing this article.

REFERENCES

1. Gower E, Estes C, Blach S, et al. Global epidemiology and genotype distribution of the hepatitis C virus infection. J Hepatol 2014;61(1 Suppl):S45–57.
2. World Health Organization. Global report on access to hepatitis C treatment - focus on overcoming barriers. Geneva (Switzerland): World Health Organization; 2016.
3. U.S. Department of Health and Human Services. National viral hepatitis action plan. US Department of Health and Human Services; 2017.
4. Horberg M, Hurley L, Towner W, et al. The HIV care cascade measured over time and by age, sex, and race in a large national integrated care system. AIDS Patient Care STDs 2015;11:582–90.
5. Raymond B, Wheatley B. Toward better HIV care: a thought leader interview. Perm J 2018;22:100–5.
6. U.S. Preventive Services Task Force. Final recommendation statement hepatitis C: screening. US Preventive Services Task Force; 2013.
7. Centers for Disease Control and Prevention. Testing recommendations for Hepatitis C virus infection. Available at: https://www.cdc.gov/hepatitis/hcv/guidelinesc.htm. Accessed August 25, 2017.
8. The Hepatitis C Trust. Hepatitis C information for MSM. Available at: http://www.hepctrust.org.uk/information/living-hepatitis-c/hepatitis-c-and-msm. Accessed August 25, 2017.
9. Joy JB, McCloskey RM, Nguyen T, et al. The spread of hepatitis C virus genotype 1a in North America: a retrospective phylogenetic study. Lancet Infect Dis 2016;16(6):698–702.
10. Smith BD, Morgan RL, Beckett GA, et al. Hepatitis C virus testing of persons born during 1945-1965: recommendations from the centers for disease control and prevention. Ann Intern Med 2012;157(11):817–22.
11. Healthcare.gov. Preventive health services. Available at: https://www.healthcare.gov/coverage/preventive-care-benefits/. Accessed August 25, 2017.
12. Afdhal NH, Bacon BR, Patel K, et al. Accuracy of Fibroscan, compared with histology, in analysis of liver fibrosis in patients with hepatitis B or C: a United States multicenter study. Clin Gastroenterol Hepatol 2015;13(4):772–9.e1–3.
13. Lurie Y, Webb M, Cytter-Kuint R, et al. Non-invasive diagnosis of liver fibrosis and cirrhosis. World J Gastroenterol 2015;21(41):11567–83.
14. Lucero C, Brown RS Jr. Noninvasive measures of liver fibrosis and severity of liver disease. Gastroenterol Hepatol 2016;12(1):33–40.
15. Bonder A, Afdhal N. Utilization of FibroScan in clinical practice. Curr Gastroenterol Rep 2014;16(2):372.
16. Liang TJ, Ghany MG. Current and future therapies for hepatitis C virus infection. N Engl J Med 2013;368(20):1907–17.
17. Falade-Nwulia O, Suarez-Cuervo C, Nelson DR, et al. Oral direct-acting agent therapy for hepatitis C virus infection: a systematic review. Ann Intern Med 2017;166(9):637–48.
18. Infectious Diseases Society of America AAftSoLD. HCV Guidance: recommendations for testing, managing, and treating hepatitis C. Available at: https://www.hcvguidelines.org/. Accessed August 25, 2017.
19. Terrault NA, Zeuzem S, Di Bisceglie AM, et al. Effectiveness of ledipasvir-sofosbuvir combination in patients with Hepatitis C virus infection and factors associated with sustained virologic response. Gastroenterology 2016;151(6):1131–40.e5.

20. Ioannou GN, Beste LA, Chang MF, et al. Effectiveness of sofosbuvir, ledipasvir/ sofosbuvir, or paritaprevir/ritonavir/ombitasvir and dasabuvir regimens for treatment of patients with Hepatitis C in the veterans affairs national health care system. Gastroenterology 2016;151(3):457–71.e5.

21. Edlin BR, Kresina TF, Raymond DB, et al. Overcoming barriers to prevention, care, and treatment of hepatitis C in illicit drug users. Clin Infect Dis 2005; 40(Suppl 5):S276–85.

22. Armstrong GL, Wasley A, Simard EP, et al. The prevalence of hepatitis C virus infection in the United States, 1999 through 2002. Ann Intern Med 2006; 144(10):705–14.

23. Centers for Disease Control and Prevention. Hepatitis C FAQs for health professionals. Available at: https://www.cdc.gov/hepatitis/hcv/hcvfaq.htm#section2. Accessed August 25, 2017.

24. Centers for Disease Control and Prevention. Viral hepatitis and young persons who inject drugs. https://www.cdc.gov/hepatitis/featuredtopics/youngpwid.htm. Accessed August 25, 2017.

25. Zibbell JE, Iqbal K, Patel RC, et al, Centers for Disease Control and Prevention. Increases in hepatitis C virus infection related to injection drug use among persons aged </=30 years - Kentucky, Tennessee, Virginia, and West Virginia, 2006-2012. MMWR Morb Mortal Wkly Rep 2015;64(17):453–8.

26. FAIR Health Inc. Peeling back the curtain on regional variation in the opioid crisis - spotlight on five key urban centers and their respective states. 2017. Available at: https://medicalresearch.com/author-interviews/peeling-back-curtain-regional-variation-opioid-crisis/35379/. Accessed August 25, 2017.

27. Jonas MC, Rodriguez CV, Redd J, et al. Streamlining screening to treatment: the Hepatitis C cascade of care at Kaiser Permanente Mid-Atlantic States. Clin Infect Dis 2016;62(10):1290–6.

28. U.S. Department of Health and Human Services. Action plan for the prevention, care, & treatment of viral hepatitis 2014-2016. Available at: https://www.hhs. gov/sites/default/files/viral-hepatitis-action-plan.pdf. Accessed August 25, 2017.

29. Rosenthal ES, Graham CS. Price and affordability of direct-acting antiviral regimens for hepatitis C virus in the United States. Infect Agent Cancer 2016;11:24.

30. Young K, Rudowitz R, Garfield R, et al. Medicaid's most costly outpatient drugs - July 2016 issue brief. San Francisco (CA): The Henry J. Kaiser Family Foundation; 2016.

31. Bruen B, Brantley E, Thompson V, et al. High-cost hepatitis C drugs in Medicaid. Washington, DC: MACPAC; 2017.

32. Centers for Medicare and Medicaid Services. Medicare drug spending dashboard 2015. 2015. Available at: https://www.cms.gov/Research-Statistics-Data-and-Systems/Statistics-Trends-and-Reports/Information-on-Prescription-Drugs/. Accessed August 25, 2017.

33. Schoenberg S. MassHealth managed care plans lost $137 million last year, report finds. 2015. Available at: http://www.masslive.com/politics/index.ssf/2015/10/masshealth_managed_care_plans.html. Accessed August 25, 2017.

34. National Institute of Diabetes and Digestive and Kidney Diseases. Definition & facts of liver transplant. Available at: https://www.niddk.nih.gov/health-information/liver-disease/liver-transplant/definition-facts. Accessed August 25, 2017.

35. Bentley TS. 2014 U.S. Organ and tissue transplant cost estimates and discussion milliman. 2014.

36. McGowan CE, Fried MW. Barriers to hepatitis C treatment. Liver Int 2012; 32(Suppl 1):151–6.

37. Clark EC, Yawn BP, Galliher JM, et al. Hepatitis C identification and management by family physicians. Fam Med 2005;37(9):644–9.
38. Neff GW, Duncan CW, Schiff ER. The current economic burden of cirrhosis. Gastroenterol Hepatol 2011;7(10):661–71.
39. Harris M, Rhodes T. Hepatitis C treatment access and uptake for people who inject drugs: a review mapping the role of social factors. Harm Reduct J 2013; 10:7.
40. Rodriguez CV, Jonas MC, Rubenstein KB, et al. Abstracts from the Kaiser Permanente 2017 National Quality Conference. Permanente J 2017;21(4).
41. Brady JE, Liftman DK, Yartel A, et al. Uptake of hepatitis C screening, characteristics of patients tested, and intervention costs in the BEST-C study. Hepatology 2017;65(1):44–53.
42. Roundtable NVH. Implementing electronic medical record prompts for baby boomer screening. Available at: http://nvhr.org/EMR. Accessed August 25, 2017.
43. Graham CS. Testing the 1945-1965 birth cohort for HCV at BIDMC/CareGroup. Available at: http://nvhr.org/sites/default/files/.users/u32/HCV_Birth_Cohort_Prompt_NVHR_3_18_14.pdf. Accessed August 25, 2017.
44. Castrejon M, Chew KW, Javanbakht M, et al. Implementation of a large system-wide hepatitis C virus screening and linkage to care program for baby boomers. Open Forum Infect Dis 2017;4(3):ofx109.
45. Konerman MA, Thomson M, Gray K, et al. Impact of an electronic health record alert in primary care on increasing Hepatitis C screening and curative treatment for baby boomers. Hepatology 2017;66(6):1805–13.
46. Denniston MM, Klevens RM, McQuillan GM, et al. Awareness of infection, knowledge of hepatitis C, and medical follow-up among individuals testing positive for hepatitis C: National Health and Nutrition Examination Survey 2001-2008. Hepatology 2012;55(6):1652–61.
47. Moorman AC, Gordon SC, Rupp LB, et al. Baseline characteristics and mortality among people in care for chronic viral hepatitis: the chronic hepatitis cohort study. Clin Infect Dis 2013;56(1):40–50.
48. Janjua NZ, Kuo M, Yu A, et al. The population level cascade of care for Hepatitis C in British Columbia, Canada: the BC Hepatitis Testers Cohort (BC-HTC). EBioMedicine 2016;12:189–95.
49. Viner K, Kuncio D, Newbern EC, et al. The continuum of hepatitis C testing and care. Hepatology 2015;61(3):783–9.
50. Holmberg SD, Spradling PR, Moorman AC, et al. Hepatitis C in the United States. N Engl J Med 2013;368(20):1859–61.
51. Howes N, Lattimore S, Irving WL, et al. Clinical care pathways for patients with Hepatitis C: reducing critical barriers to effective treatment. Open Forum Infect Dis 2016;3(1):ofv218.
52. Blackburn NA, Patel RC, Zibbell JE. Improving screening methods for Hepatitis C among people who inject drugs: findings from the HepTLC initiative, 2012-2014. Public Health Rep 2016;131(Suppl 2):91–7.
53. Liu Y, Lawrence RH, Falck-Ytter Y, et al. Evaluating a hepatitis c quality gap: missed opportunities for HCV-related cares. Am J Manag Care 2014;20(7): e257–64.
54. Lebovics E, Torres R, Porter LK. Primary care perspectives on hepatitis C virus screening, diagnosis and linking patients to appropriate care. Am J Med 2017; 130(2):S1–2.
55. Chapko MK, Dufour DR, Hatia RI, et al. Cost-effectiveness of strategies for testing current hepatitis C virus infection. Hepatology 2015;62(5):1396–404.

56. Department of Veterans Affairs - Veterans Health Administration. Reflex confirmatory testing for hepatitis C infection: VHA directive 1299 (update to VHA Directive 2009-063) In:2009, 2017. Available at: https://www.hepatitis.va.gov/provider/policy/index.asp.

57. Sena AC, Willis SJ, Hilton A, et al. Efforts at the frontlines: implementing a Hepatitis C testing and linkage-to-care program at the local public health level. Public Health Rep 2016;131(Suppl 2):57–64.

58. World Health Organization. HIV and hepatitis coinfections. Available at: http://www.who.int/hiv/topics/hepatitis/hepatitisinfo/en/. Accessed August 25, 2017.

59. Centers for Disease Control and Prevention. HIV/AIDS and viral hepatitis. Available at: https://www.cdc.gov/hepatitis/populations/hiv.htm. Accessed August 25, 2017.

60. Centers for Disease Control and Prevention. HIV and viral hepatitis fact sheet. 2014. Available at: https://www.cdc.gov/hiv/pdf/library_factsheets_hiv_and_viral_hepatitis.pdf. Accessed August 25, 2017.

61. American Association for the Study of Liver Disease. Unique patient populations: patients with HIV/HCV coinfection. Available at: http://www.hcvguidelines.org/unique-populations/hiv-hcv. Accessed August 25, 2017.

62. Scott JA, Chew KW. Treatment optimization for HIV/HCV co-infected patients. Ther Adv Infect Dis 2017;4(1):18–36.

63. Groessl EJ, Liu L, Ho SB, et al. National patterns and predictors of liver biopsy use for management of hepatitis C. J Hepatol 2012;57(2):252–9.

64. Klevens RM, Canary L, Huang X, et al. The burden of hepatitis C infection-related liver fibrosis in the United States. Clin Infect Dis 2016;63(8):1049–55.

65. Trooskin SB, Poceta J, Towey CM, et al. Results from a geographically focused, community-based HCV screening, linkage-to-care and patient navigation program. J Gen Intern Med 2015;30(7):950–7.

66. Rein DB, Wittenborn JS, Smith BD, et al. The cost-effectiveness, health benefits, and financial costs of new antiviral treatments for hepatitis C virus. Clin Infect Dis 2015;61(2):157–68.

67. Chhatwal J, Kanwal F, Roberts MS, et al. Cost-effectiveness and budget impact of hepatitis C virus treatment with sofosbuvir and ledipasvir in the United States. Ann Intern Med 2015;162(6):397–406.

68. Chahal HS, Marseille EA, Tice JA, et al. Cost-effectiveness of early treatment of hepatitis C virus genotype 1 by stage of liver fibrosis in a US treatment-naive population. JAMA Intern Med 2016;176(1):65–73.

69. Manos MM, Darbinian J, Rubin J, et al. The effect of hepatitis C treatment response on medical costs: a longitudinal analysis in an integrated care setting. J Manag Care Pharm 2013;19(6):438–47.

70. Karmarkar T, Padula WV, Watson ES, et al. Factors associated with time-to-treatment in the new direct-acting antiviral era for hepatitis C patients in an integrated health care system. International Society for Pharmacoeconomics and Outcomes. Boston (MA): 2017.

71. Arora S, Kalishman S, Thornton K, et al. Expanding access to hepatitis C virus treatment–Extension for Community Healthcare Outcomes (ECHO) project: disruptive innovation in specialty care. Hepatology 2010;52(3):1124–33.

72. Project ECHO and TeleECHO Clinics Available at: https://echo.unm.edu/nm-teleecho-clinics/hepatitis-c-community-clinic/. Accessed August 25, 2017.

73. Scott JD, Unruh KT, Catlin MC, et al. Project ECHO: a model for complex, chronic care in the Pacific Northwest region of the United States. J Telemed Telecare 2012;18(8):481–4.

74. Ball S, Wilson B, Ober S, et al. SCAN-ECHO for pain management: implementing a regional telementoring training for primary care providers. Pain Med 2017; 19(2):262–8.

75. Kattakuzhy S, Gross C, Emmanuel B, et al. Expansion of treatment for Hepatitis C virus infection by task shifting to community-based nonspecialist providers: a nonrandomized clinical trial. Ann Intern Med 2017;167(5):311–8.

76. University of Washington. Hepatitis C online - HCV Medications - sofosbuvir-velpatasvir-voxilaprevir (Vosevi). Available at: https://www.hepatitisc.uw.edu/page/treatment/drugs/sofosbuvir-velpatasvir-voxilaprevir. Accessed August 25, 2017.

77. University of Washington. Hepatitis C online - HCV medications - glecaprevir-pibrentasvir (Mavyret). Available at: https://www.hepatitisc.uw.edu/page/treatment/drugs/glecaprevir-pibrentasvir/drug-summary. Accessed August 25, 2017.

78. Hempstead K. The road ahead for prescription drug prices. 2016. Available at: http://www.rwjf.org/en/library/research/2016/08/altarum-road-ahead-for-prescription-drug-price.html. Accessed August 25, 2017.

79. Denniston MM, Jiles RB, Drobeniuc J, et al. Chronic hepatitis C virus infection in the United States, National Health and Nutrition Examination Survey 2003 to 2010. Ann Intern Med 2014;160(5):293–300.

80. Reid AE. Hepatitis C in minority populations 2010. 2017. Available at: http://www.gastro.org/news_items/hepatitis-c-in-minority-populations. Accessed August 25, 2017.

81. Konerman MA, Zhang Y, Zhu J, et al. Improvement of predictive models of risk of disease progression in chronic hepatitis C by incorporating longitudinal data. Hepatology 2015;61(6):1832–41.

82. Konerman MA, Brown M, Zheng Y, et al. Dynamic prediction of risk of liver-related outcomes in chronic hepatitis C using routinely collected data. J Viral Hepat 2016;23(6):455–63.

83. Mane K, Blank, J., Horberg, M. Visual approaches to bring population data insights at your fingertips. 22nd Annual Health Care Systems Research Network Conference. Atlanta, GA, April 14–16, 2016.

84. Mane K. Visual approaches to gather rapid insights to optimize care management and decision-making. 4th Annual Lown Institute Conference. Chicago, IL, April 15–17, 2016.

85. Mane K, Blank, J., Horberg, M. Interactive HIV reports on quality improvement efforts to improve patient care. Paper presented at: Concordium 2016. Washington, DC, September 12–13, 2016.

86. Konerman MA, Lok AS. Hepatitis C treatment and barriers to eradication. Clin Transl Gastroenterol 2016;7(9):e193.

Moving?

Make sure your subscription moves with you!

To notify us of your new address, find your **Clinics Account Number** (located on your mailing label above your name), and contact customer service at:

Email: journalscustomerservice-usa@elsevier.com

800-654-2452 (subscribers in the U.S. & Canada)
314-447-8871 (subscribers outside of the U.S. & Canada)

Fax number: 314-447-8029

Elsevier Health Sciences Division
Subscription Customer Service
3251 Riverport Lane
Maryland Heights, MO 63043

*To ensure uninterrupted delivery of your subscription, please notify us at least 4 weeks in advance of move.

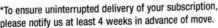
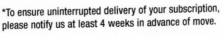